Thyroid Surgery

Preventing and Managing Complications

Dedication

"To Charles Proye,
A Friend,
A Mentor"

"To our patients,
from whom we have learned so much
after being given the privilege of caring for them".

Thyroid Surgery

Preventing and Managing Complications

EDITED BY

Paolo Miccoli MD

Professor of Surgery
University of Pisa
Pisa, Italy

David J. Terris MD, FACS

Surgical Director, Georgia Health Thyroid/Parathyroid Center
Porubsky Professor and Chairman
Department of Otolaryngology – Head and Neck Surgery
Georgia Health Sciences University
Augusta, GA, USA

Michele N. Minuto MD, PhD

Assistant Professor of Surgery
Department of Surgical Sciences (DISC)
University of Genoa
Genoa, Italy

Melanie W. Seybt

Columbia Ear, Nose and Throat Associates
Columbia, SC, USA

WILEY-BLACKWELL

A John Wiley & Sons, Ltd., Publication

This edition first published 2013, © 2013 by John Wiley & Sons, Ltd.

Wiley-Blackwell is an imprint of John Wiley & Sons, formed by the merger of Wiley's global Scientific, Technical and Medical business with Blackwell Publishing.

Registered Office
John Wiley & Sons, Ltd., The Atrium, Southern Gate, Chichester, West Sussex, PO19 8SQ, UK

Editorial Offices
9600 Garsington Road, Oxford, OX4 2DQ, UK
The Atrium, Southern Gate, Chichester, West Sussex, PO19 8SQ, UK
111 River Street, Hoboken, NJ 07030-5774, USA

For details of our global editorial offices, for customer services and for information about how to apply for permission to reuse the copyright material in this book please see our website at www.wiley.com/wiley-blackwell.

The right of the author to be identified as the author of this work has been asserted in accordance with the UK Copyright, Designs and Patents Act 1988.

Designations used by companies to distinguish their products are often claimed as trademarks. All brand names and product names used in this book are trade names, service marks, trademarks or registered trademarks of their respective owners. The publisher is not associated with any product or vendor mentioned in this book. This publication is designed to provide accurate and authoritative information in regard to the subject matter covered. It is sold on the understanding that the publisher is not engaged in rendering professional services. If professional advice or other expert assistance is required, the services of a competent professional should be sought.

The contents of this work are intended to further general scientific research, understanding and discussion only and are not intended and should not be relied upon as recommending or promoting a specific method, diagnosis or treatment by physicians for any particular patient. The publisher and the author make no representations or warranties with respect to the accuracy or completeness of the contents of this work and specifically disclaim all warranties, including without limitation any implied warranties of fitness for a particular purpose. In view of ongoing research, equipment modifications, changes in governmental regulations and the constant flow of information relating to the use of medicines, equipment and devices, the reader is urged to review and evaluate the information provided in the package insert or instructions for each medicine, equipment or device for, among other things, any changes in the instructions or indication of usage and for added warnings and precautions. Readers should consult with a specialist where appropriate. The fact that an organization or website is referred to in this work as a citation and/or a potential source of further information does not mean that the author or the publisher endorse the information the organization or website may provide or recommendations it may make. Further, readers should be aware that internet websites listed in this work may have changed or disappeared between when this work was written and when it is read. No warranty may be created or extended by any promotional statements for this work. Neither the publisher nor the author shall be liable for any damages arising herefrom.

Library of Congress Cataloging-in-Publication Data

Thyroid surgery : best practice and managing complications / edited by Paolo Miccoli ... [et al.].
   p.   cm.
  Includes bibliographical references and index.
  ISBN 978-0-470-65950-2 (hardback : alk. paper) – ISBN 978-1-118-44469-6 (epub) – ISBN 978-1-118-44470-2 (mobi) – ISBN 978-1-118-44471-9 (epdf/ebook) – ISBN 978-1-118-44483-2 (obook) 1. Thyroid gland–Surgery. 2. Thyroid gland–Diseases–Treatment. 3. Thyroid gland–Diseases–Prevention. I. Miccoli, Paolo, MD.
  RD599.T498 2013
  617.5'39–dc23

2012030208

A catalogue record for this book is available from the British Library.

Wiley also publishes its books in a variety of electronic formats. Some content that appears in print may not be available in electronic books.

Cover image: iStock © Janulla
Cover design by Andy Meaden

Set in 9/12 pt Minion by SPi Publisher Services, Pondicherry, India
Printed and bound in Malaysia by Vivar Printing Sdn Bhd

1 2013

Contents

Contributors, vii
Foreword, xi
Preface, xiii
About the companion website, xv

Part I Epidemiology and Acceptable Rates of Complications Following Thyroid and Parathyroid Surgery

1 Incidence of Morbidity Following Thyroid Surgery: Acceptable Morbidity Rates, 3
   Paolo Miccoli, Michele N. Minuto and Mario Miccoli

2 Medical Malpractice and Surgery of the Thyroid and Parathyroid Glands, 13
   Daniel D. Lydiatt and Robert Lindau

3 Extent of Thyroidectomy and Incidence of Morbidity: Risk-appropriate Treatment, 19
   Dana M. Hartl and Martin Schlumberger

4 Thyroid Surgery in Paediatric Patients, 33
   Scott A. Rivkees, Christopher K. Breuer and Robert Udelsman

Part II Best Practices in Thyroid Surgery

5 How to Perform a 'Safe' Thyroidectomy: 'Tips and Tricks', 45
   Elliot J. Mitmaker and Quan-Yang Duh

6 Minimally Invasive Video-assisted Thyroidectomy, 53
   Paolo Miccoli, Michele N. Minuto and Piero Berti

7 Robotic Thyroid Surgery, 61
   Michael C. Singer and David J. Terris

8 Extensive Surgery for Thyroid Cancer: Central Neck Dissection, 67
   Emad H. Kandil, Salem I. Noureldine and Ralph P. Tufano

9 Extensive Surgery for Thyroid Cancer: Lateral Neck Dissection, 79
   Dana M. Hartl, Haïtham Mirghani and Daniel F. Brasnu

10 Surgery for Retrosternal/Upper Mediastinal Thyroid/Parathyroid Disease, 93
   Jeffrey J. Houlton and David L. Steward

11 Reoperative Thyroid Surgery, 105
   N. Gopalakrishna Iyer and Ashok R. Shaha

12 How to Use Energy Devices and their Potential Hazards, 111
   Paolo Miccoli and Michele N. Minuto

Part III Intraoperative Complications: The 'Classic' Issues

13 The Recurrent Laryngeal Nerve, 119
   David Goldenberg and Gregory W. Randolph

14 The Superior Laryngeal Nerve, 129
   Tammy M. Holm and Sara I. Pai

15 The Parathyroid Glands in Thyroid Surgery, 137
   Maisie Shindo

16 Cosmetic Complications, 145
   Melanie W. Seybt and David J. Terris

Part IV Intraoperative Complications: The Rare Ones

17 Management and Prevention of Laryngotracheal and Oesophageal Injuries in Thyroid Surgery, 153
   Eran E. Alon and Mark L. Urken

18 Injury of the Major Vessels, 161
   Lourdes Quintanilla-Dieck and Neil D. Gross

19 Lesions Following Lateral Neck Dissection:
    Phrenic, Vagus and Accessory Nerve Injury,
    and Chyle Leak, 169
    Clive S. Grant

20 Amiodarone-induced Thyrotoxicosis
    and Thyroid Storm, 179
    *Fausto Bogazzi, Luca Tomisti, Piero Berti
    and Enio Martino*

**Part V Postoperative Complications Requiring
Urgent Treatment**

21 Respiratory Failure Following Extubation, 191
    Moran Amit and Dan M. Fliss

22 Postoperative Bleeding, 199
    Richelle T. Williams and Peter Angelos

23 The Occurrence and Management of Pneumothorax
    in Thyroid Surgery, 209
    Kamran Samakar, Jason Wallen and Alfred Simental

Part VI Postoperative Complications

24 The Recurrent Laryngeal Nerve, 221
    Michele P. Morrison and Gregory N. Postma

25 The Parathyroids, 227
    Claudio Marcocci and Luisella Cianferotti

26 The Rare Ones: Horner's Syndrome, Complications
    from Surgical Positioning and Post-sternotomy
    Complications, 237
    Lukas H. Kus and Jeremy L. Freeman

27 Late Complications of Thyroid Surgery, 249
    Dennis R. Maceri

28 Post-thyroidectomy Distress: Voice and Swallowing
    Impairment Following Thyroidectomy, 257
    Mira Milas and Zvonimir Milas

**Part VII New Issues: Complications Following
Minimally Invasive and Robotic Techniques**

29 Minimally Invasive Techniques Performed Through
    the Neck Access, 271
    *Paolo Miccoli, Michele N. Minuto and Valeria
    Matteucci*

30 Minimally Invasive Techniques Performed Through
    Other Accesses, 275
    Kee-Hyun Nam and William B. Inabnet III

31 Complications of Robotic Thyroidectomy, 285
    David J. Terris and Michael C. Singer

**Part VIII Iatrogenic Hypothyroidism, Metabolic
Effects of Post-thyroidectomy Thyroid Hormone
Replacement, and Quality of Life after
Thyroid Surgery**

32 Iatrogenic Hypothyroidism and Its Sequelae, 293
    Paolo Vitti and Francesco Latrofa

33 Quality of Life after Thyroid Surgery, 305
    Alessandro Antonelli and Poupak Fallahi

Index, 311

Contributors

Eran E. Alon MD
Attending Physician
Department of Otolaryngology Head and Neck Surgery
Chaim Sheba Medical Center
Tel Hoshomer, Israel

Moran Amit
Department of Otolaryngology
Head and Neck Surgery, and Maxillofacial Surgery
Tel Aviv Sourasky Medical Centre
Tel Aviv, Israel

Peter Angelos MD, PhD
Professor and Chief of Endocrine Surgery
Department of Surgery
University of Chicago Medical Center
Chicago, IL, USA

Alessandro Antonelli MD
Assistant Professor of Internal Medicine
University of Pisa
Pisa, Italy

Piero Berti MD
Associate Professor of Surgery
University of Pisa
Pisa, Italy

Fausto Bogazzi MD, PhD
Associate Professor of Endocrinology
Department of Endocrinology and Metabolism
University of Pisa
Pisa, Italy

Daniel F. Brasnu MD
Professor of Otolaryngology Head and Neck Surgery
University of Paris René Descartes
Chief of Otolaryngology Head and Neck Surgery and Head of
the Cancer Pole
Georges Pompidou European Hospital
Paris, France

Christopher K. Breuer MD
Department of Surgery, Yale University School of Medicine
Yale Pediatric Thyroid Center, Yale University School of
Medicine
New Haven, CT, USA

Luisella Cianferotti MD, PhD
Research and Clinical Assistant
Department of Endocrinology
Unit of Endocrinology and Bone Metabolism
University of Pisa
Pisa, Italy

Quan-Yang Duh MD, FACS
Veterans Affairs Medical Center
San Francisco, CA, USA

Poupak Fallahi MD
Research and Clinical Assistant
University of Pisa
Pisa, Italy

Dan M. Fliss MD
Professor and Chairman
Department of Otolaryngology
Head and Neck Surgery, and Maxillofacial Surgery
Tel Aviv Sourasky Medical Centre
Tel Aviv, Israel

Jeremy L. Freeman MD, FRCSC, FACS
Professor of Otolaryngology – Head and Neck Surgery
Professor of Surgery, University of Toronto
Temmy Latner/Dynacare Chair in Head and Neck Oncology
Otolaryngologist-in-Chief, Mount Sinai Hospital
Toronto, ON, Canada

David Goldenberg MD, FACS
Professor of Surgery and Oncology
Director of Head and Neck Surgery
Division of Otolaryngology – Head and Neck Surgery
Pennsylvania State University
Milton S. Hershey Medical Center
Hershey, PA, USA

Clive S. Grant MD
Professor of Surgery
College of Medicine
Mayo Clinic
Rochester, MN, USA

Neil D. Gross MD, FACS
Associate Professor
Department of Otolaryngology Head and Neck Surgery
Oregon Health and Science University
Knight Cancer Institute
Portland, OR, USA

Dana M. Hartl MD, PhD
Chief, Thyroid Surgery Unit
Department of Head and Neck Oncology
Institut Gustave Roussy
Villejuif, France

Tammy M. Holm MD, PhD
Resident
Department of General Surgery
Brigham and Women's Hospital
Harvard Medical School
Boston, MA, USA

Jeffrey J. Houlton MD
Department of Otolaryngology – Head and Neck Surgery
University of Cincinnati Academic Health Center
Cincinnati, OH, USA

William B. Inabnet III MD
Eugene W. Friedman Professor of Surgery
Chief, Division of Metabolic, Endocrine and Minimally
Invasive Surgery
Mount Sinai Medical Center
New York, NY, USA

N. Gopalakrishna Iyer MBBS, PhD, FRCS
Consultant Head and Neck Surgeon
Department of Surgical Oncology
National Cancer Centre, Singapore

Emad H. Kandil MD, FACS
Edward G. Schlieder Chair in Surgical Oncology
Assistant Professor of Surgery, Otolaryngology and Medicine
Chief, Endocrine Surgery Section
Division of Endocrine and Oncological Surgery
Department of Surgery
Tulane University, School of Medicine
New Orleans, LA, USA

Lukas H. Kus MD, MSc
Resident Physician, PGY3
Department of Otolaryngology – Head and Neck Surgery
University of Toronto
Toronto, ON, Canada

Francesco Latrofa MD
Department of Endocrinology and Metabolism
University Hospital of Pisa
Pisa, Italy

Robert Lindau MD
Assistant Professor, Division of Head and Neck Surgical
Oncology University of Nebraska Medical Center and
Methodist Estabrook Cancer Center
Omaha, NE, USA

Daniel D. Lydiatt DDS MD, FACS
Professor, Division of Head and Neck Surgical Oncology
University of Nebraska Medical Center and
Methodist Estabrook Cancer Center
Omaha, NE, USA

Dennis R. Maceri MD
Associate Professor
Department of Otolaryngology
Head and Neck Surgery
Keck School of Medicine
University of Southern California
Los Angeles, CA, USA

Claudio Marcocci MD
Professor of Endocrinology
Department of Endocrinology
Unit of Endocrinology and Bone Metabolism
University of Pisa
Pisa, Italy

Enio Martino MD
Professor of Endocrinology
Department of Endocrinology and Metabolism
University of Pisa
Pisa, Italy

Valeria Matteucci MD
Surgical Resident
Department of Surgery
University of Pisa
Pisa, Italy

Mario Miccoli DSTAT, PhD
Department of Experimental Pathology
University of Pisa
Pisa, Italy

Mira Milas MD
Professor of Surgery
Director, The Thyroid Center
Department of Endocrine Surgery
Endocrinology and Metabolism Institute
Cleveland Clinic
Cleveland, OH, USA

Zvonimir Milas MD
Assistant Professor of Surgery
Department of Head and Neck Surgery
University of Texas M.D. Anderson Cancer Center
Orlando, FL, USA

Haïtham Mirghani MD
Thyroid Surgery Unit
Department of Head and Neck Oncology
Institut Gustave Roussy
Villejuif, France

Elliot J. Mitmaker MD, MSc, FRCSC
Assistant Professor of Surgery
Department of Surgery
McGill University Health Centre
McGill University
Montreal, QC, Canada

Michele P. Morrison DO
Commander, MC, USN
Department of Otolaryngology–Head and Neck Surgery
Naval Medical Center Portsmouth
Portsmouth, VA, USA

Kee-Hyun Nam MD, PhD
Associate Professor
Department of Surgery
Yonsei University College of Medicine
Seoul, Korea

Salem I. Noureldine MD
Clinical Research Fellow
Division of Endocrine and Oncological Surgery
Department of Surgery
Tulane University, School of Medicine
New Orleans, LA, USA

Sara I. Pai MD, PhD, FACS
Associate Professor
Departments of Otolaryngology – Head and Neck Surgery and Oncology
Johns Hopkins School of Medicine
Baltimore MD, USA

Gregory N. Postma MD
Director, Center for Voice, Airway and Swallowing Disorders
Professor, Department of Otolaryngology
Georgia Health Sciences University
Augusta, GA, USA

Lourdes Quintanilla-Dieck MD
Resident
Department of Otolaryngology Head and Neck Surgery
Oregon Health and Science University
Portland, OR, USA

Gregory W. Randolph MD, FACS
Director, General and Thyroid Surgical Divisions
Massachusetts Eye and Ear Infirmary
Member Endocrine Surgical Service
Massachusetts General Hospital
Associate Professor Otolaryngology Head and Neck Surgery
Harvard Medical School
Boston, MA, USA

Scott A. Rivkees MD
Department of Pediatrics
University of Florida
Gainesville, FL, USA

Kamran Samakar MD
Department of Surgery
Loma Linda University School of Medicine
Loma Linda, CA, USA

Martin Schlumberger
Chief, Radiodiagnostics
Nuclear Medicine and Endocrine Oncology
Institut Gustave Roussy
Villejuif, France

Ashok R. Shaha
Professor of Surgery and Jatin P. Shah Chair in Head and Neck Surgery
Head and Neck Service
Department of Surgery
Memorial Sloan-Kettering Cancer Center
New York, NY, USA

Maisie Shindo MD
Professor of Otolaryngology
Department of Otolarygnology
Director of Head and Neck Endocrine Surgery
Director of Thyroid and Parathyroid Center
Oregon Health and Science University
Portland, OR, USA

Alfred Simental MD, FACS
Department of Otolaryngology Head Neck Surgery
Loma Linda University School of Medicine
Loma Linda, CA, USA

Michael C. Singer MD
Department of Otolaryngology – Head and Neck Surgery
Georgia Health Sciences University
Augusta, GA, USA

David L. Steward MD
Professor of Otolaryngology
Department of Otolaryngology – Head and Neck Surgery
University of Cincinnati College of Medicine
Cincinnati, OH, USA

Luca Tomisti MD
Assistant Professor
Department of Endocrinology and Metabolism
University of Pisa
Pisa, Italy

Ralph P. Tufano MD, FACS
Associate Professor, Otolaryngology – Head & Neck Surgery
Director of Thyroid and Parathyroid Surgery
Division of Head and Neck Cancer Surgery
Department of Otolaryngology – Head and Neck Surgery
Johns Hopkins School of Medicine
Baltimore MD, USA

Robert Udelsman MD
Department of Surgery, Yale University School of Medicine
Yale Pediatric Thyroid Center, Yale University
School of Medicine
New Haven, CT, USA

Mark L. Urken MD, FACS
Professor of Otolaryngology
Department of Otorhinolaryngology – Head and Neck Surgery
Albert Einstein College of Medicine
Director of Head and Neck Surgery
Continuum Cancer Centers of New York
Department of Otolaryngology – Head and Neck Surgery
Beth Israel Medical Center
New York, NY, USA

Paolo Vitti
Professor of Endocrinology
Department of Endocrinology and Metabolism
University Hospital of Pisa
Pisa, Italy

Jason Wallen MD, FACS, FCCP
Department of Cardiovascular and Thoracic Surgery
Loma Linda University School of Medicine
Loma Linda, CA, USA

Richelle T. Williams MD
Surgery Resident
Department of Surgery
University of Chicago Medical Center
Chicago, IL, USA

Foreword

Paolo Miccoli is a pioneer. He stepped into new and unknown territory well ahead of his time, sharing the sentiment of adventure and scientific rigor that surrounds any surgical innovation: in his hands, thyroid surgery shifted away from major surgical intervention towards minimally invasive techniques.

Paolo is an old friend and a brother from Hippocratic genealogy: we both participated in the surgical paternal mentorship of the lamented master, Charles Proye, whose memory this book is dedicated.

When he informed me about the project of writing a textbook specifically dedicated to the joy and pain of thyroid and parathyroid surgery, I expressed to him my support and interest, and it was a pleasure to be the first to appreciate the final product.

Paolo Miccoli knows what he is talking about, something that emanates from the solid rock of his experience. Furthermore, the contributors to this textbook have been carefully chosen from among the finest internationally renowned experts in the field, which, I bet, are new to very few readers.

This book encapsulates, into a concentrated nutshell, everything that the literature may offer on thyroid and parathyroid surgery, with state-of-the-art discussions around hot topics. Chapters are diligently organized and linked to each other in order to collectively drive the reader's attention.

The format is elegant, agile and easy to read, with both excellent iconography and videos illustrating new technologies and techniques, such as robotic and remote site (transaxillary, retroauricolar) thyroidectomy.

Take time to read it carefully; and appreciate the construct of the book as a snapshot of a surgeon's life: the basic epidemiological and statistical studies, the words of wisdom on how to read between the lines when studying the literature and critically reviewing the published evidence, the juvenile enthusiasm with which novel technologies and techniques are embraced, the reflections of the mature surgeon when reviewing his/her experience, and the overt discussions on the most inevitable certitude of our job ... the surgical complications.

Jacques Marescaux
MD, FACS, (Hon) FRCS, (Hon) FJSES

Preface

After faithful adherence to the surgical principles described by Theodor Kocher more than a century ago, the field of endocrine neck surgery has witnessed monumental change over the past 15 years. Fundamental technological advances (including the introduction of high-resolution endoscopy, nerve monitoring and advanced energy devices, to mention but a few) have been coupled with some subtle and some more substantial modifications in the approach to surgical thyroid disease.

While the safety of a thyroidectomy has steadily improved (both with regard to mortality as well as nerve injuries and parathyroid dysfunction), there continue to be unanticipated and unwanted adverse outcomes at the hands of well-meaning surgeons. In addition, the proliferation of novel approaches, particularly those that employ remote access points, has introduced new potential complications, some of which may be serious.

The pursuit of a text exclusively focused on the prevention and management of complications associated with thyroid and parathyroid surgery is therefore timely and appropriate. This represents the first such undertaking, and is made all the more robust by the dual-national editorship, and the multi-national authorship, which includes thought leaders from most of the important endocrine centers from around the world. Each of these authors has embraced this project with tremendous enthusiasm, reflecting the widespread consensus that this book is certain to have relevance within the scope of the average surgeon's endocrine practice. Thoughtful comments and wisdom derived from many decades of collective experience are supplemented by superior artwork and photographs, and professional-quality videos.

We trust you will find many pearls and clinically meaningful suggestions which will be both enlightening and serve to reinforce existing techniques. All of the editors welcome formal or informal feedback about this book, so that future editions will be even more useful to practitioners across the globe.

About the Companion Website

This book is accompanied by a companion website:

www.wiley.com/go/miccoli/thyroid

The website includes 20 videos showing procedures described in the book.

All videos are referenced in the text where you see this logo:

List of video clips

Video 5.1:   Conventional near-total thyroidectomy, 45

Video 5.2:   Total thyroidectomy with intraoperative nerve monitoring, 49

Video 6.1:   Near-total right lobectomy, 55

Video 6.2:   Step 1: Incision and access to the right thyroid bed, 55

Video 6.3:   Step 2: Section of the upper pedicle, 57

Video 6.4:   Identification of the recurrent nerve and the parathyroids, 57

Video 6.5:   Extraction of the thyroid lobe outside the neck and completion of the lobectomy, 58

Video 6.6:   How to recognize the 'triangle of Miccoli–Berti', 58

Video 6.7:   Suture of the access, 59

Video 6.8:   Real-time total thyroidectomy with the MIVAT technique, 59

Video 7.1:   Robot-assisted transaxillary thyroidectomy, 62

Video 7.2:   Robotic facelift thyroidectomy, 64

Video 8.1:   Video-assisted central neck dissection, 71

Video 9.1:   Left selective neck dissection levels III–IV, 81

Video 9.2:   Modified right lateral neck dissection, 81

Video 12.1:   Total lobectomy with the Ligasure Small Jaw™, 111

Video 12.2:   Total thyroidectomy with radiofrequency-based technology, 111

Video 12.3:   Total thyroidectomy with the Harmonic Focus®, 112

Video 13.1:   Unusual presentations of inferior laryngeal nerves, 124

Video 29.1:   Intraoperative management of a bleeding from a right upper pedicle during a MIVAT procedure, 266

PART I

Epidemiology and Acceptable Rates of Complications Following Thyroid and Parathyroid Surgery

CHAPTER 1

Incidence of Morbidity Following Thyroid Surgery: Acceptable Morbidity Rates

Paolo Miccoli,[1] *Michele N. Minuto*[2] *and Mario Miccoli*[3]

[1] Department of Surgery, University of Pisa, Pisa, Italy
[2] Department of Surgical Sciences (DISC), University of Genoa, Genoa, Italy
[3] Department of Experimental Pathology, University of Pisa, Pisa, Italy

Introduction

The issue of complications in surgery is a very difficult topic to deal with. Few surgeons speak openly about their problems, many are tempted to under-rate their own incidence, and even debates in the most important international circles about complications may fail to fully encompass the scope of the problem.

Unfortunately, since the dawn of surgery, complications have been inescapable, although undesired, elements of the surgical discipline but they have also allowed surgery itself to constantly improve.

In the new century, surgeons should deal with patients undergoing surgery under their care in a completely different way. The road leading to the operation itself starts well before surgery, when the patient is informed about his operation, the way it will be performed and the possibility and incidence of relevant complications. The number of complications that a surgeon generally shares with the patient before surgery requires judgement; informed consent should be obtained after a thorough discussion of the common problems that might occur after surgery, starting from the possibility of a keloid scar

(an event that is usually not related to the surgeon) to intraoperative or postoperative death, more often unrelated to surgery but due to other co-morbidities.

In between these two exceptional events, there is the real intraoperative complication that is directly or indirectly caused by the surgeon (iatrogenic) but that is not necessarily due to negligence.

Modern surgeons should be aware of how to deal with the complication and therefore instruct and start to treat the patient themselves or, at the very least, to correctly refer the patient to a relevant specialist.

In thyroid surgery, complications that may arise after surgery may vary from those that might be immediately life-threatening but resolve after proper treatment, often leaving no sequelae, to relatively minor problems that are immediately evident and can therefore cause significant impairment of the patient's quality of life. The management of those patients experiencing post-thyroidectomy sequelae can be difficult, and this book contains suggestions to help every surgeon properly manage their own patients both intra- and postoperatively, helping them to determine the possible options to deal with a selected complication.

Thyroid Surgery: Preventing and Managing Complications, First Edition. Edited by Paolo Miccoli, David J. Terris, Michele N. Minuto and Melanie W. Seybt.
© 2013 John Wiley & Sons, Ltd. Published 2013 by John Wiley & Sons, Ltd.

Morbidity of thyroid surgery

Every experienced surgeon is aware that the incidence of intra- or postoperative complications in thyroid surgery is relatively common, starting from the 'frequent' postoperative hypoparathyroidism (transient in the vast majority of cases) that in some reports has a frequency as high as 53% [1, 2].

The relative rarity is also dependent upon the method of analysis: although the single morbidity (e.g. permanent recurrent nerve injury) may be uncommon, when looking at the total incidence of the complications as a whole, the incidence of morbidity rises sharply. The rarity of a complication is also strictly related to the overall activity of the surgical practice (and therefore to the experience of the surgeon); a surgeon performing 10 thyroidectomies every week may see an injury of the recurrent nerve more often than another good surgeon who performs 60 thyroidectomies per year, even if the first is unquestionably more experienced than the latter.

The literature contains many series with an almost 0% incidence of complications that cannot be considered straightforward. How can this happen? Every experienced thyroid surgeon is perfectly aware of the issues behind such a low incidence of complications, but an inexperienced one might be misled by the results, and legal operators and lawyers might use them to manipulate facts, twisting the relatively common events and turning them to an evidence of malpractice.

We would therefore like to address the complications issue in a different way than that of a single experience reported in literature, aiming to show every surgeon how to interpret the commonly reported results, and how a sound and thorough study of complications should be conceived, in our opinion.

• When dealing with a specific complication of thyroid surgery, it is necessary to contrast our own incidence of the single event with the general incidence as reported in literature; this comparison should be made with series that are similar in terms of numbers. Going deeper into the issue, a 0% incidence of a selected complication in a series of 100 patients is a good result indeed, but if the event in question has a very low incidence, this does not represent a significantly different result from that obtained by another surgeon who reports a single one.

• This leads to the issue of statistically significant numbers, which will be better developed later in this chapter. Due to the fact that a complication is a relatively uncommon event, when analysing the results reported by other authors, the series should have sufficient numbers to have statistical relevance. It is easy to understand that a 0% incidence of permanent recurrent nerve lesions, reported in a prospective series of 33 patients in a study designed to investigate the oncological thoroughness of minimally invasive video-assisted thyroidectomy versus conventional thyroidectomy, cannot be interpreted as a statement that the rate of recurrent nerve palsy in thyroid surgery for cancer should be 0, for example. Since the paper was not planned to investigate the incidence of complications, the numbers are clearly too limited for this. Nevertheless, it was necessary to report this result in the paper, since it has an important clinical (but no statistical) value.

Further in this chapter, we give the readers some information about how to interpret statistical data from the literature, and introduce some basic statistical notions on uncommon events such as surgical complications. These simple concepts should be the basis of any audit conducted within a surgical unit.

Acceptable rates of thyroid surgery complications

We will hereafter deal only with the two principal complications of this surgery: recurrent nerve injury (RNI) and hypoparathyroidism. All other issues will be thoroughly analysed in the relevant chapters. The data reported will be drawn from the most important experiences (strictly in terms of number of patients analysed) available from the literature.

Injury of the inferior laryngeal/recurrent nerve

This complication is generally considered the worst for its potential impact on the patient immediately after surgery and for its significant consequences on the patient's future quality of life. The event causes a major impairment in one of two situations: the voice (with the onset of typical dysphonia) or the ventilation, and the related symptoms are generally present in an inverse ratio. When analysing the incidence reported by various authors, the reader should be aware of the following parameters.

- The series should take into consideration a significant number of patients (see after in this chapter), and one should be aware that the incidence reported can be obtained from the total number of patients in the study or from the total number of nerves at risk (that may double the sample, if only patients undergoing a total thyroidectomy have been selected for the analysis).
- Is the series mixing cases of thyroidectomies for benign and malignant diseases and primary and reoperative surgery? The incidence of a RNI (as well as of hypoparathyroidism) is invariably higher when a thyroidectomy for cancer (possibly associated with a central neck dissection) is performed or when the operation comes after a previous surgery. The morbidity is also significantly increased when performing a thyroidectomy for a particularly aggressive cancer subtype; the more aggressive the tumor, the higher the possibility of RNI, as described by a multicentre study that includes almost 15,000 patients [3].
- Have the authors reported whether their results were calculated on the basis of routine postoperative laryngoscopy or only on the basis of the postoperative discomfort or voice alteration of the patient? It is well known that a RNI can exist also in the presence of a remarkably normal voice. Also, a preoperative laryngoscopy should be performed in every patient undergoing thyroidectomy, since evidence of preoperative paralysis of a vocal cord is present in as many as 1.8% of patients; although in the majority of them it relates to previous surgery, the rate of this unexpected finding is still significant (six out of 14 patients without any previous surgery in the series described by Echternach et al.) [4]. When either pre- or postoperative laryngoscopy is absent, the real incidence of RNI will be significantly affected, decreasing when a postoperative laryngoscopy is not routinely performed and, on the other hand, unjustly assigning complications to the surgeon when such a preoperative examination has not been done.
- Finally, when reporting the incidence of RNI, one should always check if the patients have been followed up for at least 6 (or 12) months, to have the possibility of dividing the transient lesions (that last for 12 months at the longest and then spontaneously resolve, leaving no sequelae) from the permanent ones.

An analysis of selected papers dealing with more than 500 cases [3–12] is summarized in Table 1.1. These represent the most reliable papers dealing with the incidence of

Table 1.1 Reported incidence of transient and permanent RNI in studies considering more than 500 patients.

Author	Patients/ nerves at risk	RNI (transient/ permanent)
Lo et al. [11]	500/787	5.2/0.9
Toniato et al. [7]†	504/1008	2.2
Chiang et al. [10]	521/704	5.1/0.9
Steurer et al. [12]	608/1080	3.4/0.3 (benign disease) 7.2/1.2 (malignant disease)
Lefevre et al. [9]§	685/n.a.	n.a./1.5
Efremidou et al. [6]*	932/1864	1.3/0.2
Echternach et al. [4]	1001/1365	6.6
Bergamaschi et al. [5]	1163/2010	2.9/0.3
Thomusch et al. [8]*	7266/13436	2.1/1.1
Rosato et al. [3]	14934/n.a.	3.4/1.4

*Only patients undergoing surgery for benign diseases.
†Only patients undergoing surgery for malignant diseases.
§Only patients undergoing surgery for recurrent thyroid disease.
n.a., not analysed.

complications following thyroid surgery. These published data allow one to show either a high or a low incidence of RNI following thyroid surgery; it is immediately evident that the results demonstrate wide variability in the incidence reported by experienced thyroid surgeons.

Recurrent nerve injury has an incidence ranging from 0.3% described by Bergamaschi et al. [5] to 6.6% reported by Echternach et al. [4]. When we analyse their results more carefully, we can observe that Bergamaschi et al. report on a huge series (1192 operations and 2010 nerves at risk), dominated by benign disease (>90%) and reflecting a majority of patients who underwent less than total thyroidectomy (622), an operation that is less morbid than a total thyroidectomy. In contrast, the series reported by Echternach et al. reveals a significantly higher rate of RNI, but this result does not take into account the rate of transient and permanent lesions, since it does not have laryngoscopy follow-up 6 months after the operation, and therefore it cannot be used for a proper analysis of permanent RNI. In between these two extremes, the real and expected incidence of RNI exists.

When we consider the different series homogeneously, we can see how the reported incidence of RNI is similar for any experienced thyroid surgeon. In the studies reporting exclusively on benign diseases, the incidence appears very low (0.2% according to Efremidou et al. [6], who report their results on almost 2000 nerves at risk), whereas Toniato *et al.* [7], who describe surgeries for thyroid cancer only, report a 2.2% incidence of the same complication. To our knowledge, no study including a significant number of patients undergoing thyroid surgery for any indication (arguably consisting of more than 1000 nerves at risk, according to the authors of this chapter) reports a global incidence of RNI of less than 1%, whereas series electively dealing with surgery for benign non-recurrent thyroid diseases can obtain (but do not necessarily achieve) significantly better results. This result can be associated with a more or less aggressive surgery demanded by the nature of the disease itself. To support this speculation, we can observe that many large series still report a high incidence of less than total thyroidectomies performed when benign thyroid disease is preoperatively diagnosed, whereas when describing surgery for thyroid cancer not only are total thyroidectomies performed but they can be variously associated with central neck dissections. The results obtained by Rosato *et al.* [3] describe a significantly higher incidence of RNI when surgery is performed for an aggressive cancer (papillary and follicular < medullary < anaplastic), confirming the idea that the more aggressive the surgery is, the higher the possibility of an iatrogenic lesionis.

In conclusion, the incidence of RNI is indeed very low when a thyroidectomy is performed for a benign thyroid disease (generally less than 1%), but higher-risk groups exist that contribute to a significant rise in its incidence. These groups, as demonstrated by large experiences, include patients undergoing surgery for thyroid malignancy and those undergoing surgery for any recurrent thyroid disease. In these populations, the incidence of RNI is generally over 1% and can be as high as 2.2%. This is particularly true for postoperative hypoparathyroidism, which is well supported by results obtained from the literature.

Hypoparathyroidism

As for RNI, some general points should be raised before thoroughly analysing the incidence of this complication.
• Temporary hypoparathyroidism is not an uncommon event, especially in selected situations such as surgery for thyroid cancer, often associated with central lymph node dissection, or surgery for Graves' disease. Therefore, one should determine whether the experience reported is composed of patients selected for a certain diagnosis or if the

Table 1.2 Reported incidence of transient and permanent hypoparathyroidism in studies considering more than 500 patients.

Author	Patients	Hypoparathyroidism (transient/permanent)
Toniato *et al.* [7][†]	504	6.3
Lefevre *et al.* [9][§]	685	5/2.5
Efremidou *et al.* [6][*]	932	7.3/0.3
Bergamaschi *et al.* [5]	1163	20/4
Thomusch *et al.* [8][*]	7266	6.4/1.5
Rosato *et al.* [3]	14934	8.3/1.7

*Only patients undergoing surgery for benign diseases.
†Only patients undergoing surgery for malignant diseases.
§Only patients undergoing surgery for recurrent thyroid disease.

different indications have been co-mingled, significantly affecting the true incidence of the event.
• Many papers dealing with complications fail to distinguish between different types of surgeries such as lobectomy and total thyroidectomy, alone or associated with various neck dissections: this is another important issue to verify since, as already stated, different operations have significantly different results.
• How do the authors define the term 'hypoparathyroidism'? Do they refer to a biochemical finding (this significantly increases the incidence of the problem) or to the symptoms triggered by the hypocalcaemia (a rarer circumstance)?
The results obtained from the most important papers published in the literature [3,5–9] are summarized in Table 1.2.

Hypoparathyroidism, including both its transient and permanent forms, is a more common issue following thyroid surgery than RNI, and can therefore be better analysed through series less important in strictly numerical terms. Its occurrence is reported to be between 0.3% and 6.3% (permanent hypoparathyroidism), and between 5% and 22% (transient hypoparathyroidism).

The lowest incidence of permanent hypoparathyroidism in recent literature has been described in the study by Efremidou *et al.* [6], that focuses exclusively on patients with benign thyroid disease, whereas the highest (6.6%), reported by Toniato *et al.* [7], considers only patients undergoing surgery for malignant disease. In between these extreme results lies the true incidence of this complication, that is generally present in more than 1% of cases and is described to be significantly higher in some specific groups (higher-risk groups), such as patients undergoing more extensive surgery than total thyroidectomy alone (e.g. when central neck dissection is performed) and in patients undergoing reoperations.

A thorough analysis of the literature can easily demonstrate many studies reporting an incidence of permanent hypoparathyroidism close to 0%. These studies generally aim at demonstrating the efficacy of the parathyroid autograft in preventing permanent hypocalcaemia (dealt with in Chapter 15), and include insufficient patients from which to draw conclusions on the true incidence of this morbidity. In older studies reporting a very low incidence of permanent hypoparathyroidism, this result may be affected by a high incidence of less than total thyroidectomies, that were performed with the purpose of obtaining a lower complication rate than that obtained with a thorough extracapsular total thyroidectomy.

In conclusion, when a comprehensive analysis of the results reported in the literature is performed, the evidence is that every experienced thyroid surgeon, treating every kind of thyroid pathology, cannot obtain a complication rate of less than 1% for either permanent RNI or hypoparathyroidism. The literature can also demonstrate that the incidence rate of such complications can be higher than 6%, in particular situations, even for the experienced thyroid surgeon.

After this review of the literature, aimed at ascertaining the average incidence of the most specific adverse events after thyroid surgery, we give below a quick explanation of the basis of a proper statistical analysis, and how it should be conducted, when dealing with an uncommon or rare event.

Statistical and epidemiological analysis to study the complications of thyroid surgery

Surgical complications are relatively uncommon and this should be kept in mind when a study is designed to analyse the outcome of an operation, but also when a comparison between surgical techniques is needed. Even the rarest events should be analysed through the inferential statistics and/or a thorough epidemiological analysis, that can be more or less complicated. For example, when two different techniques need to be compared, one should consider epidemiological data (gender, age of patients), temporal

circumstances influencing surgery (different surgeons operating, different techniques or instruments), and other factors. A sporadic event should never be statistically analysed on the grounds of its rarity; on the contrary, a more careful and precise analysis is needed to obtain reliable results.

What is immediately evident to the expert's eye is the absence of a correct analysis of the statistical power in the vast majority of studies published in the common literature, that are therefore generally lacking any analysis on the numbers necessary to correctly draw statistically relevant conclusions on the results reported. In the same way, only a few studies report analysis of the correct mathematical functions needed to correctly investigate the issue being studied.

What exactly is the 'statistical power' of the study? To answer this question, it is necessary to introduce the 'type II error', the error of failing to reject a null hypothesis when the alternative hypothesis is true (in less technical but more friendly words, it is the possibility of obtaining a 'false-negative' result). The opposite of this situation, or 'the right conclusion on the correct statistical significance', is strictly related to the statistical power of the analysis, that defines when the right conclusions can be drawn ('true positive' or, more technically, when the null hypothesis can be correctly rejected).

In strictly mathematical systems, the type II error is labelled with the β symbol, and has a value between 0 and 1. The statistical power is its complementary, as expressed by the formula:

$$\text{Statistical power} = 1 - \beta$$

The statistical power is conventionally considered adequate when $1-\beta \geq 0.8$, and can be calculated in two different ways: *ex-ante* (Latin for 'before') or *ex-post* (after).

The analysis *ex-ante* allows determination of the number of subjects necessary to draw statistically relevant conclusions for a planned experiment or study before this has started. This analysis gives important information to the investigators about the feasibility of the research, and the time and resources needed for the study to be completed. On the other hand, the *ex-post* analysis is made after the enrollment of the subjects once the study has finished, and its rationale is to verify if the sample in analysis is sufficient to guarantee an appropriate statistical result.

The statistical power can be obtained using either nominal variables (e.g. the presence or absence of an anticipated complication) or continuous variables (e.g. operative time, incision length). The different statistical tests have their own formulas to determine the statistical power.

Examples of how to calculate the statistical power

We will assess the statistical power of an analysis performed to evaluate whether two different surgical techniques have significantly different complications.

A preliminary evaluation revealed that the expected incidence of complications for the two different techniques is 2% for the traditional operation and 1% for the new one. When dealing with such rare events, the number needed for a thorough statistical analysis will be extremely high. Different tests can be used to determine the statistical power for our study, and we will use in this example the free software 'R', version 2.12.1, available from the following internet address: www.r-project.org/.

The lowest power requested is 0.8, the lowest statistical threshold is generally 0.05, and the expected complications for the two different operations are 1 (p1) and 2 (p2)%, respectively.

On the 'R' software we will insert the following instructions:

power.prop.test (p1 = 0.01, p2 = 0.02,
    sig.level = 0.05, power = 0.8)
Two-sample comparison of proportions power
    calculation
n = 2318.165
p1 = 0.01
p2 = 0.02
sig.level = 0.05
power = 0.8
alternative = two.sided
NOTE: n is number in *each* group

The result obtained is n = 2318.165, which means that 2319 patients are needed *in each group* to draw reliable conclusions on the significant results that might be obtained by the statistical analysis performed.

Let's now assume that, during the study period, the *real* incidence of complications of the two techniques was revealed to be 27 out of 2319 when patients were operated on with the new technique, and 52 out of 2319 patients undergoing surgery with the traditional one. Through a simple chi-square analysis we obtain the following result:

prop.test (c(27,52),c(2319,2319))
2-sample test for equality of proportions with
    continuity correction
data: c(27, 52) out of c(2319, 2319)
X-squared = 7.4175, df = 1, p-value = 0.006459
alternative hypothesis: two.sided
95% confidence interval:
−0.018653104 −0.002907914
sample estimates:
prop 1 prop 2
0.01164295 0.02242346

The p-value obtained by this analysis is 0.006459, a significant result (<0.05) that allows one to draw conclusions about the incidence rate of complications, in favour of the most innovative technique over the traditional one. This result expresses that the possibility of error we can make when asserting that the two techniques are significantly different in terms of complication rate is low, since this result has been obtained through a statistically robust experience.

Let's now assume that, for example, the two populations studied had been lower and the complication rate had been 19 with the innovative technique and 35 with the traditional one. We would have obtained the following result:

prop.test (c(19,35),c(1500,1500))
2-sample test for equality of proportions with
    continuity correction
data: c(19, 35) out of c(1500, 1500)
X-squared = 4.243, df = 1, p-value = 0.03941
alternative hypothesis: two.sided
95% confidence interval:
−0.0208406889 −0.0004926444
sample estimates:
prop 1 prop 2
0.01266667 0.02333333

This result would also have indicated a statistically significant result (p <0.05): let's now verify the statistical power of the study with such results with a *'post hoc'* test:

power.prop.test (p1 = 0.0127, p2 = 0.0233,
    sig.level = 0.05, n = 1500)
Two-sample comparison of proportions power
    calculation
n = 1500
p1 = 0.0127
p2 = 0.0233

sig.level = 0.05
power = 0.588493
alternative = two.sided
NOTE: n is number in *each* group

The result of this test indicates that even though a statistically significant threshold has been reached with the previous test (p-value = 0.03941), the population enrolled in the analysis is not relevant enough to obtain a statistically reliable result, since a 42% possibility of error (when the power is 0.58) exists to commit a type II error when considering accurate this p-value.

From a statistical point of view the *ex-post* and *ex-ante* tests have the same validity.

The tests analysed can obviously be used also when the groups compared are more than two or composed of different numbers of subjects.

The previous examples show that when there is the need to perform a statistical analysis on rare events and on groups that can be similar, it is necessary to enroll a huge number of cases to demonstrate significant results. This is generally the case for studies dealing with surgical complications, that need an analysis with sufficient statistical power. On the other hand, when critically analysing a study about the complications issue, it is necessary to verify its statistical power to find out if the results are reliable.

When further considering the complications issue, it is necessary to introduce other statistical considerations, that can appear slightly more complicated in the beginning, but can be easily managed by every reader.

The studies on surgical complications tend to be performed through statistical tests based on nominal variables (a nominal variable is one that has two or more categories, without intrinsic ordering to the categories), such as the chi-square, the odds ratio or the logistic regression.

Various theorems of the central limit (e.g. the DeMoivre–LaPlace law) state that when the size of the sample tends to infinity, the sum of the random variables tends to lot as a normal casual one. These theories, although complicated, are particularly useful when considering rare events that need extremely large samples for a correct statistical analysis. Their final result is to allow the use of statistical tests that are used to study continuous Gaussian variables. This means that, in particular situations, a t-test can be used to evaluate the rare events in an analysis instead of a non-parametric

test, or a multiple linear regression instead of a multiple logistic one. It is obviously not mandatory to use a test used for the evaluation of Gaussian variables in the presence of large samples; a statistician can decide to ignore the possibility given by the central limit theory and use instead a test for nominal variables.

It is necessary here to reiterate that the statistical power should also be calculated in these situations, since there are formulas available to evaluate it when using multivariate analysis.

When a project is set up to study a continuous variable (e.g. evaluating the severity of complications, the operative time, the length of an incision) and a sample of sufficient size to allow the use of the central limit theory cannot be obtained, it will be necessary to evaluate whether the variable in analysis shows a Gaussian distribution or not. This preliminary analysis can be done either graphically or by using a preliminary test, such as the Bartlett test, Fligner–Killeen test, Brown–Forsyth test, Hartley test, Cochran method or Levene test. When the desired variable does not follow a normal distribution, the power test will be a non-parametric test, such as the Mann–Whitney or Kruskal–Wallis.

It is not possible to show here every power test that can be used in different analyses, but it is worth noting that every statistical software program contains all the tests necessary for different situations.

Finally, it is important to underline the necessity of a preliminary statistical analysis when evaluating the desired aims of a study. During this preliminary analysis, it is essential to determine whether is necessary to demonstrate if a statistically significant difference is present or if an anticipated result is not different among the different samples. For example, if a researcher wants to demonstrate that the operative times of two different surgical operations are not statistically different, the aim of the study will be to demonstrate an equivalence and not a difference.

In such a project, it is not adequate to use a simple t-test aimed at demonstrating the absence of a significant difference (p <0.05), since in this case the absence of a statistically significant difference only states that we do not have enough encounters to conclude that the two operations have different results; a situation identical to that of a suspect who is discharged for lack of evidence: the verdict does not necessarily mean that he is 100% innocent.

When a researcher wants to demonstrate the similarity of different treatments, a *test for therapeutic equivalence*

Table 1.3 Example of a meta-analysis (see text).

Studies	Complications	Non-events**	Complications	Non-events
	(TS*)	(TS)	(IS***)	(IS)
Study 1	2	96	1	102
Study 2	2	51	0	55
Study 3	3	170	1	120
Study 4	2	60	2	95
Study 5	1	50	1	50
Study 6	4	215	1	117
Study 7	0	70	1	70
Study 8	1	42	0	57
Study 9	3	315	1	321
Study 10	1	73	0	76
Study 11	3	418	2	433
Study 12	1	83	1	96
Study 13	1	36	1	49
Study 14	1	162	1	187
Study 15	1	84	1	97
Study 16	2	126	1	157
Study 17	1	53	0	55
Study 18	1	89	1	117
Study 19	1	97	1	109
Study 20	2	213	1	217

*TS, traditional technique;
**Non-events, number of operations without complications;
***IS, innovative technique.

should be used; on the other hand, a *non-inferiority test* can be used when trying to demonstrate that one treatment is not less effective than another. Those tests are often used for pharmacological studies but can also be used in different fields of medical research. A test of equivalence does not refer to a confidence interval but to an equivalence interval and the rules are different from those used for the tests that have been previously discussed. The power tests that should be used are also different from those previously examined, although the rationale is exactly the same.

The MBESS package available for the most recent versions of the 'R' software (www.r-project.org/) contains the equivalence tests and allows expert statisticians to perform the relative power analyses.

It is necessary to point out that in the scientific literature, the tests for therapeutic equivalence are not commonly used to demonstrate an equivalence between two different surgical operations, and the tests that are generally, and erroneously, used are the more 'traditional statistical tests' (the t-test, Mann–Whitney test, etc.).

How to perform a meta-analysis

Proper evaluation of statistically rare events (demanding extremely rich samples) is aided by the use of a meta-analysis, which will include many different studies published in the literature, thus reaching a significant sample size. When none of the studies published in the literature reaches a significant sample by itself, the studies can be considered together, thus obtaining a proper number of cases. However, this target cannot be reached simply by adding the samples from all the different studies; the rules for creating a meta-analysis are given below.

Let's suppose, once again, that a surgeon needs to compare the outcomes of two distinct operations, a traditional one (TS) and an innovative counterpart (IS), in terms of morbidity. First, it is necessary to build a table that summarizes the number of complications (or 'events') of the surgeries, and the number of operations without morbidity (or non-events). The different studies considered should be relatively homogeneous in terms of number of cases analysed, and the final number should reach that of an adequate sample, according to the result obtained by an *ex-ante* power test.

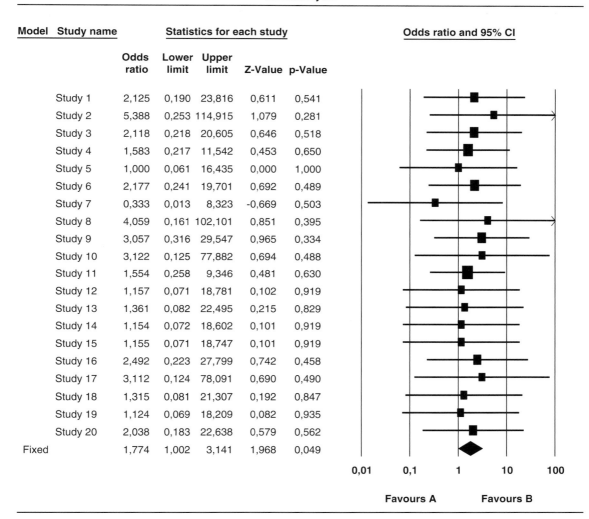

Meta Analysis

Model	Study name	Odds ratio	Lower limit	Upper limit	Z-Value	p-Value
	Study 1	2,125	0,190	23,816	0,611	0,541
	Study 2	5,388	0,253	114,915	1,079	0,281
	Study 3	2,118	0,218	20,605	0,646	0,518
	Study 4	1,583	0,217	11,542	0,453	0,650
	Study 5	1,000	0,061	16,435	0,000	1,000
	Study 6	2,177	0,241	19,701	0,692	0,489
	Study 7	0,333	0,013	8,323	-0,669	0,503
	Study 8	4,059	0,161	102,101	0,851	0,395
	Study 9	3,057	0,316	29,547	0,965	0,334
	Study 10	3,122	0,125	77,882	0,694	0,488
	Study 11	1,554	0,258	9,346	0,481	0,630
	Study 12	1,157	0,071	18,781	0,102	0,919
	Study 13	1,361	0,082	22,495	0,215	0,829
	Study 14	1,154	0,072	18,602	0,101	0,919
	Study 15	1,155	0,071	18,747	0,101	0,919
	Study 16	2,492	0,223	27,799	0,742	0,458
	Study 17	3,112	0,124	78,091	0,690	0,490
	Study 18	1,315	0,081	21,307	0,192	0,847
	Study 19	1,124	0,069	18,209	0,082	0,935
	Study 20	2,038	0,183	22,638	0,579	0,562
Fixed		1,774	1,002	3,141	1,968	0,049

Figure 1.1 The results of the meta-analysis obtained by the 'R' software.

Table 1.3 summarizes an example of a meta-analysis. When all the patients in the 20 studies are considered, we obtain a significant population, which may demonstrate an adequate statistical power.

If we consider p1 and p2 values of, respectively, 0.01 and 0.02, the two samples are indeed 'strong' enough to be considered for a sound statistical analysis, since from the first example the sample needed was 2319, and the number of subjects here obtained is over 2500.

The statistical software www.meta-analysis.com will obtain the results summarized in Figure 1.1. It is easy to

see that all the studies considered in the meta-analysis show p-values >0.05, and therefore are not statistically significant. The legend at the bottom of the figure represents the final result of the statistical analysis that takes into consideration all the 20 studies, demonstrating a p-value of 0.049 and an odds ratio of 1.774.

In conclusion, this meta-analysis works out the major issue of the size of the samples needed for a sound and powerful statistical analysis and, although contradicting the results of every single study, it represents their expression as a whole.

References

1 Pattou F, Combemale F, Fabre S, *et al.* Hypocalcemia following thyroid surgery: incidence and prediction of outcome. World J Surg 1998; 22(7): 718–24.

2 Olson JA, DeBenedetti MK, Baumann DS, Wells SA. Parathyroid autotransplantation during thyroidectomy: results of long-term follow-up. Ann Surg 1996; 223: 472.

3 Rosato L, Avenia N, Bernante P, *et al.* Complications of thyroid surgery: analysis of a multicentric study on 14,934 patients operated on in Italy over 5 years. World J Surg 2004; 28(3): 271–6.

4 Echternach M, Maurer CA, Mencke T, *et al.* Laryngeal complications after thyroidectomy: is it always the surgeon? Arch Surg 2009; 144(2): 149–53.

5 Bergamaschi R, Becouarn G, Ronceray J, Arnaud JP. Morbidity of thyroid surgery. Am J Surg 1998; 176(1): 71–5.

6 Efremidou EI, Papageorgiou MS, Liratzopoulos N, Manolas KJ. The efficacy and safety of total thyroidectomy in the management of benign thyroid disease: a review of 932 cases. Can J Surg 2009; 52(1): 39–44.

7 Toniato A, Boschin IM, Piotto A, *et al.* Complications in thyroid surgery for carcinoma: one institution's surgical experience. *World J Surg* 2008; 32(4): 572–5.

8 Thomusch O, Machens A, Sekulla C, *et al.* Multivariate analysis of risk factors for postoperative complications in benign goiter surgery: prospective multicenter study in Germany. World J Surg 2000; 24(11): 1335–41.

9 Lefevre JH, Tresallet C, Leenhardt L, *et al.* Reoperative surgery for thyroid disease. Langenbecks Arch Surg 2007; 392(6): 685–91.

10 Chiang FY, Wang LF, Huang YF, *et al.* Recurrent laryngeal nerve palsy after thyroidectomy with routine identification of the recurrent laryngeal nerve. Surgery 2005; 137(3): 342–7.

11 Lo CY, Kwok KF, Yuen PW. A prospective evaluation of recurrent laryngeal nerve paralysis during thyroidectomy. Arch Surg 2000; 135(2): 204–7.

12 Steurer M, Passler C, Denk DM, *et al.* Advantages of recurrent laryngeal nerve identification in thyroidectomy and parathyroidectomy and the importance of preoperative and postoperative laryngoscopic examination in more than 1000 nerves at risk. Laryngoscope 2002; 112(1): 124–33.

CHAPTER 2

Medical Malpractice and Surgery of the Thyroid and Parathyroid Glands

Daniel D. Lydiatt and Robert Lindau

Division of Head and Neck Surgical Oncology, University of Nebraska Medical Center and Methodist Estabrook Cancer Center, Omaha, NE, USA

Introduction

Medical malpractice occurs in every corner of the world but the degree to which it affects patients and the manner in which it is pursued vary greatly. The USA has the greatest problem and the level of prosecution has reached crisis proportions, affecting healthcare delivery and patient access to that care. This crisis began in the 1970s and became progressively more costly over the years. By 2001, St Paul Companies, the largest malpractice insurer in the United States, had stopped providing malpractice insurance [1]. Insurance premiums became progressively more expensive, with a 1995 study by the General Accounting Office estimating that insurance premiums cost medical providers between $4.86 and $9.2 billion annually [2]. Additionally, defensive medicine costs the healthcare industry between $4.2 and $12.7 billion a year [2].

Possibly even more pernicious is the effect it has had on the manner in which physicians practise medicine. Alarmingly, in a Harris poll of practising physicians in the USA, 79% admitted to ordering unnecessary test for legal protection rather than medical reasons [3]. In the milieu of spiralling healthcare costs and attempts at healthcare reform, physicians of all specialties are uncertain about how to control costs. The decision to hold the line on expensive tests is weighed against the possible ramifications of doing a disservice to our patients and placing ourselves at unnecessary risk for litigation.

When we consider thyroid and parathyroid surgery in this light, some special considerations also come to the forefront. The rates of thyroid surgery and the incidence of thyroid carcinomas seem to be increasing in the United States. In 1997, 48,000 partial or complete thyroidectomies were done in the United States; by 2007 the number was over 58,000 [4]. Litigation concerning the thyroid has also risen and the costs associated with prevention as well as the awards received by plaintiffs have sky-rocketed. In response to this rise, surgeons and other physicians have attempted to better understand these phenomena and to promote malpractice reform as one form of controlling costs and protecting ourselves and our patients.

Malpractice reform has made some minimal headway in some states but has been frustrated in many others. It has definitely been a non-starter on a national level. Frustrated with the lack of tort reform, healthcare personnel have begun looking for ways to prevent litigation through education, litigation analysis and risk management strategies. One method of developing these risk management and education strategies is by analysing data compiled by professional legal services from past litigation summaries. These data are used by attorneys to review precedents of previous suits and to assess the value of potential suits. They can also be used to understand the causes of litigation to determine how we can improve our practice patterns to prevent the litigation in the first place. This can only lead to better care for our patients

Thyroid Surgery: Preventing and Managing Complications, First Edition. Edited by Paolo Miccoli, David J. Terris, Michele N. Minuto and Melanie W. Seybt.

and cost savings from that portion of the healthcare dollar that is spent on malpractice. When one considers the 79% ordering unnecessary tests and procedures, this is not inconsiderable.

Studies evaluating litigation have been done for several head and neck sites, as well as the thyroid and parathyroid [5, 6]. The endocrine studies have identified some similarities and some unique differences with other head and neck studies. We highlight these features and attempt to identify the extent of the problem and identify possible solutions. We report these data here to highlight areas of concern and areas of potential risk management and prevention strategies.

Methods and results

The computerized legal database WESTLAW (West Publishing Co., St Paul, MN) compiles data from 14 sources and searches all 50 of the United States, including all civil state and federal trials involving malpractice and the thyroid. We abstracted from these cases data on plaintiff and defendant demographics, expert witness demographics, allegations including delays in treatment, laryngeal nerve injury, postoperative hypothyroidism or respiratory embarrassment, whether nerve monitors were documented, if tracheotomies were done, medical complications and verdict outcomes. We also evaluated allegations of misdiagnosis, failure to perform fine needle aspiration (FNA), informed consent issues and whether clinical guidelines played any role in causing or preventing litigation. We had 30 cases of litigation for thyroid surgery and added these to Kern's 36 cases [6].

The results of the two studies were slightly different but revealed some interesting conclusions and presented some possibilities for prevention. The patients were overwhelmingly female (80% and 90% from the two studies). Failure to diagnose a cancer was seen to be a very common allegation, with many patients complaining that an FNA should have been but simply was not done. Allegations of recurrent laryngeal nerve injury occurred as expected but with some interesting nuances as well. Interesting, postoperative hypoparathyroidism also occurred but again was not a commonly alleged problem. The phenomenon of a 'bad outcome' which we have discussed in the literature previously was also seen in both

the Lydiatt and Kern studies [5,6]. We highlight each of these findings, document the extent of the problem with each and discuss ways in which this information could be used to educate us and promote risk management and prevention strategies.

Poor outcome

It seems trite to say that patients with a poor outcome are more likely to bring litigation. The American legal system recognizes that medicine is not an exact science. Unsatisfactory results and errors occur in medicine but a bad outcome is not enough to show malpractice. To establish malpractice, the plaintiff must satisfy a four-part test. The defendant must have a duty to the plaintiff, a breach of that duty must have occurred, the plaintiff was injured, and the breach of duty was the proximate cause of the injury. The duty and the injury are usually readily acknowledged in medical malpractice, and an injured patient in the postoperative period makes an obvious and compelling case. Plaintiff attorneys, of course, emphasize these often devastating injuries. The breach of the duty, however, as a deviation from the established standard of care is a harder fact to establish.

Reviewing the thyroid data from our study and that of Kern, we found poor outcome to play a significant, even surprising role. In the Lydiatt study, 15 of 30 (50%) plaintiffs had a bad outcome. Nine of 30 were dead, four of 30 had severe neurological defects, one was blind, and one alive with cancer. Kern found 15% of the plaintiffs suffered from anoxic brain injury. These are all devastating injuries and doubtlessly make compelling cases, but do not necessarily imply a breach of duty and thus malpractice.

We found that a bad outcome was associated frequently in litigation involving other sites in the head and neck. In cancers of the larynx, 47% of the plaintiffs were either dead or alive with cancer [7]. In the oral cavity, 47% of plaintiffs were dead [8]. In cancer of the skin, of those for whom the oncological outcome was known, 60% were dead at the time of trial [9].

Plaintiff awards for these devastating injuries also tend to be large. In seven awards for patients with respiratory complaints, five were for greater than $1 million. A 2011 award in Washington for $4.1 million adds some chilling facts to contemplate [10]. The patient had an unrecognized postoperative bleed with haematoma formation and subsequent respiratory distress with anoxic brain injury, ultimately leading to death. The plaintiff attorneys argued understandably that the patient was not monitored properly, but alleged that the surgeon was negligent in part for not placing a surgical drain at the time of surgery. In this age of outpatient surgery, with many surgeons not placing drains at all in thyroidectomy patients, this is especially worrisome. For a jury of laypeople to be making multi-million dollar decisions about whether surgeons should have used a drain or not is inane in the extreme. Monitoring of patients after thyroid and parathyroid surgery is obviously important and the airway must be secure before any attempt to discharge the patient. Although we typically watch our patients overnight after surgery, we recognize that many surgeons send their patients home as outpatients and this has a proven safety record in their hands. We also recognize that many surgeons do not use drains after thyroid or parathyroid surgery and this has also been a safe practice.

Why then do these patients sometimes bring litigation and sometimes win large settlements? Our studies seem to show that the outcome of litigation frequently hinges on the poor outcome alone, supplemented with testimony that implicates any perceived error of commission or omission to have 'caused' the injury, rather than following the purported theory of the law. Further outcome studies and litigation analysis need to be done and physicians must be a part of this process. The law is not immutable and has changed, although slowly, in response to scientific knowledge. This process of understanding our surgical decisions and the role they play in litigation can help in the development of guidelines. These guidelines can ultimately help to improve patient care and possibly decrease litigation. The understanding may also play a role in much needed tort reform, in which physicians must play an active and intelligent part.

Diagnostic delays

Combining the two studies, 17 of 21 (81%) patients with cancer of the thyroid claimed a delay in treatment. In four of the 21 (19%) thyroid cancer patients, an FNA was done but failed to diagnose a cancer. However, in 15 of the 21 (71%), the patient alleged that an FNA should have been but was not done.

Failure to diagnose a cancer and a delay in this diagnosis are common allegations provoking litigation. Misdiagnosis of cancer costs nearly $200 million each year, approximately 30% of the money paid out for medical malpractice [8]. In our studies of various sites within the head and neck, we found a delay in diagnosis alleged in 83% of patients with cancer of the larynx, 86% in cancer of the oral cavity and 54% in skin cancers [7–9]. In many of the studies with delay in diagnosis, the problem is an error of omission in that the physician was faulted for not taking a biopsy.

The utility of FNA in diagnosing thyroid cancer has been well established [11]. FNA has been shown to have a diagnostic sensitivity of between 89% and 98%, and a specificity of 92% [11]. Ultrasound (US)-guided FNA has added to the accuracy and dependability of diagnosis [12]. The non-invasive nature and the availability of ultrasound units in hospitals, surgical and endocrinology clinics, and elsewhere have made the use of this modality widespread in the United States.

Once a nodule has been discovered in the thyroid, either by physical exam or incidentally with another scan, a thyroid-stimulating hormone level is obtained to rule out hyperthyroidism. If hyperthyroidism is ruled out, the next step in the guidelines of the American Thyroid Association and the National Comprehensive Cancers Network (NCCN) is an FNA [13,14]. Although errors in the diagnosis can and are made, most guidelines call for follow-up ultrasounds in managing the patients. Enlarging nodules call for a repeat FNA or removal of the thyroid lobe. In either event, guidelines call for an initial FNA and should be followed. Although some are reluctant to biopsy nodules, this is a common allegation prompting litigation. We found that a full 60% of plaintiffs suing dentists in oral cavity suits claimed that a biopsy should have been but was not done [8]. Head and neck surgeons, endocrinologists, endocrine surgeons or other groups routinely managing these patients should advance the policy of educating physicians about these guidelines. The guidelines are available and should be followed. These guidelines, if followed, will likely help prevent errors of omission, delays in diagnosis, harm to the patient and subsequent litigation. Following the established guidelines may also provide some protection in the legal system if litigation does occur, although this has yet to be established.

Recurrent laryngeal nerve injury

Injury to the recurrent laryngeal nerve is a prevalent concern for surgeon and patient alike. The incidence of permanent nerve injury is estimated to be around 2%. With 58,000 thyroidectomies done yearly in the United States, this is a relatively common injury. Allegations in medical malpractice and the thyroid gland vary, but in Kern's study of litigation occurring between 1985 and 1991, 60% of the patients cited recurrent laryngeal nerve damage [6]. In Lydiatt's study from 1987 to 2000, 27% alleged injury [5]. In a 2010 review of recurrent laryngeal nerve injury using a similar method but a different search engine, Abadin reviewed 1989–2009 and found 45% alleging injury to this nerve [4]. In every study it was a major concern. Additionally, in the Lydiatt study, one-third of the patients who sustained a recurrent laryngeal nerve injury complained that the injury was bilateral.

Methods of dealing with this risk include a thorough discussion between surgeon and patient to reach informed consent prior to operation. Although it is difficult to imagine not fully informing patients of the risk of recurrent laryngeal nerve injury preoperatively, in the Lydiatt study, 78% of patients with injury also alleged they had not been informed [5]. Studies show that patients only recall a portion of the information given, ranging from 35% to 57% [15,16]. In a study of informed consent for head and neck operations, Hekkenberg *et al.* found a recall rate of 48% in patients undergoing thyroidectomy, parathyroidectomy or parotidectomy [16]. Establishing good rapport with the patient preoperatively and providing written consent documents may be all we can hope for in preventing this allegation as a cause of malpractice.

Technical measures to prevent the actual occurrence of recurrent laryngeal nerve injury have also been pursued. Nerve monitors have become popular and their use in preventing injury and subsequent litigation has been studied [17–19]. Between 40% and 45% of general-surgical and otolaryngology-trained surgeons use nerve monitors in some or all cases [19]. Chan *et al.* did not find a difference in incidence of recurrent laryngeal nerve injury in operations with or without nerve monitors, but did find a higher incidence of injury in patients with cancer [18]. Shindo and Chheda also found similar incidence in injury rates with (2.09%) and without (2.96%) nerve monitors. They indicated in their paper that the monitors

might produce early warning and lessen neuropraxic injuries, but warn that they imply increased cost and may produce a feeling of false security if the nerve has not been accurately visualized [17]. They also describe how the monitor can be used to quickly facilitate initial localization of the nerve by turning up the stimulus intensity to 1.0–1.5 mA and 'searching' for the nerve. Direct visualization must ultimately be used to confirm the presence of the nerve. Nerve monitors can also be used to aid in tracing the nerve out with intermittent stimulation of the nerve. The final use is in postoperative documentation of an anatomically intact nerve.

The International Monitoring Study Group reviewed the literature and cumulative experience with intraoperative neural monitoring during thyroid and parathyroid surgery over a 15-year span [19]. It states: 'Intraoperative neural monitoring during thyroid and parathyroid surgery has gained widespread acceptance as an adjunct to the gold standard of visual nerve identification'. Further, it indicates that, 'this guideline is at its forefront, quality driven; it is intended to improve the quality of neural monitoring, to translate the best available evidence into clinical practice to promote best practices'. The paper provides many technical details to help with monitoring that seem useful to adopt. We do not believe that utilization of nerve monitoring is the 'standard of care' at this time. We do, however, find that the routine use of monitors to assist in localization of the nerve probably lessens operative time, and provides useful documentation of nerve function at the end of surgery. Abadin *et al.* did not find any mention of the presence or absence of nerve monitoring in the patients who claimed to have had a recurrent laryngeal nerve injury. This study examined patients from 1989 to 2009 and may have reflected the limited use of monitors during the study period [4]. As we mentioned earlier, the law is not immutable and does follow the scientific community, albeit very slowly.

Postoperative hypoparathyroidism

Postoperative hypocalcaemia is an established complication of thyroid and parathyroid surgery, and studies have demonstrated it as the most common adverse effect of a total thyroidectomy [20,21]. Acute parathyroid insufficiency is believed to be the reason behind postoperative hypocalcaemia, and the risk is increased with the extent of surgery, especially when a total thyroidectomy is performed and/or a central neck dissection is performed. Both procedures increase the risk of removal of the parathyroids or devascularizing one or multiple glands.

Postoperative hypocalcaemia has been reported to be anywhere from 13% to 83%. Sitges-Serra *et al.* found that 50.2% of their patients who underwent total thyroidectomy developed hypocalcaemia, with 62% developing normal calcium levels at 1 month, giving an overall prevalence of protracted hypoparathyroidism of 18.1% [22]. Glinoer *et al.* found a 1.2% incidence of permanent hypoparathyroidism at 1 year in patients who had a total thyroidectomy but 25% of the patients who had undergone a staged procedure had permanent hypoparathyroidism over the same time span. Both of these groups required calcium supplementation [21].

Although a common complication, Kern's study found 13% of the patient's alleged hypoparathyroidism occurring postoperatively as the reason to bring litigation and Lydiatt's study found 7% [5,6]. The trend downward over a decade is interesting and possibly demonstrates better techniques for recognition and more aggressive treatment of this common complication. But this does remain a concern for surgeons and endocrinologists because long-term hypocalcaemia is very devastating for the patient, so protocols and monitoring paradigms have been created.

Prevention of this complication begins in surgery with meticulous dissection, and autotransplantation of any abnormal parathyroid glands. Malignant disease, extent of surgery and number of glands preserved *in situ* were associated with hypocalcaemia in the study performed by Sitges-Serra *et al.* [22]. They also established that lymph node dissection and *in situ* preservation of fewer than three parathyroid glands were found to be risk factors associated with protracted hypoparathyroidism [22].

After surgery is performed, monitoring the patient both biochemically and clinically may be important, with prevention of devastating neurological consequences as the goal. Sabour *et al.* looked at postoperative parathyroid hormone (PTH) levels compared to observation and routine supplementation. They reported a rate of hypocalcaemia at 35% in the observation group, versus 14% in patients who had their calcium replaced based on postoperative PTH levels, compared to 4.5% of patients who were automatically given calcium supplementation. The rate of significant hypocalcaemia was 9.8% in the observational group, 2.3% in the selective PTH supplementation groups, and 0% in the routine supplementation group. Interestingly, there was also a 4.5% incidence of hypercalcaemia in the routine supplementation group [23]. Multiple studies have cited the routine use of postoperative PTH as a basis for calcium replacement, but the studies differ in protocols such as when to draw the lab and at what level to replace. They are, however, consistent in demonstrating the benefit of this approach for routine postoperative monitoring and care.

Despite best surgical technique and postoperative management, complications will arise. It is important that the surgeon address the issue of hypocalceamia up front with the patient prior to surgery when obtaining the informed consent. In the postoperative setting, it is equally important to maintain proper communication as well as appropriate follow-up to prevent any adverse sequelae of hypoparathyroidism or its treatment.

Conclusion

Medical malpractice concerns are a major contributor to practice patterns and costs in the United States. Litigation reform has not occurred in most states and has certainly not kept pace with the upward spiralling costs. Thyroid and parathyroid surgery carries its own risks and has a nuanced set of allegations that are known and fairly well studied. Methods of study include evaluation of past verdicts and allegations to help develop risk management protocols and to hopefully prevent the errors that lead to the litigation in the first place. We found delay in diagnosis, with the omission of a timely FNA, recurrent laryngeal nerve injury, and a poor outcome to be very prevalent in this group of plaintiffs. Hypoparathyroidism occurring in the postoperative period is a devastating risk, but litigation arising from this allegation did not occur with great frequency in our review. As with all malpractice, the establishment of good rapport preoperatively is often the best risk management and preventive strategy.

References

1 Mello MM, Studdert D, Brennan T. The new medical malpractice crisis. N Engl J Med 2003; 348(23): 2281–4.
2 United States General Accounting Office. Medical Liability: impact on hospital and physician costs extends beyond insurance. Available at: www.gao.gov/archiv/1995/ai95169.pdf.

3 Taylor H. Most doctors report fear of malpractice liability has harmed their ability to provide quality care: caused them to order unnecessary tests, provide unnecessary treatment and make unnecessary referrals. Available at: www.harrisinteractive.com/harris_poll/index.asp?PID=300.

4 Abadin SS, Kaplan EI, Angelos P. Malpractice litigation after thyroid surgery: the role of recurrent laryngeal nerve injuries, 1989–2009. Surgery 2010; 148(4): 718–23.

5 Lydiatt D. Medical malpractice and the thyroid gland. Head Neck 2003; 25: 429–31.

6 Kern KA. Medicolegal analysis of errors in diagnosis and treatment of surgical endocrine disease. Surgery 1993; 114: 1167–74.

7 Lydiatt DD. Medical malpractice and cancer of the larynx. Laryngoscope 2002; 112: 1–4.

8 Lydiatt DD. Cancer of the oral cavity and medical malpractice. Laryngoscope 2002; 112: 816–19.

9 Lydiatt DD. Medical malpractice and cancer of the skin. Am J Surg 2004; 187(6): 688–94.

10 Lawsuit over death of thyroidectomy patient yields $4.1 million settlement. Outpatient Surgery. Available at: www.outpatientsurgery.net/news/2011/02/11.

11 Pinchot SN, Al-Wagih H, Schaefer S, Sippel R, Chen H. Accuracy of fine-needle aspiration biopsy for predicting neoplasm or carcinoma in thyroid nodules 4 cm of larger. Arch Surg 2009; 144(7): 649–55.

12 Robitschek J, Straub M, Wirtz E, Klem C, Sniezek J. Diagnostic efficacy of surgeon-performed ultrasound-guided fine needle aspiration: a randomized controlled trial. Otolaryngol Head Neck Surg 2010; 142(3): 306–9.

13 National Comprehensive Cancer Network guidelines. Available at: www.thyroidcancer.ru/med/literature/guides/thyroid_nccn.pdf.

14 American Thyroid Association guidelines. Available at: www.thyroidguidelines.net/.

15 Lydiatt DD. Medical malpractice and facial nerve paralysis. Arch Otolaryngol Head Neck Surg 2003; 129: 50–3.

16 Hekkenberg RJ, Irish JC, Rotstein LE, Brown DH, Gullane PJ. Informed consent in head and neck surgery: how much do patients actually remember? J Otolaryngol 1997; 26: 155–9.

17 Shindo M, Chheda NN. Incidence of vocal cord paralysis with and without recurrent laryngeal nerve monitoring during thyroidectomy. Arch Otolaryngol Head Neck Surg 2007; 133: 481–6.

18 Chan W-F, Lang BH, Lo C-Y. The role of intraoperative neuromonitoring of recurrent laryngeal nerve during thyroidectomy: a comparative study of 1000 nerves at risk. Surgery 2006; 140: 866–73.

19 Randolph GW, et al. for the International Intraoperative Monitoring Study Group. Electrophysiologic recurrent laryngeal nerve monitoring during thyroid and parathyroid surgery: international standards guideline statement. Laryngoscope 2011; 121: S1–S16.

20 Wingert D, Friesen S, Illopoulus J, Pierce G, Thomas J, Hermreck A. Post-thyroidectomy hypocalcemia: incidence and risk factors. Am J Surg 1986; 152: 606–10.

21 Glinoer D, Andry G, Chantrain G, Samil N. Clinical aspects of early and late hypocalcaemia after thyroid surgery. Eur J Surg Oncol 2000; 26: 571–7.

22 Sitges-Serra A, Ruiz S, Girvent M, Manjon H, Duenas J, Sancho J. Outcome of protracted hypoparathyroidsm after total thyroidectomy. Br J Surg 2010; 97: 1687–95.

23 Sabour S, Manders E, Steward D. The role of rapid PACU parathyroid hormone in reducing post-thyroidectomy hypocalcaemia. Otlaryngol Head Neck Surg 2009; 141: 727–9.

CHAPTER 3

Extent of Thyroidectomy and Incidence of Morbidity: Risk-appropriate Treatment

Dana M. Hartl[1] and Martin Schlumberger[2]

[1] Department of Head and Neck Oncology
[2] Department of Nuclear Medicine and Endocrine Oncology, Institut Gustave Roussy, Villejuif, France

Introduction

Surgery requires the conscientious evaluation of the risk/benefit ratio to inform the patient of the potential complications, their frequency and the means of managing them. All surgery carries some risk, with wound infection and postoperative bleeding common to all types of surgery, although with varying rates and degrees of severity. Most risks are unpredictable, with a minimum risk rate for any surgeon in any circumstance. Many of these risks can be minimized, however, with various surgical techniques, surgical experience and technological advances.

In the past, less than total or 'subtotal' thyroidectomy was considered one means of minimizing surgical morbidity. Today, this is no longer the case, whether for benign or malignant lesions. The aim of this chapter is to identify and quantify the different risks of thyroidectomy, discuss the current evidence-based indications for lobectomy versus total thyroidectomy and, finally, to discuss means of minimizing these risks and optimizing outcomes.

Rate of complications in thyroid surgery

Unilateral recurrent laryngeal nerve paralysis

Unilateral recurrent laryngeal nerve paralysis (URLNP) causing dysphonia is one of the first complications that comes to mind when informing patients of the risks of thyroid surgery. The RLN is in close contact to the thyroid gland, and any thyroid surgery in most cases implies a dissection of the nerve, the extent of nerve dissection varying with the anatomy of the patient and the thyroid pathology being treated. The physiopathology of URLNP is not well understood. The mechanism of injury may be linked to the mechanical surgical trauma of the nerve during dissection, surgical devascularization, electric injury, local inflammatory processes or, more rarely, partial or complete transsection of the nerve. Neuropraxia, according to Sunderland's classification of nerve lesions, is a temporary blockade of axonal transmission, without anatomical alterations of the perineurium, endoneurium or axons [1]. This type of nerve lesion is probably the

Thyroid Surgery: Preventing and Managing Complications, First Edition. Edited by Paolo Miccoli, David J. Terris,
Michele N. Minuto and Melanie W. Seybt.
© 2013 John Wiley & Sons, Ltd. Published 2013 by John Wiley & Sons, Ltd.

most frequently observed lesion, because spontaneous recovery of voice occurs in the majority of patients.

From a phylogenetic standpoint, the larynx is above all a sphincter, protecting the airway from aspiration, the passage of food, liquids or saliva into the airway [2]. The recurrent laryngeal nerve is a branch of the vagus nerve and is a mixed motor, sensate and autonomous nerve. It innervates both adductor muscles and abductor muscles. However, the action of these muscles is not quite as distinct as it may seem. In normal larynges, for example, the principal abductor muscle (the posterior cricoarytenoid muscle) shows activity that is simultaneous with adductor muscles during certain laryngeal gestures in speech and singing [3]. Thus, the adjustments of laryngeal configuration during phonation are complex and the variability of the position of the paralysed vocal fold may be due in part to this complexity. URLNP causes insufficient laryngeal closure during swallowing, cough and phonation, and may cause dyspnea during exertion (due to the absence of normal inspiratory abduction of the paralysed vocal fold). Aspiration related to URLNP can be severe and poorly tolerated, especially in patients with compromised pulmonary function. The glottal air leak on phonation causes a breathy and rough voice quality, with a decrease in the effectiveness of communication, especially on the telephone or in a noisy environment, leading to a decrease in quality of life [4].

The definitive position of the paralysed vocal fold and thus voice quality are related to the degree of denervation, the extent of spontaneous axonal regrowth, synkinesis of antagonistic muscles, reinnervation from the uninjured side of the larynx, reinnervation of motor endplates from autonomous nerve endings and/or, finally, from muscular activity stemming from the normal bilateral innervation of the interarytenoid muscles [5–7]. Laryngeal improvement can take up to 12 months to become apparent. A favourable functional outcome is defined as serviceable voice or good voice quality, no aspiration, and good voice-related quality of life. An unfavourable functional outcome is the persistence of a breathy, bitonal or rough voice, an increased vocal effort, dyspnea on exertion, aspiration, laryngeal spasms, and/or altered voice-related quality of life.

Reported rates of transient URLNP in thyroid surgery are 1–10%, with a median of 3–4%. Rates of permanent URLNP (dysphonia persisting after 12 months) are 0–3%, with a median of 1–2% (Table 3.1). Higher rates are commonly reported in cases of surgery for thyroid cancer, large multinodular goitres, hyperthyroidism, reoperations and in cases of extralaryngeal branching of the RLN [10,12,13,16,20,21].

Bilateral recurrent laryngeal nerve paralysis

Bilateral RLNP (BRLNP) may also occur after thyroid surgery but to a much rarer extent, and the clinical manifestations and management are completely different. Voice is generally normal, due to the paramedian or median position of the vocal folds. Dyspnoea at rest or on exertion, however, is frequent, and may require tracheotomy. Aspiration is rare in cases of BRLNP. Reported rates of temporary BRLNP range from 0.2% to 0.6%, with even lower rates of permanent paralysis [16,21,22]. The physiopathological basis is similar to that of URLNP. However, although the voice can completely recover in URLNP even without complete remobilization of the paralysed vocal fold, breathing may not recover in the same fashion in BRLNP, and laryngeal surgery (partial arytenoidectomy, posterior cordotomy or vocal fold lateralization) may be necessary to improve breathing and/or decannulate patients requiring a temporary tracheotomy. Patients should be referred to specialized laryngologists to optimize management.

Other voice disorders

Intubation trauma (vocal fold edema, inflammation, granuloma, haematoma) is relatively frequent. These lesions were visible in 31% of patients prospectively examined pre- and postoperatively by Echternach *et al.*, for example [10]. These lesions resolve spontaneously without permanent dysphonia, but healing of the vocal folds may take several weeks to months. Risk factors for postintubation laryngeal granuloma include diabetes, immunosuppressant therapy, renal insufficiency and gastro-eosophageal reflux.

Injury to the external branch of the superior laryngeal nerve can occur during ligation of the superior thyroid vessels and may lead to paralysis of the corresponding cricothyroid muscle, responsible for tensing the vocal fold to increase vocal pitch and/or intensity. Voice complaints include a lower-pitched voice, an inability to sing, produce high-pitched sounds or ask questions, and vocal fatigue. Laryngoscopic diagnosis is difficult due to non-specific signs. Invasive electromyography of the cricothyroid

Table 3.1 Some reported rates of transient and permanent unilateral recurrent laryngeal nerve paralysis (URLNP) without nerve monitoring.

Study	Number of nerves at risk	Transient URLNP (%)	Permanent URLNP (%)
Thomusch et al. [8]	12486	2.8	0.7
Dralle et al. [9]	5517	2.61	0.89
Echternack et al. [10]	1365	6.6	n.a.
Barczynski et al. [11]	1000	3.8	1.2
Lo et al. [12]	787	3.3	0.9
Chiang et al. [13]	704	5.1	0.9
Chan et al. [14]	499	4.0	1.2
Shindo et al. [15]	372	3.0	0.3
Casella et al. [16]	195	4.1	2.1
Robertson et al. [17]	120	4.2	2.5
Brauchkhoff et al. [18]	84	2.6	1.3
Yarbrough et al. [19]	79	10.1	1.3

n.a., not analysed.

muscles remains the gold standard for diagnosis, and thus the exact incidence of this problem is difficult to ascertain. Systematic identification of the nerve, eventually with neurostimulation, and low ligation of the vessels, close to the thyroid, are recommended to limit injury to the nerve [22]. In the absence of nerve identification, superior laryngeal nerve injury can occur in up to 28% of cases, which may be temporary or permanent, as for URLNP [22].

Voice complaints with no visible laryngoscopic abnormalities have been reported to occur in 37–47% of patients in the early postoperative period, and to persist at 3 months for approximately one-sixth of patients [23]. The etiology is unknown but this problem may be due to scarring of the infrahyoid or cricothyroid muscles, vascular or lymphatic laryngeal modifications or subclinical laryngeal paresis. These symptoms will have generally subsided after 1 year in all patients [24].

Hypocalcaemia

A calcium level requiring treatment after total thyroidectomy is defined as a calcaemia less than 2 mM or 8 mg/dL [25,26]. Transient hypocalcaemia due to hypoparathyroidism occurs in up to 50% of cases after total thyroidectomy, and is permanent, persisting after 12 months, in up to 13% of cases. Most series, however, report a rate of permanent hypoparathyroidism of 1–2%. Permanent hypoparathyroidism does not occur after lobectomy but only after bilateral surgery (total, near-total or 'subtotal') thyroidectomy. Higher rates are seen in cases of large or substernal goitres, Graves' disease, reoperations, cancer and central compartment neck dissection. Female patients are more at risk than males [21,27–32].

Local complications

Postoperative haematoma has been reported to occur in up to 3% of cases, regardless of the extent of thyroidectomy [21, 33]. Bergenfelz et al. found that older age and male gender increased this risk, with odds ratios of 1.04 and 1.90, respectively [21].

Seroma formation has been reported in up to 6% of thyroid operations, and is more prevalent after total thyroidectomy and after surgery for substernal goitre [21].

Wound infection occurs in 1–2% of cases, regardless of the extent of surgery. For Bergenfelz et al., this risk was increased by an odds ratio of 8.18 if neck dissection was associated [21]. Reoperative surgery also carries a higher risk for infection [9,13].

Permanent anaesthesia of the skin of the neck and/or upper thorax is very rare, but temporary anaesthesia and paraesthesia are common and may last for several postoperative months. Permanent anaesthesia of the earlobe may occur if lateral neck dissection is performed. Chronic pain, persisting after one postoperative year, is very rare but also possibly under-reported in the context of thyroidectomy.

Finally, an unaesthetic scar may occur in less than 1% of patients, more often in children and adolescents, dark-skinned patients and patients with a history of keloids [33].

Lobectomy versus total thyroidectomy

Total (or near-total) thyroidectomy is defined as removal of 'all grossly visible thyroid tissue, leaving only a small amount (<1 g) of tissue' [34]. 'Subtotal' thyroidectomy, no longer recommended, is the removal of both thyroid lobes leaving more than 1 g of thyroid tissue behind. Lobectomy carries no risk of transient or permanent hypocalcaemia as compared to a total, near-total or subtotal thyroidectomy. Despite the decreased risk for lobectomy, total thyroidecotmy is still recommended in adults and children for many thyroid diseases.

• *Benign multinodular goitre.* Total thyroidectomy is to be preferred over subtotal thyroidectomy, due to a lower recurrence rate. The rate of permanent complications is similar between total and less than total thyroidectomies. Reoperation for recurrence, however, is associated with higher complication rates [35,36].

• *Solitary nodules.* A total thyroidectomy is currently recommended for either solitary nodules over 4 cm with indeterminate or suspicious cytology, or a nodule in the context of a history of neck irradiation in childhood or adolescence, and/or family history of thyroid cancer [34]. A lobectomy may be performed for smaller solitary nodules with indeterminate or suspicious cytology or large hyperfunctioning solitary nodules, when the contralateral lobe is normal on preoperative ultrasound.

• *Graves' disease.* A total thyroidectomy is currently the recommended procedure when surgery is chosen as the definitive treatment. Less than total thyroidectomies carry a higher rate of recurrence, with similar complication rates as compared to a total thyroidectomy in experienced hands [37–39].

• *Thyroid cancer.* Total thyroidectomy is currently the treatment of choice for most thyroid cancers. Lobectomy may be sufficient only for unifocal classic papillary cancers 10 mm or less without histopathological signs of aggressiveness and in the absence of a history of neck irradiation in childhood or adolescence [34,40].

Complications in central neck dissection for thyroid cancer

Current guidelines recommend therapeutic central compartment (level VI) neck dissection in the presence of known lymph node metastases, detected preoperatively or intraoperatively, due to an improvement in sur-

vival rates compared to historic controls [34]. However, prophylactic or elective neck dissection remains controversial in the absence of high-level evidence showing an improved disease-free survival rate compared to thyroidectomy alone followed by radioactive iodine. Disease-free survival is excellent regardless of neck dissection for patients in the low-risk category, and low-level evidence suggests that central neck dissection carries a higher rate of permanent hypoparathyroidism compared to total thyroidectomy alone [41]. Furthermore, if needed, a secondary central neck dissection can be performed by experienced surgeons without an increase in morbidity compared to a primary central neck dissection [42,43].

The proponents of prophylactic neck dissection rely on it for accurate staging, prognosis and postoperative radioiodine dosing, keeping in mind that 40–80% of patients will have occult nodal metastases found when prophylactic neck dissection is performed [41,44–46]. For these patients, prophylactic neck dissection may decrease postoperative thyroglobulin levels and decrease the total dose of radioiodine needed for biological cure. Furthermore, prophylactic neck dissection may be beneficial for the subgroup of patients with tumours that do not exhibit radioiodine uptake.

Low-level evidence indeed suggests that prophylactic central neck dissection increases the rate of permanent hypoparathyroidism and unintentional recurrent nerve paralysis, with rates of 0–14% (median 2.3%) and 0–5.7% (median 2.4%), respectively, in the literature review published by White *et al.* [47]. However, other reports have not shown a higher morbidity, with reported rates of permanent hypoparathyroidism and recurrent nerve paralysis of less than 2% [42–45]. Comparative studies have been unable to show a significant difference in permanent recurrent nerve paralysis between thyroidectomy with and without central neck dissection [48]. Most studies have also been unable to show a significant difference in terms of permanent hypoparathyroidism, but several studies have demonstrated that adding a central neck dissection does increase the rate of transient hypoparathyroidism [46,48]. As for thyroidectomy, experience and a precise surgical technique are mandatory [49]. Systematic reimplantation of devascularized parathyroids is highly recommended. Preservation of the thymic remnants also optimizes preservation of parathyroid function [50].

Minimizing risks

Role of surgical experience in minimizing complications

High-level evidence has shown that surgeons with more experience in thyroid surgery and surgeons in high-volume centres have a lower rate of complications [9]. Several studies with a high evidence level have shown that the rate of permanent hypoparathyroidism is reduced for surgeons who have performed over 100 thyroidectomies [28,51]. In highly specialized centres, completion thyroidectomy may not carry a higher rate of complications compared to primary surgery [52].

Risks according to patient characteristics

Children

Total thyroidectomy and lobectomy is performed safely with a low rate of complications by experienced surgeons [38,39,53]. Children in general, and those aged 0–6 years in particular, suffer from a higher rate of complications than adults, with a longer hospital stay [54]. Permanent hypoparathyroidism is more frequent than in adults, as are keloid scars [38,39]. These interventions should be performed by experienced thyroid surgeons, whether they be paediatric surgeons or not, and in centres authorized to manage paediatric surgery.

Elderly patients

Patients over 65 years of age, and especially those over 80, have significantly more complications and a longer hospital stay than younger patients [55]. Older patients have a greater risk for transient vocal fold paralysis and haematoma than other adult patients, with odds ratios of 1.04 and 1.92, respectively, in the study by Bergenfelz *et al.* [21]. Vitamin D deficiency is also more prevalent in elderly patients and has been shown to be a risk factor for transient postoperative hypoparathyroidism [25,56]. This issue should be addressed preoperatively when treating elderly patients.

Reoperation

Traditionally, reoperative surgery carries a slight but significant increase in local complications, URLNP and hypoparthyroidism. Studies conducted in highly specialized centres, however, have shown that completion thyroidectomy does not necessarily carry a higher risk of complications compared to primary surgery [52,57,58]. Reoperation still should be avoided when possible (which is why total thyroidectomy is now recommended instead of subtotal resections) and should always be performed in specialized centres [59].

Pre-existing unilateral RLNP

Preoperative laryngoscopic examination is fundamental to thyroid sugery, especially for reoperative surgery or if malignancy is suspected [60]. A pre-existing URLNP increases the risk of BRLNP in cases of dissection of the sole functioning nerve. This issue must be discussed with patients prior to the intervention, and may lead to modifications in the surgical strategy. If malignancy is suspected, and the involved nerve is known to be non-functional preoperatively, it may be sacrificed.

Prior radiation therapy to the neck

Radiation therapy to the neck may alter tissue trophicity, vascularization and lymphatic drainage, predisposing patients to local complications. The effects of radiation therapy are dose dependent but the threshold for late radiation effects is also patient dependent.

Cancer

Surgery for thyroid cancer carries a higher risk of temporary and permanent vocal fold paralysis [9,13,61]. A higher rate of temporary and permanent hypoparathyroidism is also observed if central neck dissection is performed [21].

Recurrent nerve paralysis

Systematic intraoperative visualization of the recurrent nerve is the gold standard for thyroid surgery due to the decrease in URLNP with this technique as compared to a 'blind' approach [9,61,62]. Despite a large number of prospective randomized trials, the bulk of the literature has failed to show that intraoperative nerve monitoring decreases the rate of transient or permanent URLNP, compared to nerve visualization [8,9,14,15,19,63]. Only one recent prospective randomized trial with 1000 nerves at risk in each group found that intraoperative neurophysiological monitoring (IONM) significantly reduced the risk of transient URLNP, but not the risk of permanent URLNP [11]. One recent non-randomized trial also found a decrease in transient URLNP using intraoperative nerve monitoring for multinodular goitre [64]. There are, however, other advantages to nerve monitoring, such as aid in identification and dissection of the nerve in difficult cases and reoperations, and the high negative predictive value of a normal evoked waveform at the end of the resection [65].

Systematic preoperative and postoperative laryngeal examination is highly recommended, not necessarily to decrease the incidence of postoperative URLNP but to diagnose invasive disease and pre-existing laryngeal conditions [60]. URLNP diagnosed preoperatively is a risk factor for BRLNP, and this complication should be discussed with patients preoperatively. A preoperative diagnosis of unilateral vocal fold paralysis may signify invasive disease requiring more extensive surgery. Diagnosis of other voice disorders pre- or postoperatively may require appropriate management before thyroidectomy. Postoperative laryngoscopy may reveal asymptomatic vocal fold paralysis, and allows for the diagnosis of vocal complaints not related to vocal fold paralysis [61].

Surgical treatment of URLNP with vocal fold medialization (Figure 3.1), vocal fold injection (Figure 3.2) or reinnervation is beneficial for patients with aspiration, poor voice quality, increased vocal effort and decreased quality of life due to these symptoms [4]. Patients with vocal complaints should be referred to a specialized laryngologist to optimize care for this complication of thyroid surgery [7].

Preoperative written information about recurrent nerve paralysis and early referral to a laryngology specialist if needed will not decrease the incidence of vocal fold paralysis, but efficient management of these patients can only be beneficial and may possibly decrease the risk of litigation [66].

Hypoparathyroidism

There is high-level evidence demonstrating several key steps to minimize hypoparathyroidism.

Identification

Knowledge of parathyroid anatomy is indispensable (Figures 3.3, 3.4) [29]. Surgeons with an experience of over 100 thyroidectomies have lower rates of hypoparathyroidism [30,51]. A meticulous technique with identification of at least two parathyroid glands has been shown to significantly reduce the rate of permanent hypoparathyroidism compared to identification of no or

only one parathyroid gland [27]. The use of surgical loupes significantly improved identification in the study by Pata et al. [67]. The high level of right–left symmetry (80% for the superior glands and 70% for the inferior glands) can also aid in locating and identifying the parathyroid glands [68]. The chance of finding an intrathyroidal parathyroid gland on definitive pathology is 1–2% [69,70]. The risk of postoperative hypoparathyroidism is not increased in cases of intrathyroidal parathyroid, however [51].

Intravenous methylene blue has been used in the past as a selective stain to identify parathyroid glands, particularly in reoperative surgery. There are recent reports, however, of severe encephalopathy secondary to the administration of methylene blue, which has biochemical properties similar to those of monoamine oxidase inhibitors [71]. The association of methylene blue with drugs enhancing central serotonin transmission (certain antidepressants) seems to be the cause of this severe complication. Extreme precaution must be taken when using methylene blue, and some teams have abandoned its use altogether [72].

Preservation

It has been shown that a technique using distal ligation of the vessels at the thyroid capsule instead of a proximal ligation decreases the rate of transient and permanent hypoparathyroidism [27]. Dissection and preservation of the thymic remnant and the thyrothymic ligament may also aid in minimizing hypoparathyroidism. Akerström et al. located an inferior parathyroid in the thyrothymic ligament in 25% of cases [68] and Pellitteri et al. found that 2–5% of the inferior parathyroids are actually intrathymic [70].

The Harmonic® technology (Ethicon, USA) has been recently developed as a means of ligating vessels reliably and quickly, avoiding ligatures and clips in endoscopic and open surgery. Transient hypocalcaemia has been shown to be reduced by an average of 31% with the Harmonic® technology compared to classic thyroidectomy [73].

Autotransplantation

Treat each parathyroid as if it were the only one. Systematic autotransplantation of devascularized or traumatized parathyroid glands has been shown to decrease the rate of permanent hypoparathyroidism (Figure 3.5)

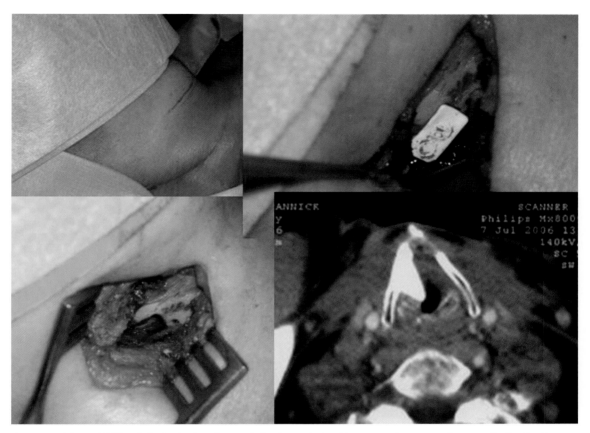

Figure 3.1 Right vocal fold medialization by thyroplasty under local anaesthesia, with postoperative computed tomography showing the implant in place.

[74,75]. The reimplanted parathyroid starts to function at 2–4 weeks, and complete function is obtained after 6–8 weeks. High rates of successful autotransplantation ranging from 83% to 100% have been reported [74,75].

Prediction

A descending slope for calcaemia levels measured successively on postoperative days 1, 2 and 3 is predictive of hypocalcaemia needing treatment. Earlier prediction of hypocalcaemia may be obtained by measuring postoperative parathormone levels. Postoperative parathormone levels measured at any time from 10 min to 20 h will provide accurate information, due to the short biological half-life of parathormone [26,76,77]. Only 7% of patients with normal postoperative parathormone levels developed hypocalcaemia in a large Australian study, and hypocalcaemia was generally mild and self-limiting in

this group [26,78]. Thus, measuring parathormone postoperatively can help stratify patients according to the risk of hypocalcaemia and lead to supplementation when necessary, keeping in mind that the accuracy is less than 100% and that even when postoperative levels are normal, hypocalcaemia may still occur in 5–10% of patients.

Supplementation

A recent prospective study found that preoperative vitamin D deficiency (vitamin D3 <10 ng/mL) was a risk factor for transient postoperative hypocalcaemia and extended hospital stay [25]. This suggests that preoperative dosing of vitamin D and supplementation in cases of deficiency may improve outcomes and reduce the rate of transient hypocalcaemia. Several prospective randomized studies have also shown that systematic postoperative supplementation in calcium and/or vitamin D

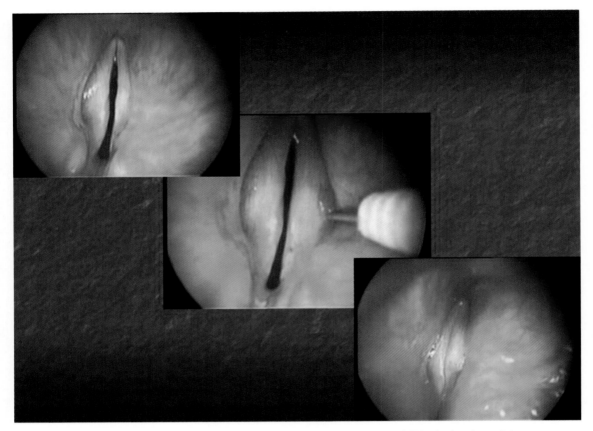

Figure 3.2 Right vocal fold medialization for unilateral recurrent nerve paralysis by direct intracordal injection (autologous fat).

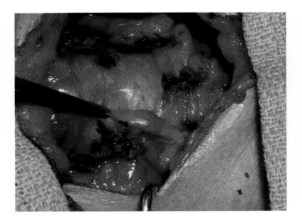

Figure 3.3 Right inferior parathyroid gland at the distal end of the thymic remnant.

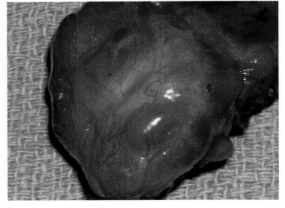

Figure 3.4 Left subcapsular inferior parathyroid after removal of a large multinodular goitre.

(a)

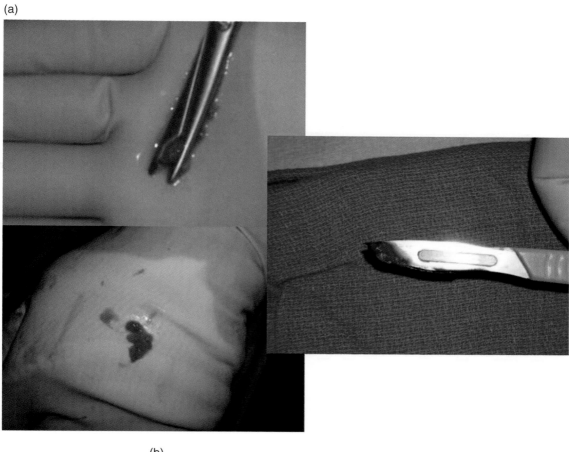

(b)

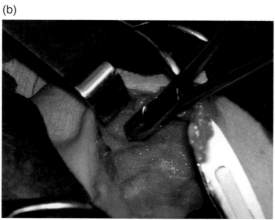

Figure 3.5 Parathyroid reimplantaion: the parathyroid is minced (a) and reimplanted in a pocket in the sternomastoid muscle (b).

decreases the rate of symptomatic and asymptomatic hypocalcaemia [79–81].

Local complications

High-level evidence from prospective randomized trials has shown that drains do not decrease the risk of haematoma formation [82,83]. Drains do not decrease the rate of seroma but avoid repeated needle aspiration to drain the seroma [84]. Finally, drains do not decrease or increase the risk of infection. Prophylactic antibiotics do not decrease the risk of infection and are not indicated for thyroidectomy. These local complications are rare and only a meticulous surgical technique can reduce the risk to a minimum, without, however, completely abolishing the risk.

Scar

One aim of minimally invasive thyroid surgery is to reduce or hide the scar, and several different approaches have been reported. Minimally invasive open surgery is basically the same procedure as that described over 100 years ago by Professor Theodor Kocher, but the incision is less than 7 cm. This approach is facilitated by new haemostatic technologies which allow minimally invasive haemostasis, reduce the length of the operating procedure and can even reduce overall cost [85–87].

Minimally invasive video-assisted thyroidectomy (MIVAT) is a combined endoscopic and open approach that reduces the scar to 1–2 cm [88]. High-level evidence (prospective randomized trials) has shown that the complication rate is not higher than that of conventional thyroidectomy and that postoperative pain is reduced and patient satisfaction increased by this technique [89,90]. The main limitation of this technique is the size of the thyroid gland, since it is difficult to remove thyroid nodules larger than 35 mm by these small incisions.

Completely endoscopic approaches to thyroidectomy with breast, axillary, scalp or dorsal portals, with or without CO_2 insufflation, and with or without robotic assistance, are routinely employed by experienced teams [91–98]. These approaches aim not at minimizing the scar, nor minimizing the extent of the subplatysmal dissection, but at hiding the scar in inconspicuous areas. In experienced hands, these techniques are effective without increasing the rate of permanent complications, but surgical experience, experience of the operating room team and proper patient selection are primary.

Postoperative pain

The MIVAT technique, when applicable, has been shown to reduce postoperative pain, compared to conventional thyroidectomy [89,90]. Subjective voice and swallowing symptoms are also reduced with this technique [99]. New haemostatic technologies have also been shown to reduce postoperative pain (see below). Finally, several prospective randomized trials have shown that intraoperative subcutaneous injection of local anaesthetic (bupivacaine) reduces pain in the first postoperative hours, but also reduces the perception of pain up to and including postoperative day 2 [100,101]. Chronic pain lasting over 1 year after surgery is rare but probably under-reported. In this context, complete evaluation in a specialized pain centre should be performed and patients managed by pain specialists.

New haemostatic technologies

At the present time, there are two basic types of haemostatic devices used in thyroid surgery: LigaSure® (Covidien, USA) and Harmonic® technology (Ethicon, USA). These technologies have been developed as a means of ligating vessels reliably and quickly, avoiding ligatures and clips in endoscopic and open surgery.

Both of these technologies are routinely employed by many surgical teams throughout the world. The volume and quality of the scientific publications have lead to three different meta-analyses of the literature and an evaluation of the evidence base for the utilization of these technologies [73,86,102]. Operating time is significantly shorter by at least 20–25% (or 23 min, on average) [73]. Transient hypocalcaemia has been shown to be reduced by an average of 31% with the Harmonic® technology compared to classic thyroidectomy [102]. Blood loss is reduced by an average of 20 mL (or 30–50%), and postoperative pain and hospital stay are also significantly reduced with the Harmonic® technology [86]. The LigaSure® technology has also been shown to significantly reduce postoperative pain and hospital stay, without a significant reduction in hypocalcaemia rates or blood loss, however, compared to conventional thyroidectomy [102].

Two prospective randomized studies have compared the two technologies [87,103]. Pons *et al.* found that total thyroidectomy was on average 8 min shorter with the Harmonic® technology compared to LigaSure® (114 min versus 122 min, p=0.04, with 151 min for conventional thyroidectomy) [87]. Neither study found any difference, however, in terms of morbidity, pain, blood loss or hospital stay between the two technologies. The rate of vocal fold paralysis is not altered by the use of these technologies [104].

Conclusion

Total or near-total thyroidectomy, with the removal of all visible thyroid tissue leaving less than 1 g, is the recommended procedure for most thyroid diseases. Total thyroidectomy can be performed without more complications than subtotal thyroidectomy, and recurrence rates for goitre, Graves' disease and cancer are lower. In experienced hands, permanent recurrent nerve paralysis and permanent hypoparathyroidism occur in approximately 1–2% of patients, with higher rates according to various risk factors (notably age, large goitres, Graves'disease, reoperations and surgery for cancer). Thyroid surgeons should be knowledgeable about current technical and technological advances that aid in reducing complications.

References

1 Sunderland S. A classification of peripheral nerve injuries producing loss of function. Brain 1951; 74: 491–516.
2 Negus V (ed). The Mechanism of the Larynx. London: Heinemann, 1929.
3 Hirose H. Posterior cricoarytenoid as a speech muscle. Ann Otol Rhinol Laryngol 1976; 85: 335–42.
4 Spector BC, Netterville JL, Billante C, Clary J, Reinisch L, Smith TL. Quality-of-life assessment in patients with unilateral vocal cord paralysis. Otolaryngol Head Neck Surg 2001; 125: 176–82.
5 McCulloch TM, Hoffman HT. Medialization laryngoplasty with expanded polytetrafluoroethylene. Surgical technique and preliminary results. Ann Otol Rhinol Laryngol 1998; 107: 427–32.
6 Crumley RL. Laryngeal synkinesis: its significance to the laryngologist. Ann Otol Rhinol Laryngol 1989; 98: 87–92.
7 Hartl DM, Travagli JP, Leboulleux S, Baudin E, Brasnu DF, Schlumberger M. Clinical review: current concepts in the management of unilateral recurrent laryngeal nerve paralysis after thyroid surgery. J Clin Endocrinol Metab 2005; 90: 3084–8.
8 Thomusch O, Sekulla C, Machens A, Neumann HJ, Timmermann W, Dralle H. Validity of intra-operative neuromonitoring signals in thyroid surgery. Langenbecks Arch Surg 2004; 389: 499–503.
9 Dralle H, Sekulla C, Haerting J, et al. Risk factors of paralysis and functional outcome after recurrent laryngeal nerve monitoring in thyroid surgery. Surgery 2004; 136: 1310–22.
10 Echternach M, Maurer CA, Mencke T, Schilling M, Verse T, Richter B. Laryngeal complications after thyroidectomy: is it always the surgeon? Arch Surg 2009; 144: 149–53; discussion 53.
11 Barczynski M, Konturek A, Cichon S. Randomized clinical trial of visualization versus neuromonitoring of recurrent laryngeal nerves during thyroidectomy. Br J Surg 2009; 96: 240–6.
12 Lo CY, Kwok KF, Yuen PW. A prospective evaluation of recurrent laryngeal nerve paralysis during thyroidectomy. Arch Surg 2000; 135: 204–7.
13 Chiang FY, Wang LF, Huang YF, Lee KW, Kuo WR. Recurrent laryngeal nerve palsy after thyroidectomy with routine identification of the recurrent laryngeal nerve. Surgery 2005; 137: 342–7.
14 Chan WF, Lo CY. Pitfalls of intraoperative neuromonitoring for predicting postoperative recurrent laryngeal nerve function during thyroidectomy. World J Surg 2006; 30: 806–12.
15 Shindo M, Chheda NN. Incidence of vocal cord paralysis with and without recurrent laryngeal nerve monitoring during thyroidectomy. Arch Otolaryngol Head Neck Surg 2007; 133: 481–5.
16 Casella C, Pata G, Nascimbeni R, Mittempergher F, Salerni B. Does extralaryngeal branching have an impact on the rate of postoperative transient or permanent recurrent laryngeal nerve palsy? World J Surg 2009; 33: 261–5.
17 Robertson ML, Steward DL, Gluckman JL, Welge J. Continuous laryngeal nerve integrity monitoring during thyroidectomy: does it reduce risk of injury? Otolaryngol Head Neck Surg 2004; 131: 596–600.
18 Brauckhoff M, Gimm O, Thanh PN, et al. First experiences in intraoperative neurostimulation of the recurrent laryngeal nerve during thyroid surgery of children and adolescents. J Pediatr Surg 2002; 37: 1414–18.
19 Yarbrough DE, Thompson GB, Kasperbauer JL, Harper CM, Grant CS. Intraoperative electromyographic monitoring of the recurrent laryngeal nerve in reoperative thyroid and parathyroid surgery. Surgery 2004; 136: 1107–15.
20 Sancho JJ, Pascual-Damieta M, Pereira JA, Carrera MJ, Fontane J, Sitges-Serra A. Risk factors for transient vocal cord palsy after thyroidectomy. Br J Surg 2008; 95: 961–7.
21 Bergenfelz A, Jansson S, Kristoffersson A, et al. Complications to thyroid surgery: results as reported in a database from a multicenter audit comprising 3,660 patients. Langenbecks Arch Surg 2008; 393: 667–73.
22 Cernea CR, Brandao LG, Hojaij FC, et al. Negative and positive predictive values of nerve monitoring in thyroidectomy. Head Neck 2012; 34: 175–9.
23 Soylu L, Ozbas S, Uslu HY, Kocak S. The evaluation of the causes of subjective voice disturbances after thyroid surgery. Am J Surg 2007; 194: 317–22.

24 Lombardi CP, Raffaelli M, de Crea C, *et al.* Long-term outcome of functional post-thyroidectomy voice and swallowing symptoms. Surgery 2009; 146: 1174–81.

25 Kirkby-Bott J, Markogiannakis H, Skandarajah A, Cowan M, Fleming B, Palazzo F. Preoperative vitamin D deficiency predicts postoperative hypocalcemia after total thyroidectomy. World J Surg 2011; 35: 324–30.

26 Grodski S, Serpell J. Evidence for the role of perioperative PTH measurement after total thyroidectomy as a predictor of hypocalcemia. World J Surg 2008; 32: 1367–73.

27 Thomusch O, Machens A, Sekulla C, Ukkat J, Brauckhoff M, Dralle H. The impact of surgical technique on postoperative hypoparathyroidism in bilateral thyroid surgery: a multivariate analysis of 5846 consecutive patients. Surgery 2003; 133: 180–5.

28 Thomusch O, Machens A, Sekulla C, *et al.* Multivariate analysis of risk factors for postoperative complications in benign goiter surgery: prospective multicenter study in Germany. World J Surg 2000; 24: 1335–41.

29 Fewins J, Simpson CB, Miller FR. Complications of thyroid and parathyroid surgery. Otolaryngol Clin North Am 2003; 36: 189–206, x.

30 Zambudio AR, Rodriguez J, Riquelme J, Soria T, Canteras M, Parrilla P. Prospective study of postoperative complications after total thyroidectomy for multinodular goiters by surgeons with experience in endocrine surgery. Ann Surg 2004; 240: 18–25.

31 Delbridge L, Guinea AI, Reeve TS. Total thyroidectomy for bilateral benign multinodular goiter: effect of changing practice. Arch Surg 1999; 134: 1389–93.

32 Wilson RB, Erskine C, Crowe PJ. Hypomagnesemia and hypocalcemia after thyroidectomy: prospective study. World J Surg 2000; 24: 722–6.

33 Watkinson JC. Fifteen years' experience in thyroid surgery. Ann R Coll Surg Engl 2010; 92: 541–7.

34 Cooper DS, Doherty GM, Haugen BR, *et al.* Revised American Thyroid Association management guidelines for patients with thyroid nodules and differentiated thyroid cancer. Thyroid 2009; 19: 1167–214.

35 Agarwal G, Aggarwal V. Is total thyroidectomy the surgical procedure of choice for benign multinodular goiter? An evidence-based review. World J Surg 2008; 32: 1313–24.

36 Moalem J, Suh I, Duh QY. Treatment and prevention of recurrence of multinodular goiter: an evidence-based review of the literature. World J Surg 2008; 32: 1301–12.

37 Stalberg P, Svensson A, Hessman O, Akerstrom G, Hellman P. Surgical treatment of Graves' disease: evidence-based approach. World J Surg 2008; 32: 1269–77.

38 Scholz S, Smith JR, Chaignaud B, Shamberger RC, Huang SA. Thyroid surgery at Children's Hospital Boston: a 35-year single-institution experience. J Pediatr Surg 2011; 46: 437–42.

39 Raval MV, Browne M, Chin AC, Zimmerman D, Angelos P, Reynolds M. Total thyroidectomy for benign disease in the pediatric patient – feasible and safe. J Pediatr Surg 2009; 44: 1529–33.

40 Bilimoria KY, Bentrem DJ, Ko CY, *et al.* Extent of surgery affects survival for papillary thyroid cancer. Ann Surg 2007; 246: 375–81; discussion 81–4.

41 Soriano JV, Liu N, Gao Y, *et al.* Inhibition of angiogenesis by growth factor receptor bound protein 2-Src homology 2 domain bound antagonists. Mol Cancer Ther 2004; 3: 1289–99.

42 Alvarado R, Sywak MS, Delbridge L, Sidhu SB. Central lymph node dissection as a secondary procedure for papillary thyroid cancer: is there added morbidity? Surgery 2009; 145: 514–18.

43 Shen WT, Ogawa L, Ruan D, *et al.* Central lymph node dissection for papillary thyroid cancer. Arch Surg 2010; 145: 272–5.

44 Hughes DT, White ML, Miller BS, Gauger PG, Burney RE, Doherty GM. Influence of prophylactic central lymph node dissection on postoperative thyroglobulin levels and radioiodine treatment in papillary thyroid cancer. Surgery 2010; 148: 1100–7.

45 Hartl D, Leboulleux S, Al Ghuzlan A, *et al.* Optimization of staging of the neck with prophylactic central and lateral neck dissection for papillary thyroid carcinoma. Ann Surg 2012: 255: 777–83.

46 Moo T, McGill J, Allendorf J, Lee J, Fahey T, Zarnegar R. Impact of prophylactic central lymph node dissection on early recurrence in papillary thyroid carcinoma. World J Surg 2010; 34: 1187–91.

47 White ML, Gauger PG, Doherty GM. Central lymph node dissection in differentiated thyroid cancer. World J Surg 2007; 31: 895–904.

48 Mazzaferri E, Doherty GM, Steward DL. The pros and cons of central compartment lymph node dissection for papillary thyroid carcinoma. Thyroid 2009; 19: 683–9.

49 Hartl D, Travagli JP. Central compartment neck dissection for thyroid cancer: a surgical technique. World J Surg 2011; 35: 1553–9.

50 El Khatib Z, Lamblin J, Aubert S, *et al.* Is thymectomy worthwhile in central lymph node dissection for differentiated thyroid cancer? World J Surg 2010; 34: 1181–6.

51 Sasson AR, Pingpank JF Jr, Wetherington RW, Hanlon AL, Ridge JA. Incidental parathyroidectomy during thyroid surgery does not cause transient symptomatic hypocalcemia. Arch Otolaryngol Head Neck Surg 2001; 127: 304–8.

52 Erdem E, Gulcelik MA, Kuru B, Alagol H. Comparison of completion thyroidectomy and primary surgery for differentiated thyroid carcinoma. Eur J Surg Oncol 2003; 29: 747–9.

53 Bargren AE, Meyer-Rochow GY, Delbridge LW, Sidhu SB, Chen H. Outcomes of surgically managed pediatric thyroid cancer. J Surg Res 2009; 156: 70–3.

54 Sosa JA, Tuggle CT, Wang TS, *et al.* Clinical and economic outcomes of thyroid and parathyroid surgery in children. J Clin Endocrinol Metab 2008a; 93: 3058–65.

55 Sosa JA, Mehta PJ, Wang TS, Boudourakis L, Roman SA. A population-based study of outcomes from thyroidectomy in aging Americans: at what cost? J Am Coll Surg 2008b; 206: 1097–105.

56 Lips P. Vitamin D deficiency and secondary hyperparathyroidism in the elderly: consequences for bone loss and fractures and therapeutic implications. Endocr Rev 2001; 22: 477–501.

57 Terris DJ, Khichi S, Anderson SK, Seybt MW. Reoperative thyroidectomy for benign thyroid disease. Head Neck 2010; 32: 285–9.

58 Levin KE, Clark AH, Duh QY, Demeure M, Siperstein AE, Clark OH. Reoperative thyroid surgery. Surgery 1992; 111: 604–9.

59 Mitchell J, Milas M, Barbosa G, Sutton J, Berber E, Siperstein A. Avoidable reoperations for thyroid and parathyroid surgery: effect of hospital volume. Surgery 2008; 144: 899–906; discussion 907.

60 Randolph GW, Kamani D. The importance of preoperative laryngoscopy in patients undergoing thyroidectomy: voice, vocal cord function, and the preoperative detection of invasive thyroid malignancy. Surgery 2006; 139: 357–62.

61 Steurer M, Passler C, Denk DM, Schneider B, Niederle B, Bigenzahn W. Advantages of recurrent laryngeal nerve identification in thyroidectomy and parathyroidectomy and the importance of preoperative and postoperative laryngoscopic examination in more than 1000 nerves at risk. Laryngoscope 2002; 112: 124–33.

62 Riddell V. Thyroidectomy: prevention of bilateral recurrent nerve palsy. Results of identification of the nerve over 23 consecutive years (1946–69) with a description of an additional safety measure. Br J Surg 1970; 57: 1–11.

63 Thomusch O, Sekulla C, Walls G, Machens A, Dralle H. Intraoperative neuromonitoring of surgery for benign goiter. Am J Surg 2002; 183: 673–8.

64 Randolph GW, Shin JJ, Grillo HC, *et al.* The surgical management of goiter: Part II. Surgical treatment and results. Laryngoscope 2011a; 121: 68–76.

65 Randolph GW, Dralle H, Abdullah H, *et al.* Electrophysiologic recurrent laryngeal nerve monitoring during thyroid and parathyroid surgery: international standards guideline statement. Laryngoscope 2011b; 121(Suppl 1): S1–16.

66 Shaw GY, Pierce E. Malpractice litigation involving iatrogenic surgical vocal fold paralysis: a closed-claims review with recommendations for prevention and management. Ann Otol Rhinol Laryngol 2009; 118: 6–12.

67 Pata G, Casella C, Mittempergher F, Cirillo L, Salerni B. Loupe magnification reduces postoperative hypocalcemia after total thyroidectomy. Am Surg 2010; 76: 1345–50.

68 Akerstrom G, Malmaeus J, Bergstrom R. Surgical anatomy of human parathyroid glands. Surgery 1984; 95: 14–21.

69 Bahar G, Feinmesser R, Joshua BZ, *et al.* Hyperfunctioning intrathyroid parathyroid gland: a potential cause of failure in parathyroidectomy. Surgery 2006; 139: 821–6.

70 Pellitteri PK. Directed parathyroid exploration: evolution and evaluation of this approach in a single-institution review of 346 patients. Laryngoscope 2003; 113: 1857–69.

71 Pollack G, Pollack A, Delfiner J, Fernandez J. Parathyroid surgery and methylene blue: a review with guidelines for safe intraoperative use. Laryngoscope 2009; 119: 1941–6.

72 Han N, Bumpous JM, Goldstein RE, Fleming MM, Flynn MB. Intra-operative parathyroid identification using methylene blue in parathyroid surgery. Am Surg 2007; 73: 820–3.

73 Melck A, Wiseman S. Harmonic scalpel compared to conventional hemostasis in thyroid surgery: a meta-analysis. Int J Surg Oncol 2010; ID 396079.

74 Sierra M, Herrera MF, Herrero B, *et al.* Prospective biochemical and scintigraphic evaluation of autografted normal parathyroid glands in patients undergoing thyroid operations. Surgery 1998; 124: 1005–10.

75 Lo CY, Lam KY. Postoperative hypocalcemia in patients who did or did not undergo parathyroid autotransplantation during thyroidectomy: a comparative study. Surgery 1998; 124: 1081–6; discussion 1086–7.

76 Friedman M, Vidyasagar R, Bliznikas D, Joseph NJ. Intraoperative intact parathyroid hormone level monitoring as a guide to parathyroid reimplantation after thyroidectomy. Laryngoscope 2005; 115: 34–8.

77 Payne RJ, Hier MP, Tamilia M, Young J, MacNamara E, Black MJ. Postoperative parathyroid hormone level as a predictor of postthyroidectomy hypocalcemia. J Otolaryngol 2003; 32: 362–7.

78 Australian Endocrine Surgeons Guidelines AES06/01. Postoperative parathyroid hormone measurement and early discharge after total thyroidectomy: analysis of Australian data and management recommendations. ANZ J Surg 2007; 77: 199–202.

79 Roh JL, Park CI. Routine oral calcium and vitamin D supplements for prevention of hypocalcemia after total thyroidectomy. Am J Surg 2006; 192: 675–8.

80 Bellantone R, Lombardi CP, Raffaelli M, *et al.* Is routine supplementation therapy (calcium and vitamin D) useful after total thyroidectomy? Surgery 2002a; 132: 1109–12; discussion 1112–13.

81 Tartaglia F, Giuliani A, Sgueglia M, Biancari F, Juvonen T, Campana FP. Randomized study on oral administration of calcitriol to prevent symptomatic hypocalcemia after total thyroidectomy. Am J Surg 2005; 190: 424–9.

82 Corsten M, Johnson S, Alherabi A. Is suction drainage an effective means of preventing hematoma in thyroid surgery? A meta-analysis. J Otolaryngol 2005; 34: 415–17.

83 Pothier DD. The use of drains following thyroid and parathyroid surgery: a meta-analysis. J Laryngol Otol 2005; 119: 669–71.

84 Gourin CG JJ. Postoperative complications. In: Randolph G (ed) Surgery of the Thyroid and Parathyroid Glands. Philadelphia: Saunders, 2003: 433–43.

85 Terris DJ, Gourin CG, Chin E. Minimally invasive thyroidectomy: basic and advanced techniques. Laryngoscope 2006; 116: 350–6.

86 Ecker T, Carvalho AL, Choe JH, Walosek G, Preuss KJ. Hemostasis in thyroid surgery: harmonic scalpel versus other techniques – a meta-analysis. Otolaryngol Head Neck Surg 2010; 143: 17–25.

87 Pons Y, Gauthier J, Ukkola-Pons E, et al. Comparison of LigaSure vessel sealing system, harmonic scalpel, and conventional hemostasis in total thyroidectomy. Otolaryngol Head Neck Surg 2009; 141: 496–501.

88 Miccoli P, Berti P, Frustaci GL, Ambrosini CE, Materazzi G. Video-assisted thyroidectomy: indications and results. Langenbecks Arch Surg 2006; 391: 68–71.

89 Miccoli P, Berti P, Raffaelli M, Materazzi G, Baldacci S, Rossi G. Comparison between minimally invasive video-assisted thyroidectomy and conventional thyroidectomy: a prospective randomized study. Surgery 2001; 130: 1039–43.

90 Bellantone R, Lombardi CP, Bossola M, et al. Video-assisted vs conventional thyroid lobectomy: a randomized trial. Arch Surg 2002b; 137: 301–4; discussion 305.

91 Yeung GH. Endoscopic thyroid surgery today: a diversity of surgical strategies. Thyroid 2002; 12: 703–6.

92 Choe JH, Kim SW, Chung KW, et al. Endoscopic thyroidectomy using a new bilateral axillo–breast approach. World J Surg 2007; 31: 601–6.

93 Lee KE, Kim HY, Park WS, et al. Postauricular and axillary approach endoscopic neck surgery: a new technique. World J Surg 2009; 33: 767–72.

94 Schardey HM, Barone M, Portl S, von Ahnen M, von Ahnen T, Schopf S. Invisible scar endoscopic dorsal approach thyroidectomy: a clinical feasibility study. World J Surg 2010; 34: 2997–3006.

95 Cougard P, Osmak-Tizon L, Balestra L, Dancea R, Goudet P. [Endoscopic thyroidectomy via median approach with gas insufflation: analysis of the first 100 cases]. J Chir (Paris) 2007; 144: 297–300.

96 Kang SW, Jeong JJ, Yun JS, et al. Gasless endoscopic thyroidectomy using trans-axillary approach: surgical outcome of 581 patients. Endocr J 2009; 56: 361–9.

97 Lee J, Yun JH, Nam KH, Soh EY, Chung WY. The learning curve for robotic thyroidectomy: a multicenter study. Ann Surg Oncol 2011a; 18: 226–32.

98 Lee J, Yun JH, Nam KH, Choi UJ, Chung WY, Soh EY. Perioperative clinical outcomes after robotic thyroidectomy for thyroid carcinoma: a multicenter study. Surg Endosc 2011b; 25: 906–12.

99 Lombardi CP, Raffaelli M, d'Alatri L, et al. Video-assisted thyroidectomy significantly reduces the risk of early post-thyroidectomy voice and swallowing symptoms. World J Surg 2008; 32: 693–700.

100 Steffen T, Warschkow R, Brandle M, Tarantino I, Clerici T. Randomized controlled trial of bilateral superficial cervical plexus block versus placebo in thyroid surgery. Br J Surg 2010; 97: 1000–6.

101 Kesisoglou I, Papavramidis TS, Michalopoulos N, et al. Superficial selective cervical plexus block following total thyroidectomy: a randomized trial. Head Neck 2010; 32: 984–8.

102 Yao HS, Wang Q, Wang WJ, Ruan CP. Prospective clinical trials of thyroidectomy with LigaSure vs conventional vessel ligation: a systematic review and meta-analysis. Arch Surg 2009; 144: 1167–74.

103 Rahbari R, Mathur A, Kitano M, et al. Prospective randomized trial of ligasure versus harmonic hemostasis technique in thyroidectomy. Ann Surg Oncol 2011; 18: 1023–7.

104 Zarebczan B, Mohanty D, Chen H. A comparison of the LigaSure and harmonic scalpel in thyroid surgery: a single institution review. Ann Surg Oncol 2011; 18: 214–18.

CHAPTER 4

Thyroid Surgery in Paediatric Patients

Scott A. Rivkees,[1] *Christopher K. Breuer*[2] *and Robert Udelsman*[2]

[1] Department of Pediatrics, University of Florida, Gainesville, FL, USA
[2] Department of Surgery, Yale University School of Medicine; Yale Pediatric Thyroid Center, Yale University School of Medicine, New Haven, CT, USA

Introduction

Paediatric thyroid disease requiring surgery is uncommon and is associated with a greater risk of complications than in adults. Thyroid conditions requiring surgery in the paediatric population include Graves' disease, thyroid cancer and thyroid nodules. Each of these conditions is discussed below.

Graves' disease

Graves' disease (GD) is the most common cause of hyperthyroidism in children and adults, and occurs when the thyroid gland is stimulated by immunoglobulins [1–3]. In children, the incidence is about 1:10,000 [4]. It is estimated that there are about 8000 paediatric patients with active GD in the United States [4].

Current treatment approaches for GD include the antithyroid drugs (ATDs) propylthiouracil (PTU) and methimazole (MMI), surgery and radioactive iodine (RAI; ^{131}I), therapies that have been used for more than five decades [5–10]. The treatment of GD in children, though, remains controversial, and treatment practices vary widely among institutions and practitioners [11].

Central to considering treatment options in GD in the paediatric population is recognizing that remission occurs in a small minority of individuals. The most extensive study of this issue, involving nearly 200 children, showed that less than 20% of children treated medically achieved remission lasting greater than 2 years, despite treatment for up to 10 years in some individuals [12]. In another large series of 186 children, less than 30% of children went into remission [13]. In a recent prospective study in France, 24% of 154 children treated medically for GD went into remission after 2 years of treatment [14]. In a study from the north-west region of the US, 25% of 64 children went into remission after several years of medical therapy [15]. Remission rates are even less in prepubertal than pubertal children, reaching only 5–10% [16,17].

The persistence of active GD in children is reflective of the persistence of thyroid receptor antibodies (TRAbs, or thyroid-stimulating immunoglobulins (TSI)) in the paediatric population with GD [18]. As such, the vast majority of paediatric patients with GD will need definitive therapy.

Considering the above data, many practitioners will consider a trial of MMI for 1 or 2 years and proceed to surgery or ^{131}I therapy if remission does not occur. Practitioners may also elect to continue ATDs for many years, as long as toxic reactions and progressive thyromegaly do not occur. When continuing MMI for extended periods, practitioners should consider that the use and monitoring of thyroid function and the risk of potential side-effects, although low, may be greater than levothyroxine treatment alone following surgery or ^{131}I therapy.

Thyroid Surgery: Preventing and Managing Complications, First Edition. Edited by Paolo Miccoli, David J. Terris, Michele N. Minuto and Melanie W. Seybt.

Radioactive iodine

Radioactive iodine (RAI) therapy of GD was first introduced more than 60 years ago by Saul Hertz and co-workers at Massachusetts General Hospital, with later contributions coming from Earl Chapman and others [7,19]. It is estimated that more than 1 million individuals have been treated with ^{131}I for hyperthyroidism [7]. The use of RAI has been reported in more than 1200 children [10]. Patients as young as 1 year of age have been treated with ^{131}I with excellent outcomes [10]. Overall, studies of ^{131}I use in children report remission rates that exceed 95% [10,20,21].

The goal of ^{131}I therapy for GD is to induce hypothyroidism. Radioactive iodine should not be given to make patients euthyroid, as this results in residual, partially irradiated thyroid tissue with an associated risk of thyroid neoplasm [22,23].

Radioactive iodine doses are typically calculated to deliver the desired amount of radiation based on gland size and RAI uptake [24]. Some centers give all patients the same fixed dose of ^{131}I with excellent outcome [25]. To achieve thyroid ablation or hypothyroidism, more than 150 uCi of ^{131}I per gram of thyroid tissue should be administered [26,27]. With larger glands (30–80 g), higher administered activates of [131]I (200–300 uCi of ^{131}I per gram) may be needed [26]. Radioactive iodine is often not effective with very large glands (>80 g) [28]. Thus, surgery may be preferable to ^{131}I in these patients, although patients can be given repeated RAI treatments.

Although RAI is being used in progressively younger ages, we do not know if there is an age below which high-dose ^{131}I therapy should be avoided. Risks of thyroid cancer after external irradiation are highest in children less than 5 years of age and progressively decline with advancing age [20,29–31]. If there is residual thyroid tissue in young children after RAI treatment, there is a theoretical risk of thyroid cancer.

In addition to thyroid cancer risks, potential influences of ^{131}I therapy on other cancers need to be considered as ^{131}I therapy results in low-level whole-body radiation exposure. Several large cohorts of adults in the US and other countries have not revealed increased cancer incidence or mortality in adults treated with ^{131}I for GD [32–38].

Total-body radiation dose after ^{131}I varies with age, and the same absolute dose of ^{131}I will result in more radiation exposure to a young child than to an adolescent or adult [39,40]. Based on theoretical calculations, we feel it is prudent to avoid RAI therapy in very young children (<5 years) and to avoid >10 mCi in patients less than 10 years of age.

Surgery

Surgery is an acceptable form of therapy for GD in children [11]. When performed, near-total or total thyroidectomy is recommended, as subtotal thyroidectomy is associated with a higher relapse rate [41]. The goal of surgery is to render the patient permanently hypothyroid and eliminate the potential for recurrent hyperthyroidism. In addition, surgically induced collateral injuries to the recurrent and superior laryngeal nerves as well as to the parathyroid glands must be avoided. Surgery is preferred in young children (<5 years) when definitive therapy is required and can be performed by an experienced thyroid surgeon. In individuals with large thyroid glands (>80 g), the response to ^{131}I may be poor [28,42] and surgery is recommended for these patients.

In preparation for surgery, the child should be rendered reasonably euthyroid to prevent perioperative thyroid storm [43]. This is typically done with MMI for 1 or 2 months. Even with optimal treatment, it is typical for the child to have a suppressed serum TSH level at the time of surgery. It is also important to have an experienced paediatric anaesthesiologist to help manage these patients. Ten to 14 days before surgery, 3–10 drops t.i.d. (0.15–0.5 mL) of super saturated potassium iodine (SSKI) solution should be administered to decrease the vascularity and increase the firmness of the thyroid gland [44,45].

There are unique technical considerations. The thyroid gland in Graves' patients can be extremely vascular and prone to both intra- and postoperative bleeding. The surgeon must employ meticulous haemostasis and avoid leaving significant thyroid remnants *in vivo*. The pyramidal lobe must be completely excised as it commonly hypertrophies and if left *in situ* will recur as a midline neck mass and hyperthyroid state [46]. In addition, the parathyroid glands are vulnerable and can be easily injured when they are mobilized off a hypertrophied thyroid gland [47]. Parathyroid injury coupled with long-standing hyperthyroidism with its associated increased bone turnover render these patients at high risk for postoperative hypocalcaemia.

Postoperatively, younger children appear to be at higher risk for transient hypoparathyroidism than adolescents or adults [48]. Thus we now also routinely begin paediatric patient on calcitriol 3 days before surgery, and wean the calcitriol over the two postoperative weeks. Using this approach, we find that only 5% of patients require postoperative calcium infusions versus 40% in children without vitamin D preoperative treatment.

Data in adults show that acute complications following thyroidectomy include hypocalcaemia (40%), haematoma (2%) and recurrent laryngeal nerve paresis (2%) [48–52]. Long-term complications include hypoparathyroidism (1%) and recurrent laryngeal nerve injury (2%) [48–52]. Although surgery is performed in children with GD, relatively little is known about paediatric surgical outcomes and complication data from adults have been improperly applied to the paediatric population [11].

To address this issue, a cross-sectional analysis of Healthcare Cost and Utilization Project–National Inpatient Sample hospital discharge information from 1999 to 2005 was performed by our group. All patients who underwent thyroidectomy/parathyroidectomy were included. Bivariate and multivariate analyses were performed to identify independent predictors of patient outcomes. Data pertaining to 1199 patients, 17 years old or younger, undergoing thyroidectomy/parathyroidectomy were examined. Outcome measures included in-hospital patient complications, length of stay and inpatient hospital costs.

Children aged 0–6 years had complication rates of 22%, 7–12 years had complication rates of 11%, and 13–17 years had complication rates of 11%. These rates are higher than those seen in adults. Importantly, when surgery was performed by paediatric surgeons, the complication rate for total thyroidectomy (not for cancer) was about 15%. In comparison, the complication rate for high-volume (>30 thyroidectomies per year) thyroid surgeons was about 4% (p <0.01). We also found that most of the thyroid surgery operations in children in the US were performed by paediatric surgeons. Thus, surgery may not be an optimal option for some paediatric patients with GD, especially in young children.

Considering these data, in circumstances where local paediatric thyroid surgery expertise is not available, referral of a child with GD to a high-volume thyroid surgery center of excellence that also has paediatric experience is indicated. A multidisciplinary healthcare team that includes paediatric endocrinologists and experienced thyroid surgeons and anaesthesiologists is also very important. At the Yale Pediatric Thyroid Center, which we estimate performs at least 50% of the thyroidectomies in young children in the United States, we pair a high-volume 'adult' thyroid surgeon with a paediatric thyroid surgeon on every case, resulting in excellent outcomes.

Thyroid cancer

Paediatric thyroid cancer is a rare and treatable disease with an excellent prognosis [53]. The thyroid cancer types in children are papillary (PTC) in 60%, follicular variant of papillary in 23%, follicular in 10% (FTC) and medullary in 5% (MTC) [53]. Compared with adults, children with differentiated thyroid cancer (DTC) present with more extensive disease [54–63]. Lymph node involvement at diagnosis is seen in 40–90% of children [54–64] compared with 20–50% of adults [65]. The prevalence of distant metastases, most commonly lung, is 20–30% in children versus 2% in adults [54–63,66]. Multifocal disease is more common in children than adults and is seen in about 40% of childhood PTC cases.

In general, DTC with onset less than 10 years of age appears to have higher recurrence and mortality rates than presentation at older ages [66,67] and DTC onset older than 10 years of age behaves similar to young adults [66]. DTC is generally more widespread at presentation and more likely to recur in younger than older children [68]. Other investigators have found that DTC has similar biological properties in younger children and adolescents [69].

Nodule evaluation

Thyroid cancer needs to be suspected when thyroid nodules are detected in children and adolescents. DTC accounts for about 30% of thyroid nodules in the paediatric population in iodine-sufficient regions [70–72].

When thyroid nodules are detected, serum thyrotropin (TSH), estimated free thyroxine and thyroxine, and a neck ultrasound should be obtained. Calcitonin determination may facilitate the diagnosis of medullary thyroid cancer, which accounts for 3–5% of paediatric thyroid cancers [53,73]. If the TSH is suppressed, a radionuclide scan may identify a hyperfunctioning nodule.

Ultrasound characteristics suggestive of malignancy include microcalcifications, indistinct margins and a variable echotexture [74–76]. Ultrasound can determine the intrathyroidal location of nodules, identify additional nodules, and assess if there is lymph node involvement [74–76]. In children after Chernobyl, the most reliable ultrasound diagnostic criteria for malignancy were an irregular outline (sensitivity 70%, specificity 86%; p ≤0.01), subcapsular location (sensitivity 65%, specificity 86%; p ≤0.01) and an increased intranodular vascularization by Doppler technique (sensitivity 70%, specificity 88%; p ≤0.01) [77]. For thyroid nodules larger than 15 mm in diameter, the accuracy of ultrasound diagnosis was much lower than for smaller nodules [77]. Ultrasonographic appearance alone, though, cannot reliably distinguish between benign and malignant lesions. Thus, fine needle aspiration (FNA) is indicated for children with thyroid nodules [74].

Fine needle aspiration is the most accurate means of evaluating if a thyroid nodule is malignant [74]. Reports of FNAs performed in children describe similar specificity and sensitivity as adults [78–80]. Difficulty arises when the FNA is non-diagnostic or the cytology is 'indeterminate', as malignancy can be present up to 50% of the time with such cytological features [81]. If this occurs, the clinician may repeat the ultrasound study and FNA within 3–6 months or proceed to surgical removal. In children <10 years of age or those patients at higher risk for malignancy (e.g. prior ionizing radiation exposure, family history of thyroid cancer), prompt surgical removal following preoperative cytological evaluation is advised.

The nodule size at which FNA should be performed in children is a matter for discussion [82]. In adults, recent recommendations suggest that FNA be performed when nodule diameter reaches or exceeds 1 cm [74]. However, since about 30% of paediatric thyroid nodules are malignant, and FNA can be performed in nodules less than 1 cm, it is reasonable to biopsy smaller lesions in children if such capabilities are available, especially for nodules 0.5–1.0 cm. Ultrasound-guided FNA is recommended especially in children because of the difficulty of sampling small nodules which rarely can be palpated [83]. When FNA is performed in children, because this is an uncommon procedure, special expertise outside paediatric departments may be needed, especially with small nodules.

Surgical options

Surgical options for DTC include total, near-total or subtotal thyroidectomy, or lobectomy [84]. Anatomically,

the thyroid is divided into right and left lobes, which are connected by the isthmus. The thyroid gland is encased by a capsule. A total thyroidectomy is a complete resection of the thyroid gland via an extracapsular dissection [85,86]. If it is determined intraoperatively that a complete extracapsular dissection will result in irreversible damage to either the recurrent laryngeal nerve (RLN) or parathyroid glands, the capsule can be entered and a small amount of thyroid tissue can be left *in situ* to avoid injury to either the RLNs or parathyroid glands, a procedure referred to as a near-total thyroidectomy [85,86]. A subtotal thyroidectomy refers to removal of the contralateral lobe, the isthmus and the medial portion of the ipsilateral thyroid lobe [85,86]. The blood supply to the remaining thyroid tissue is left intact, along with the parathyroid gland, thus theoretically reducing the risk of postoperative hypoparathyroidism [85,86]. Additionally, dissection near the RLN is avoided, thus reducing the chance of damaging the nerve. The remaining thyroid tissue is vascularized and typically remains metabolically active, avoiding or reducing the need for thyroid hormone replacement. A lobectomy is an extracapsular resection of an anatomical lobe or anatomical lobe and isthmus. These operations can be performed without lymph node dissection, the selective removal of lymph nodes that appear pathological at surgery ('berry picking'), or compartmental lymph node dissection, during which all lymph nodes in a region are systematically removed *en bloc* irrespective of gross appearance [84,87].

In children, all the large cohort studies, and several of the smaller sample size studies, demonstrate increased relapse rates with lobectomy versus total thyroidectomy [54,88–91]. Welch Dinauer observed relapse rates of about 50% with lobectomy versus 14% with total thyroidectomy [54]. Handkiewicz-Junak observed relapse rates of about 20% with lobectomy versus 3% with total thyroidectomy [89]. Hay observed relapse rates of about 30% with lobectomy versus 12% with total thyroidectomy [90].

The extent of lymph node surgery has been the subject of attention [92,93]. Cancer recurrence most commonly occurs in lymph nodes in the laryngotracheal region [94]. In children and adults, the greater the lymph node involvement in recurrent disease, the greater is the risk of distant metastasis and mortality [53,58,61–63]. Lymph node metastasis is a pervasive component of DTC in children, as up to 90% of children with DTC will have nodal disease. Importantly, in up to 50% of cases, DTC involvement of lymph nodes is not detectable by preoperative ultrasonography [95,96].

An important consideration in advocating for routine central lymph node and selected lateral and contralateral lymph node compartments dissection is the increased risk of complications associated with the procedure versus total thyroidectomy alone. Potential complications include damage to the recurrent laryngeal nerves, external branches of the superior laryngeal nerves and parathyroid glands, as well as haemorrhage and infection [97].

Paediatric data summarized by Thompson and Luster revealed complication rates ranging from 0% to 40% for recurrent laryngeal nerve injury and 0–32% for permanent hypoparathyroidism [58,61]. Recent database analysis of thyroidectomy complications in the US showed that children aged 0–6 years have higher complication rates (22%) than older children (15% for 7–12 years and 11% for 13–17 years) [48]. Children had higher endocrine-specific complication rates than adults after thyroidectomy (9.1% versus 6.3%) [48]. Importantly, surgical outcome was significantly optimized when surgeries were performed by high-volume surgeons, defined as those performing 30 or more thyroid operations per year [48]. Yet even when surgery was performed by high-volume thyroid surgeons, complication rates reached 6% [48].

Another noteworthy consideration is the added complexity of reoperation when macroscopic residual or recurrent disease is detected. Reoperation at previous neck surgical sites is associated with substantially higher complication rates related to local scar tissue and altered postsurgical anatomy [98,99]. As such, for children with DTC, we recommend total or near-total thyroidectomy along with central compartment lymph node dissection as part of the initial operation. The anatomical extent of a central neck dissection was recently described and can be performed in the ipsilateral or bilateral compartments [84]. In addition, lateral compartment dissection (modified radical neck dissection) with lymph node removal is indicated when lymph node involvement is localized preoperatively by imaging studies and/or FNA. To minimize the risk of complications, surgery should be performed by high-volume thyroid surgeons.

Radioactive iodine
The majority of paediatric patients with DTC present with nodal metastases, are not low risk, and should be assumed to have micrometastases. Based on the above data, children should be treated with RAI to ablate residual disease and reduce the risk of disease recurrence. Administered ^{131}I activities to be applied should be in the range 100–200 mCi (3.7–7.4 GBq), which may be corrected for body weight (50–100 MBq, 1.35–2.7 mCi/kg). New analyses show that treatment with at least 200 MBq/kg (5.4 mCi/kg), and in most patients even much higher activities, is possible without a risk of exceeding bone marrow tolerance limits (Verburg, unpublished data).

For the uncommon low-risk paediatric patient with microcarcinoma without lymph node involvement, treatment with 30 mCi (1.2 GBq) for the purposes of remnant ablation may be administered, and additional courses given if there is thyroglobulin (Tg) persistence. Based on studies in adults [100–102], about 10% of patients administered ^{131}I for remnant ablation will have biochemical evidence of remaining thyroid tissue and will require retreatment. Alternatively, as recently suggested [103], RAI may be withheld for the child with microcarcinoma, and the patient monitored for disease persistence and recurrence with Tg level assessment and ultrasonography. If Tg levels rise in the absence of gross disease, RAI can be later administered.

Differences with American Thyroid Association (ATA) management guidelines
The ATA management guidelines for DTC are a benchmark for the evaluation, treatment and follow-up of the condition [103]. In general, these guidelines are applicable to children, with notable exceptions.

The recommendation that near-total or total thyroidectomy without central compartment neck dissection (#27) may be appropriate for T1 or T2 lesions in adults may not apply to children, who have a much higher rate of lymph node metastasis than adults. As such, central compartment dissection is recommended for T1 and T2 lesions, if surgery can be performed by a high-volume surgeon.

The TNM classification system for DTC cannot be used in children correctly, because the T-category underestimates the aggressiveness of the disease (#31). In addition, the American Joint Committee on Cancer (AJCC) staging system is of modest utility in children, where DTC mortality is low. Such mortality-based scoring systems do not reflect the risk of recurrent or persistent disease, which is a major component of paediatric DTC. It is recommended that a more paediatric-specific scoring system be developed. Alternatively, the response-to-therapy system estimating the risk of having persistent or recurrent disease recently proposed by Tuttle and co-workers might be tested on a paediatric population [104].

In adults, it is recommended (#32) that RAI be administered for T3 and T4 tumours but used selectively for T1 and T2 tumours. In children, considering high rates of lymph node involvement, higher rates of recurrence than adults and the complicating factor of residual thyroid tissue following surgery that confounds long-term follow-up, we recommend that RAI be used for T1 and T2 tumours. Alternatively, for small unifocal microcarcinomas, RAI may be withheld and the child monitored for disease persistence. If Tg levels are detectable or rise in the absence of gross disease, RAI should be administered.

Non-cancerous nodules

In chemically euthyroid patients, benign nodules can be observed unless there is a diagnostic dilemma or they are causing symptoms. Nodules can cause symptoms due to size or elaboration of excessive amounts of thyroid hormone. If a patient develops symptoms of compression related to mass effect, such as discomfort or pain (globus sensation), dysphagia, dysphonia or difficulty breathing, particularly when lying flat, surgery should be considered. Uninodular goitres are amenable to lobectomy, while multinodular goitres require near-total or total thyroidectomy.

Metabolically active nodules will present with increased uptake on a thyroid radioisotope scan. Toxic adenomas are autonomously functioning benign tumours that cause symptomatic hyperthyroidism. The true incidence of toxic adenomas in children is low enough to preclude epidemiological estimates [105]. In the case of children with solitary or unilobar toxic adenomas, thyroid lobectomy is the recommended procedure (or isthmusectomy if the toxic nodule is in the isthmus, which is rare) [106]. Subtotal lobectomy or nodulectomy are not adequate resections, and risk recurrence of the disease. As in the case of Graves' disease, these patients should be rendered biochemically and clinically euthyroid prior to surgery. The risk of lobectomy includes bleeding and recurrent laryngeal nerve injury.

Conclusion

Paediatric thyroid disease requiring surgery is associated with a greater risk of complications than in adults. When surgery is performed for GD, near-total or total thyroidectomy is recommended. When surgery is performed for patients with thyroid cancer, total thyroidectomy with central compartment lymph node dissection is recommended. Complication rates for thyroidectomy are considerably higher in children than adults. Therefore, paediatric patients who require thyroid surgery should be managed by an experienced thyroid team consisting of paediatric endocrinologists, paediatric and endocrine surgeons.

Acknowledgement
Supported by NIH grant 1R01FD003707 to SAR.

References

1 LeFranchi S, Mandel SH. Graves' disease in the neonatal period and childhood. In: Braverman LE, Utiger RD (eds) The Thyroid: Fundamental and Clinical Text. Philadelphia: JB Lippincott, 1995: 1237–46.

2 Rivkees SA. The treatment of Graves' disease in children. J Pediatr Endocrinol Metab 2006; 19(9): 1095–111.

3 Zimmerman D, Lteif AN. Thyrotoxicosis in children. Endocrinol Metab Clin North Am 1998; 27(1): 109–26.

4 Hepatic Toxicity Following Treatment for Pediatric Graves' Disease Meeting, October 28, 2008. Eunice Kennedy Shriver National Institute of Child Health and Human Development. Available from: http://bpca.nichd.nih.gov/outreach/index.cfm.

5 Weetman AP. Grave's disease 1835–2002. Horm Res 2003; 59(Suppl 1): 114–8.

6 Weetman AP. Graves' disease. N Engl J Med 2000; 343(17): 1236–48.

7 Chapman EM. History of the discovery and early use of radioactive iodine. JAMA 1983; 250(15): 2042–4.

8 Cooper DS. Antithyroid drugs. N Engl J Med 2005; 352(9): 905–17.

9 Gruneiro-Papendieck L, Chiesa A, Finkielstain G, Heinrich JJ. Pediatric Graves' disease: outcome and treatment. J Pediatr Endocrinol Metab 2003; 16(9): 1249–55.

10 Rivkees SA, Sklar C, Freemark M. Clinical review 99: the management of Graves' disease in children, with special emphasis on radioiodine treatment. J Clin Endocrinol Metab 1998; 83(11): 3767–76.

11 Lee JA, Grumbach MM, Clark OH. The optimal treatment for pediatric Graves' disease is surgery. J Clin Endocrinol Metab 2007; 92(3): 801–3.

12 Hamburger JI. Management of hyperthyroidism in children and adolescents. J Clin Endocrinol Metab 1985; 60(5): 1019–24.

13 Glaser NS, Styne DM. Predictors of early remission of hyperthyroidism in children. J Clin Endocrinol Metab 1997; 82(6): 1719–26.

14 Kaguelidou F, Alberti C, Castanet M, Guitteny MA, Czernichow P, Leger J. Predictors of autoimmune hyperthyroidism relapse in children after discontinuation of antithyroid drug treatment. J Clin Endocrinol Metab 2008; 93: 3817–26.

15 Glaser NS, Styne DM. Predicting the likelihood of remission in children with Graves' disease: a prospective, multicenter study. Pediatrics 2008; 121(3): e481–8.

16 Shulman DI, Muhar I, Jorgensen EV, Diamond FB, Bercu BB, Root AW. Autoimmune hyperthyroidism in prepubertal children and adolescents: comparison of clinical and biochemical features at diagnosis and responses to medical therapy. Thyroid 1997; 7(5): 755–60.

17 Lazar L, Kalter-Leibovici O, Pertzelan A, Weintrob N, Josefsberg Z, Phillip M. Thyrotoxicosis in prepubertal children compared with pubertal and postpubertal patients. J Clin Endocrinol Metab 2000; 85(10): 3678–82.

18 Smith J, Brown RS. Persistence of thyrotropin (TSH) receptor antibodies in children and adolescents with Graves' disease treated using antithyroid medication. Thyroid 2007; 17(11): 1103–7.

19 Hertz S. Assurances as to the advantages and safety of radioactive iodine treatment of hyperthyroidism. New Orleans Med Surg J 1950; 103(2): 51–62.

20 Read CH, Jr., Tansey MJ, Menda Y. A thirty-six year retrospective analysis of the efficacy and safety of radioactive iodine in treating young Graves' patients. J Clin Endocrinol Metab 2004; 89: 4229–33.

21 Levy WM, Schumacher OP, Gupta M. Treatment of childhood Graves' disease. A review with emphasis on radioiodine treatment. Cleveland Clin J Med 1988; 55: 373–82.

22 Sheline GE, McCormack KR, Galante M. Thyroid nodules occurring late after treatment of thryotoxicosis with radioiodine. J Clin Endocrinol Metab 1962; 22: 8–17.

23 Dobyns BM, Sheline GE, Workman JB, Tompkins EA, McConahey WM, Becker DV. Malignant and benign neoplasms of the thyroid in patients treated for hyperthyroidism: a report of the Cooperative Thyrotoxicosis Therapy Follow-up Study. J Clin Endocrinol Metab 1974; 38: 976–98.

24 Quimby EM, Feitelberg S, Gross W. Radioactive Nuclides in Medicine and Biology. Philadelphia: Lea and Febiger, 1970.

25 Nebesio TD, Siddiqui AR, Pescovitz OH, Eugster EA. Time course to hypothyroidism after fixed-dose radioablation therapy of Graves' disease in children. J Pediatr 2002; 141(1): 99–103.

26 Rivkees SA, Cornelius EA. Influence of iodine-131 dose on the outcome of hyperthyroidism in children. Pediatrics 2003; 111(4 Pt 1): 745–9.

27 Rivkees SA, Dinauer C. An optimal treatment for pediatric Graves' disease is radioiodine. J Clin Endocrinol Metab 2007; 92(3): 797–800.

28 Peters H, Fischer C, Bogner U, Reiners C, Schleusener H. Treatment of Graves' hyperthyroidism with radioiodine: results of a prospective randomized study. Thyroid 1997; 7(2): 247–51.

29 Boice JD Jr. Radiation and thyroid cancer – what more can be learned? Acta Oncol 1998; 34: 321–4.

30 Boice JD Jr. Thyroid disease 60 years after Hiroshima and 20 years after Chernobyl. JAMA 2006; 295(9): 1060–2.

31 Dolphin GW. The risk of thyroid cancers following irradiation. Health Phys 1968; 15: 219–28.

32 Flynn RW, Macdonald TM, Jung RT, Morris AD, Leese GP. Mortality and vascular outcomes in patients treated for thyroid dysfunction. J Clin Endocrinol Metab 2006; 91(6): 2159–64.

33 Franklyn JA, Maisonneuve P, Sheppard MC, Betteridge J, Boyle P. Mortality after the treatment of hyperthyroidism with radioactive iodine. N Engl J Med 1998; 338(11): 712–18.

34 Franklyn JA, Sheppard MC, Maisonneuve P. Thyroid function and mortality in patients treated for hyperthyroidism. JAMA 2005; 294(1): 71–80.

35 Goldman MB, Monson RR, Maloof F. Cancer mortality in women with thyroid disease. Cancer Res 1990; 50: 2283–9.

36 Holm LE, Hall P, Wiklund K, et al. Cancer risk after iodine-131 therapy for hyperthyroidism. J Natl Cancer Inst 1991; 83: 1072–7.

37 Metso S, Auvinen A, Huhtala H, Salmi J, Oksala H, Jaatinen P. Increased cancer incidence after radioiodine treatment for hyperthyroidism. Cancer 2007; 109(10): 1972–9.

38 Ron E, Doody M, Becker D, et al. Cancer mortality following treatment for adult hyperthyroidism. Cooperative Thyrotoxicosis Therapy Follow-up Study Group. JAMA 1998; 280: 347–55.

39 Toohey RE, Stabin MG, Watson EE. The AAPM/RSNA physics tutorial for residents: internal radiation dosimetry: principles and applications. Radiographics 2000; 20(2): 533–46.

40 Toohey RE, Stabin MG (eds). Comparative analysis of dosimetry parameters for nuclear medicine. ORISE Report 99–1064, 1999. Proceedings of the Sixth International Radiopharmaceutical Dosimetry Symposium, 1996. Gatlinburg, TN.

41 Miccoli P, Vitti P, Rago T, *et al.* Surgical treatment of Graves' disease: subtotal or total thyroidectomy? Surgery 1996; 120(6): 1020–4; discussion 1024–5.

42 Peters H, Fischer C, Bogner U, Reiners C, Schleusener H. Reduction in thyroid volume after radioiodine therapy of Graves' hyperthyroidism: results of a prospective, randomized, multicentre study. Eur J Clin Invest 1996; 26(1): 59–63.

43 Netterville JL, Aly A, Ossoff RH. Evaluation and treatment of complications of thyroid and parathyroid surgery. Otolaryngol Clin North Am 1990; 23(3): 529–52.

44 Ansaldo GL, Pretolesi F, Varaldo E, *et al.* Doppler evaluation of intrathyroid arterial resistances during preoperative treatment with Lugol's iodide solution in patients with diffuse toxic goiter. J Am Coll Surg 2000; 191(6): 607–12.

45 Erbil Y, Ozluk Y, Giris M, *et al.* Effect of lugol solution on thyroid gland blood flow and microvessel density in the patients with Graves' disease. J Clin Endocrinol Metab 2007; 92(6): 2182–9.

46 Delbridge L. Total thyroidectomy: the evolution of surgical technique. Aust NZ J Surg 2003; 73(9): 761–8.

47 Thomusch O, Machens A, Sekulla C, Ukkat J, Brauckhoff M, Dralle H. The impact of surgical technique on postoperative hypoparathyroidism in bilateral thyroid surgery: a multivariate analysis of 5846 consecutive patients. Surgery 2003; 133(2): 180–5.

48 Sosa JA, Tuggle CT, Wang TS, *et al.* Clinical and economic outcomes of thyroid and parathyroid surgery in children. J Clin Endocrinol Metab 2008; 93(8): 3058–65.

49 Lal G, Ituarte P, Kebebew E, Siperstein A, Duh QY, Clark OH. Should total thyroidectomy become the preferred procedure for surgical management of Graves' disease? Thyroid 2005; 15(6): 569–74.

50 Boger MS, Perrier ND. Advantages and disadvantages of surgical therapy and optimal extent of thyroidectomy for the treatment of hyperthyroidism. Surg Clin North Am 2004; 84(3): 849–74.

51 Witte J, Goretzki PE, Dotzenrath C, *et al.* Surgery for Graves' disease: total versus subtotal thyroidectomy – results of a prospective randomized trial. World J Surg 2000; 24(11): 1303–11.

52 Sosa JA, Bowman HM, Tielsch JM, Powe NR, Gordon TA, Udelsman R. The importance of surgeon experience for clinical and economic outcomes from thyroidectomy. Ann Surg 1998; 228(3): 320–30.

53 Hogan AR, Zhuge Y, Perez EA, Koniaris LG, Lew JI, Sola JE. Pediatric thyroid carcinoma: incidence and outcomes in 1753 patients. J Surg Res 2009; 156(1): 167–72.

54 Welch Dinauer CA, Tuttle RM, Robie DK, *et al.* Clinical features associated with metastasis and recurrence of differentiated thyroid cancer in children, adolescents and young adults. Clin Endocrinol (Oxf) 1998; 49(5): 619–28.

55 Reiners C, Demidchik YE. Differentiated thyroid cancer in childhood: pathology, diagnosis, therapy. Pediatr Endocrinol Rev 2003; 1(Suppl 2): 230–5; discussion 235–6.

56 Chaukar DA, Rangarajan V, Nair N, *et al.* Pediatric thyroid cancer. J Surg Oncol 2005; 92(2): 130–3.

57 Okada T, Sasaki F, Takahashi H, *et al.* Management of childhood and adolescent thyroid carcinoma: long-term follow-up and clinical characteristics. Eur J Pediatr Surg 2006; 16(1): 8–13.

58 Thompson GB, Hay ID. Current strategies for surgical management and adjuvant treatment of childhood papillary thyroid carcinoma. World J Surg 2004; 28(12): 1187–98.

59 O'Gorman CS, Hamilton J, Rachmiel M, Gupta A, Ngan BY, Daneman D. Thyroid cancer in childhood: a retrospective review of childhood course. Thyroid 2010; 20(4): 375–80.

60 Rachmiel M, Charron M, Gupta A, *et al.* Evidence-based review of treatment and follow up of pediatric patients with differentiated thyroid carcinoma. J Pediatr Endocrinol Metab 2006; 19(12): 1377–93.

61 Luster M, Lassmann M, Freudenberg LS, Reiners C. Thyroid cancer in childhood: management strategy, including dosimetry and long-term results. Hormones (Athens) 2007; 6(4): 269–78.

62 Dinauer C, Francis GL. Thyroid cancer in children. Endocrinol Metab Clin North Am 2007; 36(3): 779–806, vii.

63 Dinauer CA, Breuer C, Rivkees SA. Differentiated thyroid cancer in children: diagnosis and management. Curr Opin Oncol 2008; 20(1): 59–65.

64 Zimmerman D, Hay ID, Gough IR, *et al.* Papillary thyroid carcinoma in children and adults: long-term follow-up of 1039 patients conservatively treated at one institution during three decades. Surgery 1988; 104(6): 1157–66.

65 Zaydfudim V, Feurer ID, Griffin MR, Phay JE. The impact of lymph node involvement on survival in patients with papillary and follicular thyroid carcinoma. Surgery 2008; 144(6): 1070–7; discussion 1077–8.

66 Hung W, Sarlis NJ. Current controversies in the management of pediatric patients with well-differentiated nonmedullary thyroid cancer: a review. Thyroid 2002; 12(8): 683–702.

67 Schlumberger M, de Vathaire F, Travagli JP, *et al.* Differentiated thyroid carcinoma in childhood: long term follow-up of 72 patients. J Clin Endocrinol Metab 1987; 65(6): 1088–94.

68 Lazar L, Lebenthal Y, Steinmetz A, Yackobovitch-Gavan M, Phillip M. Differentiated thyroid carcinoma in pediatric patients: comparison of presentation and course between pre-pubertal children and adolescents. J Pediatr 2009; 154(5): 708–14.

69 Machens A, Lorenz K, Nguyen Thanh P, Brauckhoff M, Dralle H. Papillary thyroid cancer in children and adolescents does not differ in growth pattern and metastatic behavior. J Pediatr 2010; 157(4): 648–52.

70 Hung W. Solitary thyroid nodules in 93 children and adolescents. a 35-years experience. Horm Res 1999; 52(1): 15–18.

71 Fowler CL, Pokorny WJ, Harberg FJ. Thyroid nodules in children: current profile of a changing disease. South Med J 1989; 82(12): 1472–8.

72 Zimmerman D. Thyroid neoplasia in children. Curr Opin Pediatr 1997; 9(4): 413–18.

73 Cheung K, Roman SA, Wang TS, Walker HD, Sosa JA. Calcitonin measurement in the evaluation of thyroid nodules in the United States: a cost-effectiveness and decision analysis. J Clin Endocrinol Metab 2008; 93(6): 2173–80.

74 Cooper DS, Doherty GM, Haugen BR, et al. Management guidelines for patients with thyroid nodules and differentiated thyroid cancer. Thyroid 2006; 16(2): 109–42.

75 Brignardello E, Corrias A, Isolato G, et al. Ultrasound screening for thyroid carcinoma in childhood cancer survivors: a case series. J Clin Endocrinol Metab 2008; 93(12): 4840–3.

76 Corrias A, Einaudi S, Chiorboli E, et al. Accuracy of fine needle aspiration biopsy of thyroid nodules in detecting malignancy in childhood: comparison with conventional clinical, laboratory, and imaging approaches. J Clin Endocrinol Metab 2001; 86(10): 4644–8.

77 Lyshchik A, Drozd V, Demidchik Y, Reiners C. Diagnosis of thyroid cancer in children: value of gray-scale and power doppler US. Radiology 2005; 235(2): 604–13.

78 Moslavac S, Matesa N, Kusic Z. Thyroid fine needle aspiration cytology in children and adolescents. Coll Antropol 2010; 34(1): 197–200.

79 Kapila K, Pathan SK, George SS, Haji BE, Das DK, Qadan LR. Fine needle aspiration cytology of the thyroid in children and adolescents: experience with 792 aspirates. Acta Cytol 2010; 54(4): 569–74.

80 Corrias A, Mussa A, Baronio F, et al. Diagnostic features of thyroid nodules in pediatrics. Arch Pediatr Adolesc Med 2010; 164(8): 714–19.

81 Theoharis CG, Schofield KM, Hammers L, Udelsman R, Chhieng DC. The Bethesda thyroid fine-needle aspiration classification system: year 1 at an academic institution. Thyroid 2009; 19(11): 1215–23.

82 Mazzaferri EL, Sipos J. Should all patients with subcentimeter thyroid nodules undergo fine-needle aspiration biopsy and preoperative neck ultrasonography to define the extent of tumor invasion? Thyroid 2008; 18(6): 597–602.

83 Izquierdo R, Shankar R, Kort K, Khurana K. Ultrasound-guided fine-needle aspiration in the management of thyroid nodules in children and adolescents. Thyroid 2009; 19(7): 703–5.

84 Carty SE, Cooper DS, Doherty GM, et al. Consensus statement on the terminology and classification of central neck dissection for thyroid cancer. Thyroid 2009; 19(11): 1153–8.

85 Udelsman R, Lakatos E, Ladenson P. Optimal surgery for papillary thyroid carcinoma. World J Surg 1996; 20(1): 88–93.

86 Udelsman R. Thyroid cancer surgery. Rev Endocr Metab Disord 2000; 1(3): 155–63.

87 Miller BS, Doherty GM. An examination of recently revised differentiated thyroid cancer guidelines. Curr Opin Oncol 2010; 23: 1–6.

88 Demidchik YE, Demidchik EP, Reiners C, et al. Comprehensive clinical assessment of 740 cases of surgically treated thyroid cancer in children of Belarus. Ann Surg 2006; 243(4): 525–32.

89 Handkiewicz-Junak D, Wloch J, Roskosz J, et al. Total thyroidectomy and adjuvant radioiodine treatment independently decrease locoregional recurrence risk in childhood and adolescent differentiated thyroid cancer. J Nucl Med 2007; 48(6): 879–88.

90 Hay ID, Gonzalez-Losada T, Reinalda MS, Honetschlager JA, Richards ML, Thompson GB. Long-term outcome in 215 children and adolescents with papillary thyroid cancer treated during 1940 through 2008. World J Surg 2010; 34(6): 1192–202.

91 Borson-Chazot F, Causeret S, Lifante JC, Augros M, Berger N, Peix JL. Predictive factors for recurrence from a series of 74 children and adolescents with differentiated thyroid cancer. World J Surg 2004; 28(11): 1088–92.

92 Mazzaferri EL. A vision for the surgical management of papillary thyroid carcinoma: extensive lymph node compartmental dissections and selective use of radioiodine. J Clin Endocrinol Metab 2009; 94(4): 1086–8.

93 Doherty GM. Prophylactic central lymph node dissection: continued controversy. Oncology (Williston Park) 2009; 23(7): 603, 608.

94 Gimm O, Rath FW, Dralle H. Pattern of lymph node metastases in papillary thyroid carcinoma. Br J Surg 1998; 85(2): 252–4.

95 Bonnet S, Hartl D, Leboulleux S, et al. Prophylactic lymph node dissection for papillary thyroid cancer less than 2 cm: implications for radioiodine treatment. J Clin Endocrinol Metab 2009; 94(4): 1162–7.

96 Bonnet S, Hartl DM, Travagli JP. Lymph node dissection for thyroid cancer. J Visc Surg 2010; 147(3): e155–9.

97 Pereira JA, Jimeno J, Miquel J, et al. Nodal yield, morbidity, and recurrence after central neck dissection for papillary thyroid carcinoma. Surgery 2005; 138(6): 1095–100, discussion 1100–1.

98 Shindo M, Stern A. Total thyroidectomy with and without selective central compartment dissection: a comparison of complication rates. Arch Otolaryngol Head Neck Surg 2010; 136(6): 584–7.

99 Giles Y, Boztepe H, Terzioglu T, Tezelman S. The advantage of total thyroidectomy to avoid reoperation for incidental thyroid cancer in multinodular goiter. Arch Surg 2004; 139(2): 179–82.

100 Bal C, Padhy AK, Jana S, Pant GS, Basu AK. Prospective randomized clinical trial to evaluate the optimal dose of 131 I for remnant ablation in patients with differentiated thyroid carcinoma. Cancer 1996; 77(12): 2574–80.

101 Catargi B, Borget I, Deandreis D, *et al.* Comparison of four strategies of radioiodine ablation in patients with thyroid cancer with low-risk recurrence: the randomized, prospective ESTIMABL study on 753 patients. 14th International Thyroid Conference, Paris, France, 2010.

102 Mallick U, Harmer C, Clarke S, *et al.* HiLo: multicentre randomised phase III clinical trials of high vs low dose radioiodine, with or without re-combinant human thyroid stimulating hormone (rhTSH), for remnant ablation for differentiated thyroid cancer. 14th International Thyroid Conference, Paris, France, 2010.

103 Cooper DS, Doherty GM, Haugen BR, *et al.* Revised American Thyroid Association management guidelines for patients with thyroid nodules and differentiated thyroid cancer. Thyroid 2009; 19(11): 1167–214.

104 Tuttle RM, Tala H, Shah J, *et al.* Estimating risk of recurrence in differentiated thyroid cancer after total thyroidectomy and radioactive iodine remnant ablation: using response to therapy variables to modify the initial risk estimates predicted by the new american thyroid association staging system. Thyroid 2010; 20(12): 1341–9.

105 Zimmerman D. Fetal and neonatal hyperthyroidism. Thyroid 1999; 9(7): 727–33.

106 Group CPTNCS. The Canadian Pediatric Thyroid Nodule Study: an evaluation of current management practices. J Pediatr Surg 2008; 43(5): 826–30.

PART II

Best Practices in Thyroid Surgery

CHAPTER 5

How to Perform a 'Safe' Thyroidectomy: 'Tips and Tricks'

Elliot J. Mitmaker[1] *and Quan-Yang Duh*[2]

[1] Department of Surgery, McGill University Health Centre and McGill University, Montreal, Canada
[2] Veterans Affairs Medical Center, San Francisco, CA, USA

Introduction

During the French Revolution, in 1791, Pierre-Joseph Desault, a surgeon in Paris, France, performed the first published account of a successful thyroidectomy for an enlarging goitre [1]. With the passage of time, surgery on the thyroid gland has greatly expanded to include removing the thyroid not only for glandular enlargement but also for the definitive treatment of hyperfunctioning glands as well as neoplastic conditions. Operative concepts based on anatomy have evolved that assure the safe performance of a thyroid operation whatever its pathology. Whether thyroidectomy is performed for benign or malignant conditions, the goal of surgical resection is to achieve cure while minimizing morbidity. This chapter will review the steps needed to perform a 'safe' thyroidectomy as well as providing several hints that can assure safe passage through the anatomical difficulties encountered during thyroid surgery. An edited video of a total thyroidectomy can be seen at this link: Video 5.1.

Preoperative considerations

Obtaining informed consent

Prior to surgery, the surgeon must obtain informed consent from the patient. This is one of the most crucial steps of the operation as it sets the stage for patient expectations

before and after thyroidectomy. First, the diagnosis and prognosis are discussed in detail as well as what would occur if surgery is not performed. Second, a detailed discussion of the surgical technique is outlined for the patient with the aid of an anatomical thyroid model (if available) or a free-hand drawing of the thyroid and its relationship with the parathyroid glands, recurrent laryngeal nerves, trachea, oesophagus and pertinent vasculature. Finally, a detailed discussion of possible complications should take place with the patient. These complications include recurrent laryngeal nerve injury, either temporary (5%) or permanent (1%), resulting in hoarseness (if unilateral) and potential need for tracheotomy (if bilateral). Other complications include temporary or permanent injury to the parathyroid glands resulting in hypoparathyroidism and hypocalcaemia, requiring calcium and vitamin D supplements. Postoperative bleeding may require reintubation and re-exploration of the neck. Other rare complications include infection, tracheal and/or vascular injury. Investing time with the patient preoperatively while obtaining an informed consent is very important in order to match patient expectations with that of the surgeon.

Additional preoperative issues specific to thyroid surgery

Based on the patient's medical history, consultations for cardiac, respiratory, metabolic and other specialties may be necessary. Thyroid imaging studies (ultrasound, computed

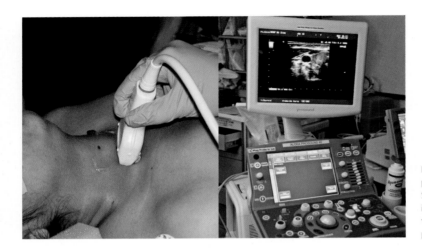

Figure 5.1 Preincision ultrasound performed before sterile draping. Surgeon-performed ultrasound helps with incision placement, confirms previous thyroid imaging and alerts the surgeon to potential unexpected findings.

tomography, magnetic resonance imaging) as well as thyroid function tests, along with specific thyroid antibodies and tumour markers (thyroid peroxidase, thyroglobulin, thyroglobulin antibody) should be considered for preoperative baseline studies. Although perioperative antibiotics are usually not indicated, some special circumstances may justify their use [2]. Finally, preoperative surgeon-performed ultrasound is a useful adjunctive measure (if available) as it helps the surgeon to visualize the thyroid gland and its pathology, and provides guidance for the incision. If the patient complains of voice problems, a preoperative laryngoscopy will be important to document vocal fold mobility.

Intraoperative considerations for thyroidectomy

Patient positioning

The patient is placed in the supine position on the operating room table with slight extension of the neck (10–15°). Neck extension can be achieved by placing a gel roll supporting the shoulder blades. It is important to verify that the neck is not hyperextended because patients may experience severe neck and upper back pain following surgery. Both arms are tucked to the patient's sides. Bilateral superficial cervical plexus blockade using a long-acting local anaesthetic (i.e. bupivacaine, ropivacaine) is performed along the midposterior border of the sternocleidomastoid muscle, thereby blocking the

anterior rami of C2–C4 nerve fibres. Additional local anaesthetic is injected subcutaneously. After positioning, the surgeon performs a neck ultrasound, which provides a roadmap of important surgical landmarks (position of superior poles, isthmus, location of tumour, etc.) and helps determine the placement of the incision (Figure 5.1). In addition, the operative strategy may change if additional pathology is found.

Incision placement

A transverse cervical incision is used most commonly for either thyroid lobectomy or total thyroidectomy. The optimal incision is at the level of the upper border of the isthmus along the nearest prominent skinfold. The upper border of the isthmus can be determined by ultrasound or by palpation; it is usually 1–2 cm caudal to the cricoid cartilage [3]. The incision is made in the direction of Langer's lines in order to minimize scarring and improve the cosmetic appearance of the scar. If there are no prominent natural skin wrinkle lines within an adequate distance of the anticipated incision, the surgeon may artificially create a symmetrical neck crease using a 0-silk suture along Langer's line (Figure 5.2).

Placing the incision near the upper border of the isthmus helps with the dissection of the superior pole. The location and size of the thyroid gland as well as the presence of lymph nodes might change the incision placement and may necessitate either a lateral extension or a new counter-incision. Perioperative surgeon-performed ultrasound is useful for placement of the incision.

(a)   (b)

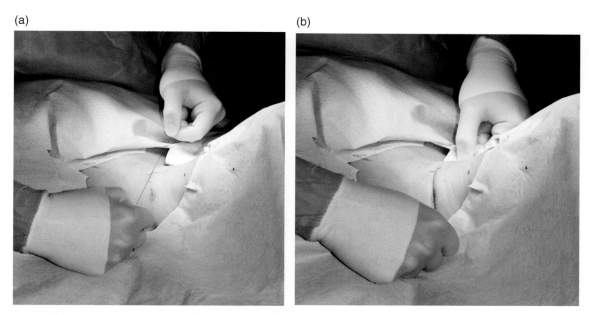

Figure 5.2 After marking the length of the skin incision (a), a 0-silk suture is used to create an artificial Langer line (b).

Raising skin flaps and mobilizing strap muscles

Incision is made with a scalpel (no. 15 blade) and then carried down past the subcutaneous fat and through the platysma muscle with an electrocautery device using a protected electrocautery tip. Straight Kelley clamps are used to grasp and retract the platysma muscle and upper and lower subplatysmal flaps are created, extending to the thyroid cartilage and sternal notch (Figure 5.3). The midline fascia between the strap muscles is divided.

> **Trick:** Exposing the cranial portion of the strap muscles allows for easier identification of the midline, especially in the case of young patients whose midline is less well defined due to well-developed strap muscles.

Once the midline fascia of the strap muscles is divided, the sternohyoid and sternothyroid muscles are separated by blunt dissection. Blunt dissection is carried out until the internal jugular vein and ansa cervicalis nerve are identified. Separating the sternohyoid from the sternothyroid muscles allows for mobilization of the thyroid through a short transverse incision without transecting the strap muscles. Thyroid Richardson retractors or lateral retractors are used to expose the thyroid gland.

Dividing the isthmus

After mobilizing the sternohyoid and sternothyroid muscles, attention is then directed to dissecting the cranial edge of the isthmus. If present, the pyramidal lobe is dissected first and freed. Next, the tissue anterior to the trachea is dissected down to the cartilaginous rings. A small vein running anteriorly on the surface of the trachea is frequently encountered, which should be ligated to prevent bleeding. The space between the undersurface of the isthmus and trachea is dissected. An energy device, such as the LigaSure™ or Harmonic® scalpel, can be used to divide the isthmus. Alternatively, the isthmus can be sharply divided between two Dandy clamps and then sutured to provide haemostasis. The divided isthmus is then grasped with Allis clamps and freed from the trachea by dissecting the medial aspect of Berry's ligament. This manoeuvre mobilizes the thyroid medially and with appropriate traction facilitates lateral dissection. After transecting the isthmus, the dissection is continued into the medio-inferior aspect of the lower pole. Although isthmus transection first facilitates subsequent lobectomy, if the isthmus contains cancer or if *en bloc* central neck dissection is planned, it should not be transected.

(a)

(b)

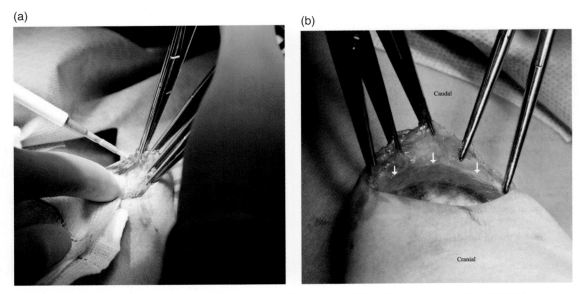

Figure 5.3 (a) Placement of straight Kelly clamps and creation of subplatysmal plane. (b) Subplatysmal plane completely dissected.

Division of the superior pole vessels

Safe dissection of the superior pole of the thyroid is critical. There are three important structures that require special attention when dissecting the superior pole: recurrent laryngeal nerve, external branch of the superior laryngeal nerve (also known as the Amelita Galli Curci nerve or opera singer's nerve) and the superior thyroid vessels.

After retracting the sternothyroid muscle superolaterally, it is necessary to identify the space of Reeve (named after T.S. Reeve of Australia), the space between the cricothyroid muscle and the medial aspect of the superior pole of the thyroid (Figure 5.4). This is an avascular plane between the cricothyroid muscle and thyroid parenchyma. The upper pole of the thyroid is grasped with a Mayo or Allis clamp. The superior pole is retracted 'down and out'. This prevents injury to the external branch of the superior laryngeal nerve. A blunt tip clamp may be used to gently sweep any remaining muscle fibres attached to the thyroid parenchyma. A right-angle clamp is used to dissect the superior thyroid artery and vein.

Tip: Careful dissection and separate ligation of the branches of the artery and vein ensure effective haemostasis and avoid inadvertent retraction of small vessels that could cause life-threatening bleeding postoperatively.

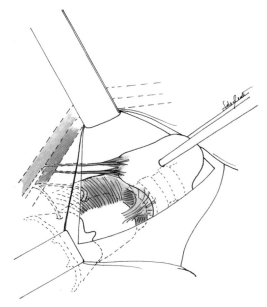

Figure 5.4 Dissection of the superior thyroid vessels with the upper pole of the thyroid being retracted in the "down and out" position to avoid injury to the external branch of the superior laryngeal nerve.

The branches of the upper pole vessels are dissected and ligated individually, mobilizing the upper pole from medial to lateral-superior.

Branches of the vessels are dissected close to the thyroid gland in order to avoid injuring the recurrent laryngeal nerve, superior laryngeal nerve and/or the upper parathyroid gland.

> **Tip:** The recurrent laryngeal nerve can loop up higher than its normal insertion into the cricothyroid muscle.

Meticulous dissection of the superior pole vessels is a critical step during thyroidectomy.

Identification of the recurrent laryngeal nerve and parathyroid glands and mobilization of the lower pole vessels

With the superior pole vessels and isthmus divided, the usual approach is to reflect the thyroid gland medially and dissect the lateral aspect of the thyroid gland and to identify the recurrent laryngeal nerve. Previous mobilization of the medial aspect of the lower pole after isthmus transection now facilitates the medial retraction of the lobe and allows the thyroid gland to be brought out through the incision with minimal traction on the recurrent laryngeal nerve. The middle thyroid vein is then ligated (see Figure 5.4), allowing for further medial retraction of the thyroid gland and aiding in the dissection of the parathyroid glands and identification of the recurrent laryngeal nerve.

There are several useful landmarks to help identify the recurrent laryngeal nerve. They include the inferior thyroid artery (most consistent landmark), the tubercle of Zuckerkandl and the relationship of the nerve to the parathyroid glands (RLN is ANTERIOR to the superior parathyroid gland and POSTERIOR to the inferior parathyroid gland).

> **Tip:** If a nerve stimulator device is used, try to map out the RLN based on its anatomical relationship to the parathyroid glands (Figure 5.5). This allows for minimal dissection around the nerve and helps prevent nerve traction injury.

The RLN is identified, either visually or by 'mapping' with a nerve-monitoring probe. The dissection is done as close as possible to the surface of the thyroid gland. A thyroidectomy procedure with intraoperative nerve monitoring is shown in Video 5.2. Dissecting the thyroid parenchyma from the loose alveolar tissue and dense

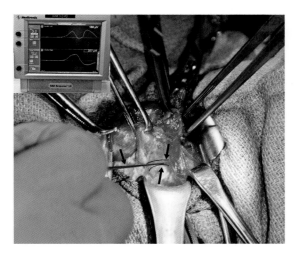

Figure 5.5 A nerve stimulator is used to map out the right recurrent laryngeal nerve while using the tubercle of Zuckerkandl and parathyroid glands as anatomical landmarks.

endocervical fascia will allow the recurrent laryngeal nerve to remain in the tracheo-oesophageal groove and help prevent traction nerve injury. In addition, when dissecting the parathyroid glands from the thyroid, it is important to ligate or clip the distal branches of the inferior thyroid artery and on the medial surface of the parathyroid gland. This allows the parathyroid glands to be gently swept laterally with a peanut dissector while maintaining blood supply from the inferior thyroid artery. Once the parathyroid glands and RLN are identified, more liberal dissection can take place with the division of the branches of the inferior pole vessels on the surface of the thyroid gland.

> **Tip:** To help retract a large goitre extending inferiorly below the clavicle, 0-chromic sutures can be placed in the thyroid parenchyma and the thyroid is retracted cranially and medially.

Dissection of the tubercle of Zuckerkandl

The tubercle of Zuckerkandl is a useful landmark to help localize the recurrent laryngeal nerve. It was originally described as the posterior horn of the thyroid and is associated with great anatomical variability. However, in the case of an identifiable tubercle of Zuckerkandl (65% of cases), it can be a useful landmark to help identify the recurrent laryngeal nerve [4]. It is important to recognize this structure because if left behind, the remnant can potentially pose a dilemma for the patient, endocrinologist and surgeon as it can make follow-up difficult while increasing the risk (5×) of injury to the RLN if reoperation becomes necessary.

Berry's ligament, haemostasis and closure

The final step before removing the thyroid is to separate the gland from the anterior surface of the trachea by dividing Berry's ligament. This can be done either by LigaSure™, electrosurgical instruments or sharply with Metzenbaum scissors or a scalpel (Figure 5.6). Usually the pyramidal lobe is dissected before transection of the isthmus and it is included with the resected lobe, if only a lobectomy is planned. In this case, a total thyroidectomy was planned and the pyramidal lobe was seen after transection of the isthmus and removal of the right lobe. Dissection of the pyramidal lobe occurred during the dissection of the left lobe (Figure 5.7).

The thyroid bed is carefully inspected for haemostasis. The ligated branches of the superior and inferior pole vessels are inspected. The trachea is gently retracted medially to inspect the tracheo-oesophageal groove. Several small vessels are often seen around the nerve and sutures and clips are rarely necessary for haemostasis. Manual pressure over these areas will usually stop the bleeding. A variety of topical haemostatic agents may also be used.

> **Tip:** You may ask the anaesthesiologist to initiate a Valsalva manoeuvre up to a pressure of 30–35 mmHg. Although this does not eliminate the risk of postoperative bleeding, it may find small vessels that might have been improperly sealed or ligated.

Closure is done in layers, which include the strap muscles, the platysma muscle and finally the skin (Figures 5.8, 5.9). Since we separated the sternohyoid and sternothyroid muscles, we reapproximate these muscles in the midline separately using two 4-0 absorbable sutures

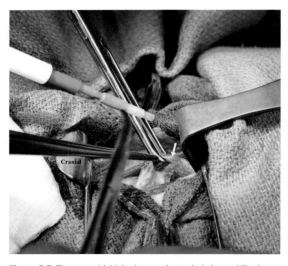

Figure 5.7 The pyramidal lobe is tented anteriorly by an Allis clamp. Dissection is carried superiorly until the pyramidal lobe tapers towards the hyoid bone. Care is taken to avoid injury to the anterior jugular veins.

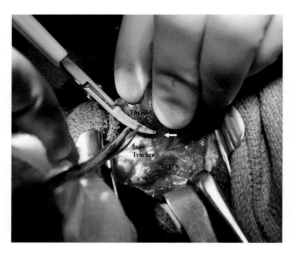

Figure 5.6 The LigaSure™ device is used to divide Berry's ligament, separating the thyroid gland from the anterior surface of the trachea.

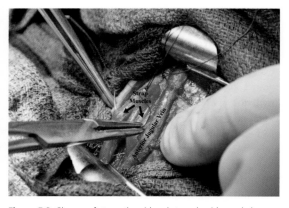

Figure 5.8 Closure of sternothyroid and sternohyoid muscle layers.

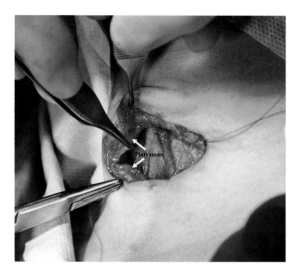

Figure 5.9 Closure of platysma muscle layer.

in the sternothyroid layer and then 4–5 4-0 absorbable sutures in the sternohyoid layer, leaving a space caudal for egress of blood in case of postoperative bleeding. The platysma is reapproximated using 4-0 absorbable sutures, making sure to align the skin markings that were made preoperatively for better cosmetic results. The skin is closed using a running 4-0 monofilament absorbable suture in a subcuticular fashion. Steri-Strips are then placed over the incision and a small dressing is applied. Alternatively, a 4-0 monofilament non-absorbable suture can be used as a holding stitch with placement of surgical glue to keep the skin edges approximated, creating a watertight seal. The suture is removed before the patient leaves the operating room.

Postoperative considerations

Patients should stay in the hospital overnight because of the risk of postoperative bleeding. Post-thyroidectomy bleeding is a surgical emergency and the majority will occur within 4–6 h after the operation [5]. Those patients who are anticoagulated preoperatively are at risk for developing a haematoma for a longer period and are instructed to go to the emergency room if they notice an expanding neck mass or experience difficulty in breathing while at home. Institution-specific protocols after thyroidectomy may include measuring neck circumference, having a tracheotomy set available at the bedside and serum calcium measurements to check for postoperative hypocalcaemia. Most patients return home the next day and are seen in follow-up approximately 2 weeks later.

Acknowledgements

We would like to thank Dr Sze Ling Wong, General Surgery Resident, Memorial University of Newfoundland, for providing the photographs for this chapter.

References

1 Welbourn RB. The History of Endocrine Surgery. New York: Greenwood Publishing Group, 1990.
2 Moalem J, Ruan DT, Farkas RL, *et al.* Patterns of antibiotic prophylaxis use for thyroidectomy and parathyroidectomy: results of an international survey of endocrine surgeons. J Am Coll Surg 2010; 210(6): 949–56.
3 Sturgeon C, Corvera C, Clark O. The missing thyroid. J Am Coll Surg 2005; 201(6): 841–6.
4 Yalçin B, Poyrazoglu Y, Ozan H. Relationship between Zuckerkandl's tubercle and the inferior laryngeal nerve including the laryngeal branches. Surg Today 2007; 37(2): 109–13.
5 Rosenbaum MA, Haridas M, McHenry CR. Life-threatening neck hematoma complicating thyroid and parathyroid surgery. Am J Surg 2008; 195(3): 339–43; discussion 343.

Videoclips

This chapter contains the following videoclips. They can be accessed at: www.wiley.com/go/miccoli/thyroid

Video 5.1   Conventional near-total thyroidectomy. (This video was recorded using the VITOM® system from Karl Storz.)
Video 5.2   Total thyroidectomy with intraoperative nerve monitoring.

CHAPTER 6

Minimally Invasive Video-assisted Thyroidectomy

Paolo Miccoli,[1] *Michele N. Minuto*[2] *and Piero Berti*[1]

[1] Department of Surgery, University of Pisa, Pisa, Italy
[2] Department of Surgical Sciences (DISC), University of Genoa, Genoa, Italy

Introduction

The impact of the endoscope, which first appeared in the late 1980s, was dramatic not only for abdominal surgery but also for other surgical fields. Thyroid surgery, in particular, had been considered a surgery with little potential for significant improvement in its quality standards but, after the first reports appeared of successful laparoscopic techniques applied to several organs, countless new minimally invasive techniques were soon proposed for neck and thyroid surgery [1,2]. In the very beginning, parathyroid surgery seemed to offer an ideal field of application for the new surgical approaches, and in 1996 the first report of a successful parathyroidectomy performed entirely endoscopically was published [3], immediately followed by the description of other videoscopic procedures for both parathyroid and thyroid glands. During the following years, several different endoscopic or video-assisted procedures were proposed for removal of the thyroid gland. These operations were initially limited to benign thyroid diseases, and later on expanded to the treatment of low-risk malignancies.

A classification of endoscopic thyroidectomies can be attempted, dividing the different techniques into two main groups [4].

1 Minimally invasive thyroidectomy performed via a cervical approach
  • Minimally invasive video-assisted thyroidectomy (MIVAT) [5]

  • Endoscopic thyroidectomy via an infraclavicular access [6]

2 Minimally invasive thyroidectomy performed via an extracervical approach
  • Endoscopic thyroidectomy performed through the axillary approach [7]
  • Endoscopic thyroidectomy performed through the breast approach [8]
  • Various combinations of the breast and axillary approaches [9–11]

Among the issues raised upon discussion of these techniques, the main one is represented by the definition of 'minimally invasive' and 'endoscopic'.

There is a great difference between the two terms, since an endoscopic operation cannot always be considered minimally invasive. Only the endoscopic procedures implying a direct cervical approach can be considered minimally invasive, whereas those performed through other access routes can be considered 'cosmetic' or 'scarless in the neck' but certainly not 'minimally invasive'. On the contrary, most of them should be considered maximally invasive since they involve longer operative time, a wider surgical dissection to reach the neck region and, as a consequence, greater postoperative pain [12].

Another initial limitation of remote access surgery is the impossibility of performing a thorough total thyroidectomy because of the lateral access. Eventually

Thyroid Surgery: Preventing and Managing Complications, First Edition. Edited by Paolo Miccoli, David J. Terris,
Michele N. Minuto and Melanie W. Seybt.

these techniques were modified to allow a bilateral operation, as in the 'axillary bilateral breast access' (ABBA) or the 'bilateral axillary breast access' (BABA). These modifications nevertheless are even more time consuming and more invasive than their original counterparts. The long operative times and the significant invasiveness of these procedures may hardly rival those of MIVAT or conventional thyroidectomy that, in expert hands, are more or less equivalent [13] and are considered as the standard for this surgery in many centres throughout the world.

Minimally invasive video-assisted thyroidectomy

In 1999, after the successful development of the minimally invasive technique for parathyroidectomy [14], an operation that had rapidly become a gold standard in the field of parathyroid surgery [15], Miccoli's technique was used to approach the thyroid gland and perform a thyroidectomy. Initially in a series of patients with small thyroid nodules [5], the first standardized MIVAT gained a large consensus offering several advantages with respect to other endoscopic techniques.
• Since it is not entirely endoscopic, it is similar to the conventional procedures.
• It utilizes mostly reusable instruments, thus not significantly raising the costs of the single procedure.
• The direct access to the thyroid gland allows for a faster learning curve.
The technique has now become the most widespread minimally invasive thyroidectomy.

Indications
Indications for correct selection of patients who may undergo a MIVAT procedure are as follows.
• Benign thyroid nodules under 35 mm in their largest diameter, or cytologically malignant (or suspicious) nodules under 20 mm, *together with*
• A thyroid volume (ultrasonographically estimated) under 25 cc
• No suspicion of metastatic lymph nodes in the central neck
• No evidence of metastatic or suspicious lymph nodes in the lateral neck
• No evidence of severe thyroiditis

Tip: When starting your own experience, try to select the easiest case possible. A small papillary thyroid cancer or indeterminate nodule, especially when the opposite lobe is normal, may represent the perfect indication with which to start. In contrast, Graves' disease, even in the presence of a small thyroid, represents an advanced indication.

Position of the patient and surgeons
The operation can be conducted under general (either with orotracheal intubation or laryngeal mask) or locoregional anaesthesia, following the surgeon's, anaesthesiologist's and/or patient's preferences.

The patient will be placed in a supine position, with the neck only slightly hyperextended. This position is in part responsible for the lesser pain that the patient will experience after the procedure when compared to those undergoing surgery with the traditional operation.

(Note: 'he', 'his' and 'him' are used for the surgeon and assistants for ease of description only.) The first surgeon will be placed on the right side of the patient, whereas his two assistants will be positioned as follows: in front of him, but slightly toward the patient's feet (camera assistant), and at the head of the patient (retractor assistant). A third assistant, or an observer, can be positioned between the two, exactly in front of the surgeon.

The monitors will be placed at both sides of the patient's head. The main monitor is in front of the first surgeon, the second being optional.

The camera assistant will always hold his instrument looking toward the patient's head, positioned slightly from the axis of the patient's midline, depending on the working side. The angled endoscope should always be confined in two main positions: looking upside-down (30° lens looking inferiorly), and downside-up (30° angle looking upward), with no intermediate positions between. This standardization allows the surgeon to always obtain the same visualization of the anatomy and the orientation of the neck, allowing the non-experienced surgeon to be orientated during all the steps of the procedure.

Tip: During the surgery, if the surgeon does have some anatomical perplexities or some difficulties in orienting himself, always check the orientations of both the endoscope and the retractors.

The technique
The MIVAT is a technique that, from its starting point, was designed to follow almost exactly the same principles of the conventional total thyroidectomy operation to avoid

unnecessary morbidity, waste of time and additional charges. In fact, all the entirely endoscopic thyroidectomies necessitate a much longer access to the gland and more time for the retrieval of the specimen through the trocar.

The basic principle is the fact that using the 20×magnification of the endoscope is useful only for the purpose of a careful and precise identification of the extremely small 'critical' structures of the neck, whereas the rest of the procedure is performed following the traditional technical points. This is the reason why the operation was called 'video-assisted' and not 'endoscopic'.

In the same way, the use of external retraction instead of CO_2 insufflation is the main principle that contributed to a faster and less morbid operation (a resident holding a retractor is unquestionably faster and safer than a vacuum needle insufflating CO_2 gas into the neck!), avoiding the negative impact of insufflation.

Finally, the same basic principles are behind the instruments dedicated to MIVAT. The specific ones are a few and almost all of them have been only slightly modified from already existing instruments that can be found in any operating room. The peculiar instruments needed are:
• a 30°, 7 or 5 mm, 29 cm long endoscope
• a single 21 cm long suction dissector (it will be necessary to avoid fogging of the endoscope due to the steam produced by the energy instrument in such small spaces)
• two 2 mm elevators of approximately the same length as the suction dissector
• small grasping forceps (15 cm long)
• small scissors (8 mm blades, 8 cm long)
• two small retractors (16 cm long)
• two conventional Army-Navy (Farabeuf) retractors.
Other useful instruments are an energy device of choice, titanium clips and conventional forceps used for thyroid surgery.

The description of the technique includes five main steps that will be developed individually.
• *Step 1.* Incision and access to the thyroid region (performed under direct vision) (see Video 6.1, 0':00' – 3':35')
• *Step 2.* Section of the upper pedicle (performed endoscopically) (Video 6.1, 3':38' – 8':18')
• *Step 3.* Identification of the critical structures: the recurrent nerve and the parathyroids (performed endoscopically) (Video 6.1, 8':22' – 9:45')
• *Step 4.* Extraction of the thyroid lobe outside the neck and completion of the near-total or total lobectomy (performed under direct vision) (Video 6.1, 9':50' – 17':10')
• *Step 5.* Suture of the access (Video 6.1, 17':57' – end).

Step 1. Incision and access to the thyroid region (Video 6.2)

The operation starts with a 2 cm median incision on a skin crease 2 cm above the sternal notch (Figure 6.1). This will help to maintain a satisfactory result in case the operation needs conversion to open surgery, when a short extension of the wound edges would convert the access to that of a conventional thyroidectomy.

> **Tip:** Always be aware that the incision length will invariably be enlarged once the whole operation is finished, so: (1) when using a slightly enlarged starting incision (strongly suggested for beginners), a surgeon might be disappointed because the final cosmetic result looks no different from that of a usual thyroidectomy performed from a very small incision, and (2) a more limited incision (1.5 cm, for example) can be used when a surgeon is skilled enough with the technique.

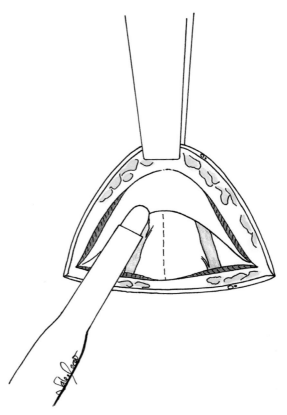

Figure 6.1 The incision is 1.5–2 cm in size, placed along the line of a conventional Kocher's incision. Only a minimal skin flap is necessary.

(a)

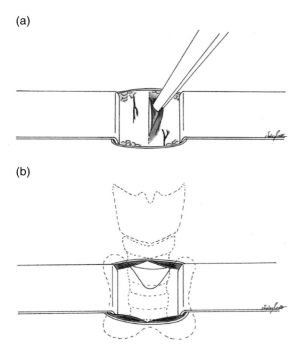

(b)

Figure 6.2 (a) The midline is found, if not evident, by palpation of the tip of the thyroid cartilage, and is opened for a short length. (b) This short dissection of the midline allows the surgeon to focus the retraction on the prethyroidal muscles, and not on the skin edges.

After the incision, the two smallest retractors should be positioned laterally on both sides (Figure 6.2a). The "Linea alba" should be carefully identified as in conventional open surgery, but with the confounding factor of the very small access; palpating the tip of the thyroid cartilage can help finding the midline and delineate it.

The midline should be dissected with conventional electrocautery for a short extent, not much larger than the edge of a conventional Army-Navy (Farabeuf) retractor. This short aperture of the strap muscles will help avoid excessive retraction on the skin edges, focusing the majority of the tension on the muscles themselves (Figure 6.2b). This allows the skin edges to remain vital and results in a good cosmetic outcome.

> **Tip:** Don't forget to protect and insulate the blade of the electrocautery, leaving only its tip exposed. This is necessary to avoid burns on the skin edges, otherwise inevitable in such a small space.

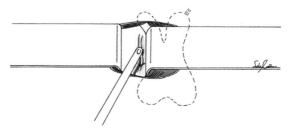

Figure 6.3 The correct position of the retractors when performing a right lobectomy: the lateral one should retract the carotid sheath laterally whereas the medial one should 'hook' the thyroid lobe medially, trying to slightly rotate it on the tracheal axis.

Enter the thyroid bed on one side with blunt dissection utilizing the spatulas. The virtual space between the strap muscles and the thyroid lobe should be progressively entered with the small retractors at first, replaced by the conventional Army-Navy after the carotid sheath is visualized.

The correct positioning of the retractors is one of the key points of this operation. The lateral one should be placed so that it laterally retracts the carotid sheath in all its elements (very important to avoid undesired lesions to those structures when the energy devices are used in such small spaces during the following steps), and the medial one should 'hook' the thyroid lobe medially, trying to slightly rotate it at the same time on the tracheal axis, almost hiding it from the view of the endoscope (Figure 6.3). The medial retractor mimics the role of the hand of the assistant during a conventional thyroidectomy. Be aware that, in this phase, the two retractors should always be placed in a symmetrical position, at the two edges of the incision.

> **Tip:** A frequently encountered problem is the correct position and movements of the retractors. Both of them should not only pull externally on the two sides, but they also need to 'load' their structures: doing this, the medial retractor will lift the thyroid lobe sufficiently to allow visualization of the region where the nerve lies (remember that since the neck is not hyperextended, the nerve lies flat on the posterior surface of our surgical field, allowing its identification. If this space is not opened, the structures will be hidden behind the thyroid lobe itself. A good trick: when inserting the endoscope, if you see the thyroid lobe 'bulging' beyond the tip of the retractor, its position is not correct. When, on the other hand, the lobe is completely hidden behind the blade of the retractor, its placement is perfect.

Step 2. Section of the upper pedicle (Video 6.3)

This is the most difficult part of the endoscopic operation, since it is the only step that is significantly different from the way it is performed in traditional surgery.

The largest retractors are still positioned on both sides of the incision. This position will be maintained throughout this entire step.

The endoscopic portion of the operation starts by inserting the tip of the endoscope inside the operative field. The endoscope is a 30°, 5 or 7 mm calibre scope that will initially be oriented with a caudal view, to check for the middle thyroid vein, that will be eventually ligated using an energy instrument or clips.

Once this quick step is done, the endoscope can be rotated downside-up and, viewing the cephalic direction, the upper pedicle will be visualized at the top of the screen. You can decide, then, to proceed in two separate ways: by cutting the pedicle in its entirety with the energy instrument or with the help of titanium clips, thus performing an *en bloc* resection (always remember that the small thyroids that are indicated for MIVAT may have a very small upper pedicle), or by selectively cutting every single vessel separately.

It was only after quite a large number of cases that we had the serendipitous evidence that the magnification of the images and the possibility to see very cephalad in the neck region allowed the visualization of the external branch of the superior laryngeal nerve in its lowest variants [16].

Before cutting the entire pedicle, the surgeon should always carefully check for the external branch of the superior laryngeal nerve, which creates a loop coming down from the medial side of the pedicle and consequently ascending on the lateral side of the cricothyroid muscle. This nerve can be visualized by gently opening the narrow space between the cricothyroid muscle and the pedicle, where the sheaths of the energy instrument will be inserted, once ready to cut the pedicle. This manoeuvre can be performed with the help of a dissector spatula pulling the pedicle laterally. When this space is opened adequately, the nerve, if present, will be put on tension and easily recognized, thus sparing it from iatrogenic lesions.

Always double-check the haemostasis of the vessels of the upper pedicle after their section, and take care of situations that look uncertain. An immediate bleed can be very hard to manage endoscopically at the very beginning of a surgeon's experience, and can lead to undesired conversions. On the other hand, a delayed bleed can cause more dangerous situations, since no drain will be left in the neck and the incision will be sealed with glue, not allowing a spontaneous evacuation of the haematoma.

> **Tip:** The key point of this step is to completely dissect the upper pedicle to the more posterior vessels. An incomplete section of the pedicle will result in difficulty in obtaining correct mobilization of the lobe, a manoeuvre that will lead to the extraction of the lobe itself without any traction on the delicate structures.

Step 3. Identification of the recurrent nerve and the parathyroids (Video 6.4)

Although it is the most important, this step is the easiest of the whole procedure. The surgeon will explore, identify and dissect the 'noble' structures of the thyroid region using delicate, blunt dissection allowed by the precise movements of the thin dissectors, partnered with the advantage of the magnification provided by the endoscopic vision.

The correct position of the whole team is the key point during this step. The retractors, in their lateral positions, should expose the space where the recurrent nerve and the parathyroids are located. The medial retractor is essential to 'load' the thyroid lobe, also lifting it in order to visualize the area between the trachea and the oesophagus, as previously described. The endoscope will always be oriented downward, only slightly looking medially.

The main branch of the recurrent nerve lies on the anterior surface of the vertebral muscles (on the right side) and on the oesophagus (left side). On each side the nerve can be easily visualized at its crossing with the inferior thyroid artery only by using a blunt dissection with the two spatulas. An additional indicator can be the visual identification of the many small lymph nodes that are almost always present in the area surrounding the recurrent nerve, and that can be easily dissected, uncovering the nerve itself. Once identified, the recurrent nerve can be easily followed and exposed until its point of insertion to the cricothyroid muscle. It is not necessary, in our opinion, to dissect it too extensively in its caudal direction.

The most frequent position of the superior parathyroid gland is at the upper pole of the thyroid lobe, laterally to the lobe itself or adherent to it. The absolutely typical shape and colour are of great help for the recognition of the gland, and these characteristics are greatly enhanced by the endoscopic vision. Once identified, the parathyroid can be gently dissected, always taking care to preserve its small pedicle, and delicately moved away from the thyroid gland, to avoid any damage to its vascular support during the mobilization and extraction of the lobe.

The inferior parathyroid gland can be identified when it is in a favourable position, thus not in particularly caudal ectopies or in the midportion of the thyroid lobe, a position where it can be hidden behind the blade of the retractor. To proceed to the next step (the extraction of the lobe outside the incision), it is necessary to identify and dissect the recurrent nerve and at least the superior parathyroid gland. If the inferior parathyroid has not been identified, the gland will be sought after the lobe is delivered outside the incision, as is usually done in conventional open surgery.

> **Tip:** The surgeon should always be aware of the position of the camera; the wrong position can be responsible for disorientation of the entire surgical team. Check in particular the following landmarks: the thyroid lobe should always be under the blade of the large retractor, almost entirely loaded and moved medially; the carotid sheath should be carefully loaded and laterally retracted, to guarantee the widest operative field in the region of the recurrent nerve. Also, it is easier to identify the recurrent nerve in its caudal position, at the level of the inferior portion of the thyroid lobe, a region that can be properly visualized when the camera is angled at almost 90° on the patient.

Step 4. Extraction of the thyroid lobe outside the neck and completion of the lobectomy (Video 6.5)

This portion of the operation is performed under direct vision, basically following the rules of the conventional open surgery.

This step starts by grasping the superior pole of the thyroid lobe, that has already been dissected, with a conventional Kelly/Crile forceps, and gently extracting it outside by rotating the entire lobe on its longest axis, taking particular care to avoid any damage to the vessels of the inferior pole, from where the vascular supply of the inferior parathyroid gland may arise. If the upper pedicle has been properly and completely dissected, the surgeon will encounter no resistance in delivering the superior pole of the lobe outside. Once the upper pole is out from the incision, it is necessary to increase the mobility of the lobe itself. This can be obtained by a step-by-step dissection, starting from the areas that are safer (with a minimal risk of creating any morbidity).

With this basic principle in mind, better mobility can be obtained by starting to dissect the lobe from the upper pole and descending toward the isthmus, dividing it. The key point of this manoeuvre, in our opinion, is to open the space between the posterior aspect of the upper pedicle (the origin of the ligament of Berry) and the isthmus itself (Figure 6.4). This area is well known among those who perform the MIVAT procedure as the 'triangle of Miccoli–Berti' (see Video 6.6), following the ideas of the surgeons who identified this as an essential step in the extraction of the thyroid lobe. It is a manoeuvre that can present some difficulties to the novice thyroid surgeon. The 'triangle' is oriented downward and composed of the posterior aspect of the upper pedicle (laterally), the pyramidal lobe (medially) and the prethyroidal muscles

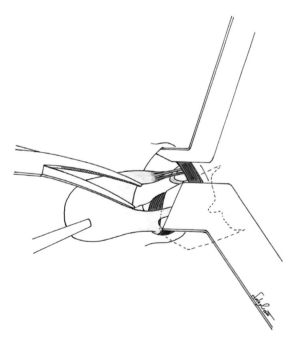

Figure 6.4 The 'triangle of Miccoli–Berti' (right side in the picture) is composed of the posterior aspect of the upper pedicle laterally, the pyramidal lobe medially and the curtain created by the retracted strap muscles upward. The section of the lobe should start from the isthmus, the safest part, in a downward direction.

(base) (see Video 6.1, 10':21'), allowing performance of a safe dissection prior to exposing the recurrent nerve and the parathyroids once again, to complete the lobectomy.

Once all the elements are identified, it is necessary to cut the isthmus in a downward direction, completely dividing it and exposing the nude tracheal surface. The lobe is now free from its superior and medial portion, and the next step is to cut the vessels of the inferior pole, taking care not to damage the vessels supporting the inferior parathyroid gland. Once this step is complete, the lobe can be completely and delicately delivered outside the incision, and the surgeon is ready to expose the lateral side of the lobe, following, once again, the previously identified recurrent nerve and both the parathyroids in the traditional way.

> **Tip:** If the thyroid lobe, freed in its upper and lower portions, cannot be delivered outside by minimal traction on the parenchyma, consequently risking rupture of the thyroid capsule, there are some simple manoeuvres that can help. The first, when the thyroid nodule has a cystic component, is to empty the liquid content by means of a sterile syringe or by cutting a small hole in its wall. The smaller nodule will immediately be pulled outside with minimal effort.
>
> When the problem is obstruction from the strap muscles, that are tense and rigid, and/or from the non-mobility of the lobe itself that can stay very deep in the neck, not compliant with the traction manoeuvres, the suggestion is to ask the anaesthesiologist for a supplement of curarization. The following effect will allow the strap muscles to relax and the entire trachea-larynx-thyroid lobe block to be more easily mobilized.

The lobectomy will then be completed following the surgeon's own best rules, also evaluating the extension to give the lobectomy (total or near-total), according to his preferences and the nature of the thyroid disease itself.

> **Tip:** It may seem unnatural to some surgeons to divide the thyroid in two lobes, but this is, in our opinion, necessary to obtain the best and safest exposure of the lateral side of the gland, where the dissection should be careful and precise. If the isthmus is not cut, the lobe will not be able to be completely rotated and therefore one cannot pull it completely outside the incision. This makes working on the lateral side uncomfortable, since the region will not be completely exposed. Nevertheless, this is a situation that follows the single surgeon's experience and preference.

A complete total thyroidectomy will be performed by repeating the same steps to the opposite side, knowing that if the surgeon has started from the largest (or affected) lobe, as we always suggest, the opposite (generally performed on a normal lobe) lobectomy can be performed faster than the previous one.

A frequent and debated issue is whether it is possible to perform an oncologically radical operation with the MIVAT technique or not. In our opinion, a thorough extracapsular total thyroidectomy can be performed with the MIVAT, since the extension of the surgery is decided in the final part of the operation that is performed under direct vision, in exactly the same way as for traditional thyroidectomy. The fact that we tend to perform a near-total lobectomy/thyroidectomy in many cases reflects our own surgical attitude, since we follow these same guidelines also in traditional open surgery in cases of benign disease or low- and/or intermediate-risk thyroid cancers [17].

Step 5. Suture of the access (Video 6.7)

Once the lobectomy/total thyroidectomy is finished, and haemostasis is carefully obtained, the surgeon should verify the noble structures on both sides for the last time. The integrity of the recurrent nerve(s) should be verified, as well as the viability of both the parathyroids, that may be autotransplanted, according to the surgeon's preference, when their vitality is uncertain. We recommend careful verification of haemostasis on the vessels of both the upper pedicles, since postoperative bleeding from there can lead to a dramatic series of events.

The closure can then be performed with one or two single stitches on the strap muscles, three single subcutaneous stitches reapproximating the skin edges, and, in our own setting, surgical glue on the skin (a running suture can always be performed as an alternative).

> **Tip:** Great attention should be paid to verification of the vitality of the skin edges; the use of 'hot' instruments during the whole operation, in such a narrow space, may lead to mild or severe burn damage to the skin. In these cases we always suggest removing the burned edges, suturing on the vital skin. This is described more fully in Chapter 16.

A complete MIVAT procedure with a few non-significant video edits (therefore almost in real time) can be seen in Video 6.8.

References

1 Mattioli FP, Cagnazzo A, Varaldo E, Bianchi C, Spigno L, Gasparini C. [An application of mini-invasive surface surgery: the thyroid]. Ann Ital Chir 1996; 67(4): 535–6.

2 Hüscher CS, Chiodini S, Napolitano C, Recher A. Endoscopic right thyroid lobectomy. Surg Endosc 1997; 11(8): 877.

3 Gagner M. Endoscopic subtotal parathyroidectomy in patients with primary hyperparathyroidism. Br J Surg 1996; 83(6): 875.

4 Miccoli P, Minuto MN. Minimally invasive thyroidectomy: state of the art. Minerva Chirurg 2009; 64(6): 545–50.

5 Miccoli P, Berti P, Conte M, Bendinelli C, Marcocci C. Minimally invasive surgery for thyroid small nodules: preliminary report. J Endocrinol Invest 1999; 22(11): 849–51.

6 Gagner M, Inabnet WB 3rd. Endoscopic thyroidectomy for solitary thyroid nodules. Thyroid 2001; 11(2): 161–3.

7 Ikeda Y, Takami H, Sasaki Y, Kan S, Niimi M. Endoscopic neck surgery by the axillary approach. J Am Coll Surg 2000; 191(3): 336–40.

8 Ohgami M, Ishii S, Arisawa Y, et al. Scarless endoscopic thyroidectomy: breast approach for better cosmesis. Surg Laparosc Endosc Percutan Tech 2000; 10(1): 1–4.

9 Choe JH, Kim SW, Chung KW, et al. Endoscopic thyroidectomy using a new bilateral axillo-breast approach. World J Surg 2007; 31(3): 601–6.

10 Bärlehner E, Benhidjeb T. Cervical scarless endoscopic thyroidectomy: axillo-bilateral-breast approach (ABBA). Surg Endosc 2008; 22(1): 154–7.

11 Lee KE, Kim HY, Park WS, et al. Postauricular and axillary approach endoscopic neck surgery: a new technique. World J Surg 2009; 33(4): 767–72.

12 Henry JF. Minimally invasive thyroid and parathyroid surgery is not a question of length of the incision. Langenbecks Arch Surg 2008; 393(5): 621–6.

13 Terris DJ, Angelos P, Steward DL, Simental AA. Minimally invasive video-assisted thyroidectomy. a multi-institutional North American experience. Arch Otolaryngol Head Neck Surg 2008; 134(1): 81–4.

14 Miccoli P, Pinchera A, Cecchini G, et al. Minimally invasive, video-assisted parathyroid surgery for primary hyperparathyroidism. J Endocrinol Invest 1997; 20(7): 429–30.

15 Miccoli P, Monchik JM. Minimally invasive parathyroid surgery. Surg Endosc 2000; 14(11): 987–90.

16 Berti P, Materazzi G, Conte M, Galleri D, Miccoli P. Visualization of the external branch of the superior laryngeal nerve during video-assisted thyroidectomy. J Am Coll Surg 2002; 195(4): 573–4.

17 Minuto MN, Berti P, Miccoli M, et al. Minimally invasive video-assisted thyroidectomy: an analysis of results and a revision of indications. Surg Endosc 2012; 26(3): 818–22.

Videoclips

This chapter contains the following videoclips. They can be accessed at: www.wiley.com/go/miccoli/thyroid

Video 6.1 Near-total right lobectomy. The procedure is almost in real time. This clip shows the procedure in its entirety with only minor edits. Operators: Paolo Miccoli, Piero Berti, Michele N. Minuto.

Video 6.2 Step 1: Incision and access to the right thyroid bed. This step is performed under direct vision.

Video 6.3 Step 2: Section of the upper pedicle. The 30° of the endoscope is rotated upward. Notice the almost immediate visualization of the superior parathyroid.

Video 6.4 Identification of the recurrent nerve and the parathyroids. The 30° of the endoscope is rotated downward.

Video 6.5 Extraction of the thyroid lobe outside the neck and completion of the lobectomy. This part of the operation, performed under direct vision, is done following the conventional rules of a near-total or total thyroidectomy.

Video 6.6 How to recognize the 'triangle of Miccoli–Berti. This step is essential to obtain correct mobility of the thyroid lobe, allowing it to be delivered out of the neck. Always dissect the pyramidal lobe-isthmus side first.

Video 6.7 Suture of the access. The midline is closed with a single resorbable stitch, and the subcuticular tissue with three stitches of the same suture. Surgical glue is used to seal the incision.

Video 6.8 Real-time total thyroidectomy with the MIVAT technique. Operators: Paolo Miccoli and Piero Berti.

CHAPTER 7

Robotic Thyroid Surgery

Michael C. Singer and David J. Terris
Department of Otolaryngology – Head and Neck Surgery, Georgia Health Sciences University,
Augusta GA, USA

Introduction

There have been dramatic changes in the techniques of thyroid surgery over the last decade. With a number of crucial technological and procedural advancements, thyroidectomy has matured into a procedure that can be performed in both a minimally invasive and minimal incision manner on an outpatient basis. The culmination of these developments was the minimally invasive video-assisted thyroidectomy (MIVAT) technique described and perfected by Paolo Miccoli and his colleagues [1]. While this technique is safe and effective, abbreviates the recovery time and results in an incision as small as 1.5 cm, there is nonetheless a conspicuous cervical scar.

In an effort to completely obviate the need for a cervical incision, surgeons have sought to develop techniques that allow removal of the thyroid gland through remote (non-cervical) incisions. Particularly in Asian countries, where cervical scars are anathema and patients often have a predilection for hypertrophic scarring, remote access techniques have commanded significant attention. A number of remote access endoscopic approaches [2,3] have been described utilizing portals which have included presternal, inframammary, circumareolar, postauricular and transaxillary locations. These procedures tend to be lengthy and technically challenging. Woong Youn Chung in Seoul, South Korea, enhanced remote-access thyroidectomy techniques by introducing a robot-assisted, gasless transaxillary procedure (RAT) which uses a fixed retractor system [4]. Chung and his colleagues have performed more than a thousand of these thyroidectomies with excellent outcomes and low complication rates.

More recently, the robotic facelift thyroidectomy (RFT) technique has been described, which was designed to be easier to perform safely in North American patients. This chapter will focus on these techniques and discuss appropriate indications.

Robotic-assisted transaxillary thyroidectomy technique

As previously noted, a transaxillary approach was one of the favoured endoscopic remote-access thyroidectomy techniques. However, due to its technical complexity, gas insufflation was required for extended periods of time. By pioneering the use of a fixed retractor to maintain the working space, Dr. Chung was able to eliminate the need for gas insufflation. However, this gasless transaxillary approach was still surgically demanding, was restricted to the use of straight endoscopic instruments and relied on a hand-held endoscope for visualization. To overcome these challenges, Dr. Chung and his colleagues integrated the surgical robot into the procedure. The robot's strengths matched the obstacles presented by the gasless approach.

Thyroid Surgery: Preventing and Managing Complications, First Edition. Edited by Paolo Miccoli, David J. Terris,
Michele N. Minuto and Melanie W. Seybt.
© 2013 John Wiley & Sons, Ltd. Published 2013 by John Wiley & Sons, Ltd.

In the RAT approach exact patient positioning is essential in order to facilitate crossing the clavicle during dissection. While the precise methods vary, this generally involves extending the arm over the head for the duration of the procedure, potentially placing the brachial plexus under significant stress. In order to assess the extent of traction caused by this positioning during the surgery, some surgeons use intraoperative electromyographic monitoring of the muscles supplied by the brachial plexus.

This procedure begins with a 6–8 cm incision along the posterior aspect of the pectoralis muscle in the axilla (see Video 7.1). Utilizing electrocautery and sequentially longer hand-held retractors, a suprapectoral plane is created. Development of an adequate skin, subcutaneous tissue and platysmal muscle flap is critical to ensure sufficient working space. Dissection of this flap is carried beyond the clavicle. A subtle, avascular space between the sternal and clavicular heads of the sternocleidomastoid muscle is then sought. This space is then exploited to reach the thyroid compartment by division or retraction of the omohyoid muscle and elevation of the sternohyoid and sternothyroid muscles. The superior pole of the ipsilateral thyroid gland is then exposed and the fixed retractor is placed and used to maintain the operative working space. The da Vinci surgical system (Intuitive Surgical Inc., Sunnyvale, California) is then docked.

Several variations for deployment of the four robotic arms have been described. In the original technique, two of the robotic arms and the robotic camera are introduced through the axillary incision. A second 8 mm incision is then placed superior and medial to the ipsilateral nipple. This second port allows for the introduction of the third instrument arm into the surgical field. In a second approach, all four arms are placed through the axillary incision [5].

A 30° endoscope (facing downward), a Harmonic® device, a Maryland dissector and a forceps are used to perform the surgery. The forceps are used to retract the superior pole of the thyroid gland, which is then dissected free from the surrounding tissues. The Harmonic® device is used to divide the superior pole vessels. The inferior aspect of the gland is then dissected off the trachea. The gland is then retracted ventrally and medially. The recurrent laryngeal nerve is then visualized and traced. The attachments medial to the nerve are then divided and the specimen removed. At the end of the case an active drain is placed, the wound is closed and the patient is observed in the hospital.

Robotic facelift thyroidectomy

Rationale for development

Despite the success of the transaxillary technique in Korea, there have been significant challenges during its introduction into North America [6]. A number of noteworthy complications have occurred in patients undergoing RAT in the United States. These include temporary arm paralysis, injury to the oesophagus and trachea, and significant loss of blood during surgery. As this technique has been performed so successfully in Korea, the question arises as to the cause of the increased incidence of complications in North America. This likely can be at least partially attributed to the body morphology of North American patients versus Korean patients who tend to be on average significantly thinner and shorter [7]. Additionally, the average size of the nodular disease treated in Korea is markedly less than that typically addressed surgically in North America [8].

Given the occurrence of these complications and the technically challenging nature of RAT, the RFT technique was designed and implemented clinically [9,10]. A modified facelift incision, frequently utilized during parotid surgery, and the subsequent dissection along the anterior aspect of the sternocleidomastoid muscle represent anatomy that is more familiar to many head and neck surgeons. The RFT technique is a hybrid approach that integrates important components of traditional thyroid surgery with several innovative principles, including use of the modified facelift incision, integration of the da Vinci robot, and use of a fixed retractor system as described by Chung to avoid gas insufflation. RFT seems to decrease the chance of complications in a number of ways. Avoiding the need for special positioning of the arm, as is used in RAT, eliminates the possibility of brachial plexus injury. Operating in more traditional surgical planes possibly allows for improved identification of critical structures. Additionally, as the vector of approach in RFT is more ventral in nature, the trachea and oesophagus are perhaps at less risk of injury. Importantly, with RFT there is less need to compromise on some of the tremendous progress that has occurred over the last decade in thyroid surgery as RFT does not require placement of a drain and can be performed as an outpatient procedure.

Patient selection

As with any surgical procedure, careful and appropriate patient selection is essential for surgical success and mitigation of risk. For RFT, there are both patient- and disease-specific criteria to be considered when assessing a patient for eligibility. Many of these could likely be applied to any remote-access or minimally invasive thyroidectomy technique. Patients must be committed to completely eliminating a cervical neck incision as this technique leads to more postoperative discomfort and a longer recovery time than with minimally invasive techniques. Patients should be ASA class 1 or 2 and should not be morbidly obese or have previously had neck surgery. With regard to disease-specific criteria, given current technology and techniques only a hemithyroidectomy including isthmusectomy can be performed easily through a single RFT incision. Therefore, RFT is best reserved for patients who are anticipated to require unilateral surgery only. Nodule size greater than 4 cm in greatest dimension makes remote-access excision more challenging and should be considered a size limitation. Importantly, the presence of thyroiditis, whether based on patient history or clinical appearance, is a relative contraindication to performance of this technique. Finally, absence of lymphadenopathy, substernal extension or extrathyroidal extension should be established prior to performing RFT.

Technique

In order to identify the most cosmetically appropriate positioning of the incision, the patient is marked sitting upright in the holding area. The facelift incision is placed in the postauricular crease extending into the occipital hairline [11]. The descending limb is made approximately 1 cm behind the hairline (in this area the hair is clipped at the beginning of surgery) so that this portion of the incision is completely obscured (Figure 7.1). The incision should be placed so that from the frontal view, no part of the incision can be seen. The site for a possible cervical incision, needed in the unlikely event of conversion to open surgery, is marked as well.

The patient is placed on the operating table in the supine position. An electromyographic endotracheal tube is used so that laryngeal nerve monitoring can be utilized during the procedure. The head is turned 30° away from the side requiring surgery and supported to prevent excessive rotation.

Development of the surgical pocket proceeds through a systematic progression. The first structure identified is

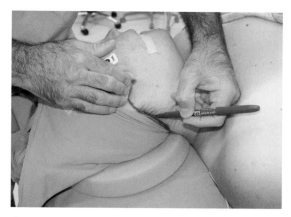

Figure 7.1 The postauricular incision extends inferiorly into the occipital hairline. The incision should not be visible from a frontal view of the patient. Reproduced from Terris *et al*. [10] with permission from Lippincott Williams and Wilkins.

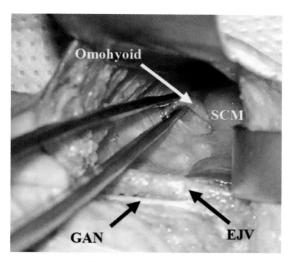

Figure 7.2 A view of a right-sided operative pocket created with open dissection, at a stage just prior to dissection beneath the strap muscles. Important landmarks include the greater auricular nerve (GAN), external jugular vein (EJV), sternocleidomastoid muscle (SCM) and omohyoid muscle. Reproduced from Terris *et al*. [10] with permission from Lippincott Williams and Wilkins.

the sternocleidomastoid muscle, followed by identification of the greater auricular nerve. The external jugular vein is then encountered and is typically reflected dorsally or can be ligated to facilitate access. Recognition of the omohyoid muscle is helpful in order to gain access to the superior pole of the thyroid gland (Figure 7.2). Deep to this muscle, the plane just above the thyroid capsule can

(a)   (b)

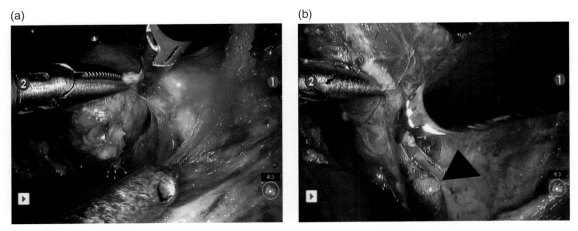

Figure 7.3 View through robotic camera. Ligation of the superior pedicle as a single bundle with ultrasonic energy (a). The superior parathyroid gland (*black arrowhead*) is reflected posteriorly (b). Reproduced from Terris *et al.* [11] with permission from Lippincott Williams and Wilkins.

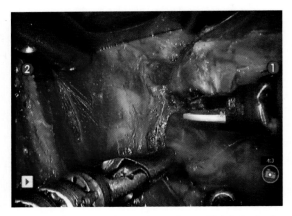

Figure 7.4 The recurrent laryngeal nerve is traced inferiorly after it is identified at its entry point underneath the inferior border of the inferior constrictor muscle. Reproduced from Terris *et al.* [11] with permission from Lippincott Williams and Wilkins.

be bluntly dissected, allowing the strap muscles to be retracted ventrally. A modified version of the Chung retractor blade (Marina Medical, Sunrise, Florida) is then used to retract the muscle and skin flap and maintain the operative pocket.

Once the fixed retractor is positioned, the daVinci surgical robotic system is deployed. The robotic pedestal is angled approximately 30° away from the operating table, with its long axis parallel to the retractor system.

Three arms are utilized: the camera arm is positioned first, holding a 30° down endoscope parallel to the retractor system, or angled slightly upward. A Maryland grasper is placed in the non-dominant arm, and a Harmonic® device (Ethicon Endosurgery Inc., Cincinnati, Ohio) is placed in the dominant arm, and these are positioned on either side of the endoscope.

Robotic resection of the gland is then performed. The superior pedicle is ligated using the Harmonic® device (Figure 7.3a). The superior pole is then reflected ventrally and blunt dissection is utilized to delineate the inferior border of the inferior constrictor muscle (the external branch of the superior laryngeal nerve can be seen running along this muscle) (see Video 7.2). In this area the superior parathyroid gland may be identified and reflected posteriorly (Figure 7.3b). At this point, exploration and identification of the recurrent laryngeal nerve at its entry underneath the inferior constrictor muscle are achieved. The nerve is then dissected inferiorly (Figure 7.4). The tissue medial to this, including the ligament of Berry, may then be safely divided using the Harmonic® device. The thyroid isthmus is transected and the middle thyroid vein is ligated. The inferior parathyroid gland is identified and dissected from the thyroid gland, and the inferior pole vessels are ligated. The thyroid gland can then be fully dissected from the trachea and retrieved.

(b)

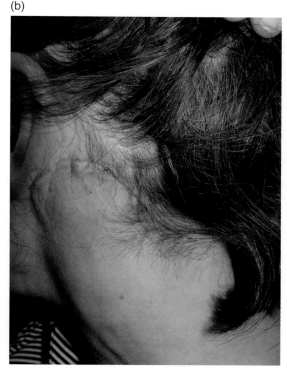

(a)

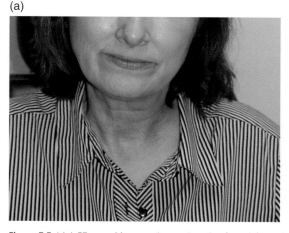

Figure 7.5 (a) A 57-year-old woman is seen 3 weeks after a left RFT for a thyroid nodule. The postauricular wound is healing appropriately with minimal surrounding oedema. (b) Note that a large part of the incision is hidden behind the hairline.

After thorough irrigation and inspection of the thyroid bed and surgical pocket, Surgicel (Ethicon Inc., Somerville, New Jersey) is placed in the thyroid compartment. The wound is then closed (Figure 7.5). No drain is placed. Patients are managed on an outpatient basis.

Conclusion

Robotic surgery of the thyroid gland is in its early phases of development. The RAT and RFT procedures both require extensive dissection to create an operative pocket sufficient to allow removal of the thyroid gland. While not minimally invasive, they completely eliminate the need for a cervical incision. Continued technological developments and innovations in surgical technique may allow these procedures to be performed more effectively and efficiently.

References

1 Miccoli P, Berti P, Conte M, *et al.* Minimally invasive surgery for thyroid small nodules: preliminary report. J Endocrinol Invest 1999; 22: 849–51.

2 Choe J, Kim SW, Chung K, *et al.* Endoscopic thyroidectomy using a new bilateral axillo-breast approach. World J Surg 2007; 31(3): 601–6.

3 Ikeda Y, Takami H, Sasaki Y, *et al.* Clinical benefits in endoscopic thyroidectomy by the axillary approach. J Am Coll Surg 2003; 196(2): 189–95.

4 Kang SW, Lee SC, Lee SH, *et al.* Robotic thyroid surgery using a gasless, transaxillary approach and the da Vinci S system: the operative outcomes of 338 consecutive patients. Surgery 2009; 146(6): 1048–55.

5 Ryu HR, Kang SW, Lee SH, *et al.* Feasibility and safety of a new robotic thyroidectomy through a gasless, transaxillary single-incision approach. J Am Coll Surg 2010; 211(3): e13–19.

6 Kuppersmith RB, Holsinger FC. Robotic thyroid surgery: an initial experience with North American patients. Laryngoscope 2011; 121(3): 521–6.

7 Landry CS, Grubbs EG, Morris GS, et al. Robot assisted transaxillary surgery (RATS) for the removal of thyroid and parathyroid glands. Surgery 2011; 149: 549–55.

8 Lee J, Nah KY, Kim RM, et al. Differences in postoperative outcomes, function, and cosmesis: open versus robotic thyroidectomy. Surg Endosc 2010; 24(12): 3186–94.

9 Singer MC, Seybt MW, Terris DJ. Robotic facelift thyroidectomy: I. Preclinical simulation and morphometric assessment. Laryngoscope 2011; 121(8): 1631–5.

10 Terris DJ, Singer MC, Seybt MW. Robotic facelift thyroidectomy: II. Clinical feasibility and safety. Laryngoscope 2011; 121(8): 1636–41.

11 Terris DJ, Singer MC, Seybt MW. Robotic facelift thyroidectomy: patient selection and technical considerations. Surg Laparosc Endosc Percutan Tech 2011; 21(4): 237–42.

Videoclips

This chapter contains the following videoclips. They can be accessed at: www.wiley.com/go/miccoli/thyroid

Video 7.1 Robot-assisted transaxillary thyroidectomy. Pocket creation and thyroid excision during a right-sided, robot-assisted transaxillary thyroidectomy.

Video 7.2 Robotic facelift thyroidectomy. Recurrent laryngeal nerve dissection and thyroid excision during a right-sided, robotic facelift thyroidectomy.

CHAPTER 8

Extensive Surgery for Thyroid Cancer: Central Neck Dissection

Emad H. Kandil,[1] *Salem I. Noureldine*[1] *and Ralph P. Tufano*[2]

[1]Division of Endocrine and Oncological Surgery, Department of Surgery, Tulane University School of Medicine, New Orleans, LA, USA
[2]Division of Head and Neck Cancer Surgery, Department of Otolaryngology – Head and Neck Surgery, Johns Hopkins School of Medicine, Baltimore, MD, USA

Introduction

The rise in the incidence of thyroid cancer is the fastest in the United States, with annual cases exceeding 48,000 patients [1]. It is the most common endocrine malignancy, accounting for over 90% of all endocrine cancers, killing approximately 1300 patients annually [2]. The management of thyroid cancer continues to evolve. Over the past 50 years we have moved toward more total thyroidectomies, evolving away from thyroid lobectomy. The rationales for total thyroidectomy include the frequent multifocal nature of the disease, ability to reduce the risk of recurrence and to facilitate radioactive iodine treatment, and the use of serum thyroglobulin levels and whole-body radioiodine scans during follow-up. Two Mazzeferri *et al.* studies suggest that total thyroidectomy reduces the recurrence of papillary thyroid cancer (PTC) and perhaps improves survival [3,4]. Most surgeons now agree that total thyroidectomy is preferred over thyroid lobectomy for the majority of patients with PTC [5].

Although the debate over the extent of thyroidectomy has largely faded, the role of neck dissection in the surgical management of PTC has become a topic of contention. Cervical lymph node metastasis occurs in up to 90% of patients with PTC, and in a lesser proportion in patients with other histotypes [6,7]. This depends not only on the actual clinical stage of disease but also on which diagnostic modalities are employed to assess for potential lymphatic metastasis [8,9].

Lymph node metastases are known to significantly correlate with both the persistence and recurrence of PTC and, potentially, survival [10]. Follicular thyroid cancer (FTC) does not commonly present with cervical lymph node metastases, and when found, a follicular variant of PTC should be considered [11]. Patients with the Hurthle cell variant of FTC may have nodal disease, which predicts a worse outcome, and should have a therapeutic central neck dissection if metastatic lymph nodes are identified [12].

The current standard of care for patients with PTC includes total thyroidectomy and a therapeutic central neck dissection for those presenting with clinically evident nodal disease. However, many surgeons advocate prophylactic central neck lymph node dissections in patients who present with no clinical or radiographic evidence of lymph node involvement [13–15]. It is controversial whether prophylactic central neck dissection (CND) is indicated when there is no evidence of pathological involvement on preoperative or intraoperative assessment [16]. Recently, the American Thyroid Association (ATA) updated and revised its original guidelines on CND for well-differentiated thyroid cancer.

Thyroid Surgery: Preventing and Managing Complications, First Edition. Edited by Paolo Miccoli, David J. Terris, Michele N. Minuto and Melanie W. Seybt.
© 2013 John Wiley & Sons, Ltd. Published 2013 by John Wiley & Sons, Ltd.

The ATA guidelines recommend that a 'prophylactic neck dissection may be performed, especially in patients with advanced primary tumors (T3 or T4)' and that a 'total thyroidectomy without prophylactic neck dissection may be appropriate for small (T1 or T2), noninvasive, clinically node negative patients' [5]. Unfortunately, the literature is still inconclusive on this subject. Herein, we discuss the surgical options for approaching CND in patients presenting with extensive thyroid cancer.

Incidence and prevalence

Papillary thyroid cancer has a tendency for cervical lymphatic spread. It occurs in 20–50% of patients when using standard pathological techniques and in 90% of those examined for micrometastases [17,18]. Thyroid tumour cells are spread through the lymphatic system in a sequential fashion that starts in the perithyroidal lymph nodes of the central neck and progresses to the lymph nodes of the lateral cervical compartments and the superior mediastinum [10,19]. Cases of 'skip' metastases to the lateral compartment without central compartment involvement are rare, but do occur. The reported frequency of skip metastases in PTC is 11.1–37.5% [20–22]. Involvement of the suprahyoid region, namely the submental and submandibular nodes, is rare [23]. The incidence of lymph node metastases is higher in young patients, with clinical involvement of 50–80% in children compared with about 15% in older patients. Only 20% of patients have isolated central lymph node metastases, while 67% have metastases in both central and lateral compartments [24]. The rate of mediastinal lymph node involvement has been reported to range between 6% and 12% [25]. It is important to note that only 10–15% of patients with micrometastases from PTC will develop macroscopic evidence of the disease [26].

The incidence of lymph node metastases in follicular thyroid cancer is 20–25% in the American population. Distant metastasis rates are reported to be 7–12% [27,28]. Patients with lymph node metastasis have higher rates of persistent and recurrent disease during postoperative surveillance [10]. However, the impact of lymph node metastasis on overall survival remains debatable [29]. Several studies have demonstrated no difference in mortality, while two large population-based studies have shown increased mortality in patients with regional lymph node metastasis [30,31].

Detection of lymph node metastasis

The first step in the management of a patient with suspected thyroid cancer is to perform a detailed examination of the thyroid that should include the cervical lymph node compartments. The classification system of cervical lymph node compartments is well defined and is important not only in identifying the location of pathological lymph nodes but also in providing an anatomical roadmap for surgical treatment, as outlined in the recent ATA guidelines for management of thyroid cancer [5,32]. The lymph node compartments of the neck are divided into six levels, each bounded by distinct anatomical borders. In particular, level VI contains the thyroid gland and lies in a central position in the neck. Its superior border is the hyoid bone, the inferior border is the suprasternal notch, and the lateral borders are the common carotid arteries. Level VI lymph nodes include pretracheal and paratracheal nodes, the precricoid (Delphian) node and the perithyroidal nodes, including nodes along the recurrent laryngeal nerves. Nodes in level VI correspond to those in the central neck compartment (Figure 8.1).

Patients with PTC occasionally present on initial assessment with cervical lymphadenopathy, which is most often located in the central neck compartment or levels III and IV of the lateral neck, usually in conjunction with an ipsilateral thyroid nodule. Cervical ultrasound (US) is often the initial imaging modality employed in the assessment since it is readily accessible, inexpensive and non-invasive. It is also an important tool for postoperative surveillance of patients with papillary thyroid cancer [5]. High-resolution ultrasonography can detect cervical nodal metastasis in up to 20% of patients with PTC, including those as small as 2–3 mm. These US findings may alter the planned surgical procedure in up to 39% of thyroid cancer patients [7,33]. Pathological lymph nodes have sonographic features that include round shape, absent hilus, calcification, intranodal necrosis, reticulation, matting, soft tissue oedema and peripheral vascularity. However, many nodal metastases demonstrate a wide variety of non-diagnostic features (Figure 8.2a) [34]. A dedicated cervical ultrasound to include nodal levels II–VI should be performed, ideally by a dedicated clinician such as the thyroid endocrinologist, the operating surgeon, or a radiologist with particular interest, to detect non-palpable lymph node metastases in patients undergoing surgical evaluation for any thyroid nodule. However, US can miss as many as 50% of the involved lymph nodes in the central neck

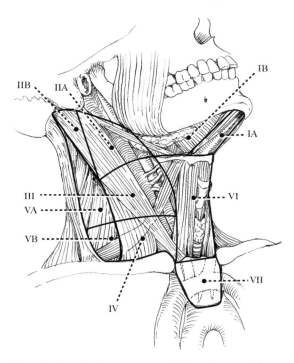

Figure 8.1 Lymph node compartments of the neck separated into levels and sublevels. Level VI and VII are included in central neck dissection, while lateral neck dissection typically includes levels II–V for treatment of papillary thyroid cancer.

because the overlying thyroid gland hinders adequate visualization [35].

Pathological lymph node metastasis detected on ultrasound may be confirmed with ultrasound-guided fine needle aspiration (FNA) [5]. The measurement of thyroglobulin (Tg) in the needle washout will confirm thyroid origin (100% sensitivity, 96.2% specificity and 100% negative predictive value) [36]. In patients with suspected mediastinal disease or with bulky cervical lymphadenopathy, cross-sectional imaging with computed tomography (CT), magnetic resonance imaging (MRI) and positron emission tomography (PET) should be considered as it can aid in the planning of neck dissection and often identifies pathological level VI and VII lymph nodes within the superior mediastinum that are not detected on cervical ultrasound or physical examination (Figure 8.3). However, the sensitivities of CT, MRI and PET for the detection of cervical lymph node metastases are relatively low (30–40%) [37,38].

A CT with iodinated contrast is considered extremely helpful in evaluating the extent of cervical and retro-oesophageal lymphadenopathy, as it can help define the extent of surgery necessary to clear all gross disease in the neck. Controversy that it can delay postoperative thyroid scanning for 4–8 weeks and can cause a subclinically hyperthyroid patient to enter thyroid storm suggests that it should be avoided [39]. However, in locally aggressive cases, the benefit of accurate surgical planning outweighs the delay in radioiodine (RAI) administration that is necessary after the use of iodinated contrast.

(a)

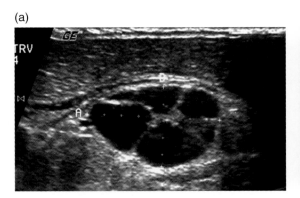

(b)

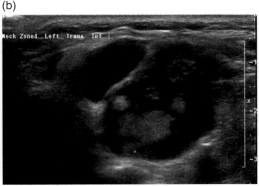

Figure 8.2 (a) Ultrasonographic appearance of a level III lymph node with papillary thyroid cancer metastasis using a 12.5 MHz linear transducer. Note the round shape, calcifications, intranodal necrosis, reticulation and lack of the normal hyperechoic hilar line.

(b) Ultrasonographic transverse appearance of a level IV lymph node with papillary thyroid cancer tall cell variant metastasis using a 12.5 MHz linear transducer. Note the atypical appearance and lack of the normal hyperechoic hilar line.

(a)

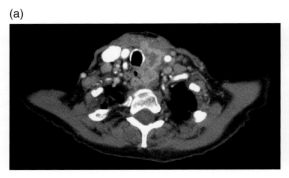

(b)

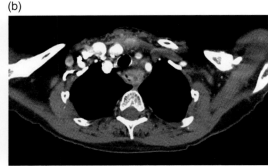

Figure 8.3 (a) Computed tomography of neck with contrast (axial). Imaging reveals a heterogeneous enhancing mass of the left neck that displaces the trachea to the right. (b) Computed tomography of chest with contrast (axial). The mass extends substernally and appears bilobed, with the posterior segment compressing the oesophagus at this level, and the anterior segment invading anteriorly to the trachea.

Operative considerations for central neck dissection

A therapeutic compartment-oriented neck dissection implies that lymph node metastases are clinically apparent (preoperative or intraoperative) or detected by imaging studies (clinically N1a). A prophylactic or elective compartment-oriented dissection implies that lymph node metastases are not detected clinically or by imaging (clinically N0). Lymph node 'berry picking' implies removal of only the clinically involved nodes rather than a complete nodal group within the compartment and is not synonymous with a selective compartment-oriented dissection [32]. There is general agreement that therapeutic node dissection should be performed in patients with PTC who have clinically involved nodes, and it should include a systemic or *en bloc* neck dissection. Isolated removal of only grossly involved lymph nodes violates the nodal compartment and may be associated with higher recurrence rates and morbidity from reoperative surgery [5]. Although cervical lymph node metastases are rare in patients with FTC, patients with the Hurthle cell variant may have nodal disease, which predicts a worse outcome, and should have a therapeutic neck dissection if metastatic lymph nodes are identified [12].

The ATA consensus statement on CND [32] emphasizes that it is important to define the terminology used to classify the procedure. It defines the central compartment neck dissection as all perithyroidal and paratracheal soft tissue and lymph nodes with borders extending superiorly to the hyoid bone, inferiorly to the innominate artery, and laterally to the common carotid arteries. The goal of defining the terminology and classification scheme for CND is to allow investigators to communicate without ambiguity and compare the efficacy of these interventions. For the first time, this consensus statement defines the extent of CND as unilateral or bilateral. Bilateral CND is preferred as the initial management of clinically involved central nodes with therapeutic intention. Nonetheless, operative reports should clearly describe the extent (unilateral versus bilateral) and the intent (elective versus therapeutic) of CND. Lack of standardized reporting has been partially responsible for the debate regarding the role of elective or prophylactic CND in PTC [29]. The inclusion of the level VII nodes in the superior mediastinum with the CND should be noted as this is often a site of persistent disease following central neck dissection [40].

The indications for lateral neck dissection are much clearer. Lateral neck dissection for PTC should be performed in a compartment-oriented manner when there is clinical or cytopathological evidence of PTC in a lateral neck lymph node (levels II–V) [5]. A bilateral CND may be included with the modified radical neck dissection to remove the presumed central neck lymph node disease based on described patterns of nodal spread [41].

Therapeutic central neck dissection

Therapeutic central neck dissection should be performed in patients with pathological lymph node involvement noted on preoperative clinical or imaging assessment [5]. The goal of removing these lymph nodes is to aid in local control, prevent recurrences and, perhaps, improve survival. Despite earlier reports of no adverse effects on survival, emerging evidence from large population-based studies demonstrates an increase in mortality with regional lymph node metastases [30,31]. Careful inspection of the central compartment lymph nodes with both physical exam and US evaluation is crucial during the preoperative assessment. The presence of pathological lymph nodes in the central compartment should also prompt a detailed comprehensive US examination of the lateral compartment for additional evidence of metastasis. Confirmation of malignancy in lymph nodes with a suspicious sonographic appearance is achieved by US-guided FNA for cytology and/or measurement of Tg in the needle washout [5]. The therapeutic lymph node dissection should include a systemic or *en bloc* neck dissection of both the ipsilateral and contralateral central compartments. However, there is controversy regarding whether the extent of central dissection needs to be ipsilateral to the thyroid tumour alone or bilateral [42,43]. Moo *et al.* [44] compared ipsilateral versus bilateral CND for PTC and concluded that an ipsilateral dissection was sufficient in tumours less than 1 cm, while larger tumours required bilateral CND based on the high incidence of contralateral central neck disease in a retrospective analysis of the pattern of nodal metastases in surgical specimens. If malignancy is present in any of the lateral neck nodes, the dissection should be extended to include an ipsilateral modified radical neck dissection to include levels II–V [45,46]. In patients undergoing thyroidectomy and lymphadenectomy for PTC, positive lateral neck lymph nodes and extensive dissection are predictive of poorer overall survival [47]. In patients with known distant metastatic disease, the debulking of cervical disease for palliative purposes is beneficial in preventing local complications [40].

The management in patients with medullary thyroid cancer (MTC) deserves special mention. MTC is a more aggressive tumour with a high incidence of lymph node metastasis and there is no role for radioiodine treatment in this type of disease [48]. Approximately 50% of patients present with lymph node metastasis, either in the jugular chain or in the lateral neck [49,50]. Patients with MTC can only be cured by surgical intervention, which at least consists of a total thyroidectomy with meticulous CND.

The adequacy of surgical resection can be assessed by stimulated calcitonin level postoperatively. If lymph node metastases are clinically apparent in the lateral neck, a modified radical neck dissection is performed to include the lymph nodes in levels II–V. Removal of all the tissues with MTC helps in long-term survival [51,52].

Prophylactic central neck dissection (see Video 8.1)

The role of prophylactic CND remains a contentious issue regarding its benefits and risks [14,53,54]. The ATA guidelines suggest that prophylactic CND may be performed for advanced primary tumours (>4 cm and/or with extrathyroidal invasion) but is not necessary for small, non-invasive papillary and most follicular thyroid cancers [5]. An essential component of any discussion on the extent of lymphadenectomy is whether patients derive any additional benefit from having a lymphadenectomy with total thyroidectomy and whether this can be done without significantly increasing the morbidity of the operation. Because microscopic nodal disease is rarely of clinical importance and subsequent radioiodine administration can ablate these occult foci, many authors argue that prophylactic CND of microscopic lymph node metastases that are not clinically identifiable at the time of surgery may not improve long-term outcome and could subject patients to more risk than benefit [55–57]. Also, if removal of subclinical metastases alone were an indication for surgery without an appreciation for the clinical significance of this disease, which certainly is debatable, then the same should theoretically apply to the lateral neck. Opponents also fear that if prophylactic CND were universally adopted by all surgeons performing thyroidectomy, the risk of parathyroid and nerve injury may increase in the absence of significant oncological benefit to the patients [53,57,58]. However, the precise role of prophylactic CND for well-differentiated thyroid cancer remains controversial because in experienced hands, this procedure can be done with minimal additional risk [13] and some studies have suggested a survival benefit in selected patients [14,15].

Proponents of prophylactic CND argue that the incidence of central neck metastases is high and the sensitivity of preoperative US in detecting pathological lymph nodes in PTC patients is higher in the lateral neck (94%)

than in the central neck compartments (53–55%) [59]. Furthermore, CND advocates argue that clearing the central neck at the initial operation removes potential sources of recurrence, increases the accuracy of staging for radioactive iodine ablation, permits accurate long-term surveillance, and avoids the potential morbidity of a reoperation [7,31,60–63]. An additional benefit of reduced postoperative Tg levels after CND was also cited [64]. Some authors have suggested that prophylactic CND be considered in patients with thyroid cancer harboring the BRAF mutation, since they have the potential to be more clinically aggressive and less responsive to RAI therapy [65]. However, additional studies are needed to demonstrate the clinical benefit of this approach. Selective neck dissection to include both the central neck and the ipsilateral neck has been recommended as necessary therapy in patients with known distant metastasis without evidence of cervical lymph node involvement, due to the high rates of nodal involvement in this subset of patients on histological examination [66].

Further large randomized studies with long-term follow-up are necessary to better define the role of prophylactic node dissection in the initial treatment of differentiated thyroid carcinoma and to establish better diagnostic modalities to identify the specific subsets of patients in whom prophylactic node dissection may have positive effects on long-term survival rates.

Reoperative surgery for persistent/recurrent disease

Regardless of the initial treatment paradigm utilized for thyroid cancer, some patients will manifest persistent or recurrent disease. Much of the persistent/recurrent disease today is detected subclinically by surveillance strategies advocated by the ATA guidelines [5,43]. High-resolution US and serum Tg assays with or without thyrotropin stimulation have lead to a new category of patients with persistent/recurrent small volume disease of uncertain clinical significance. It is also important to closely evaluate patients for the presence of additional pathological lymphadenopathy in the lateral neck and superior mediastinum, and combining cervical US and cross-sectional imaging with CT, MRI and PET scans can help to guide operative planning and to determine the necessary extent of neck dissection.

Many authors have demonstrated that reoperative surgery for this disease, especially in the central compartment, is safe [46,67,68]. We described recently a personalized approach tailoring reoperative surgery for persistent/recurrent PTC [29]. Definitions of microscopic and macroscopic nodal recurrences should help to determine which groups of patients could be observed versus those that should be offered surgery. Reasonable and realistic expectations should be set for the practitioners and patients involved. When possible, compartmental dissection of the neck nodal region involved should be performed to reduce the risk of locoregional recurrence and the morbidity of further reoperation (Figure 8.4). Many of these patients with persistent disease have undergone multiple surgeries in the central or lateral compartments. Further attempts at formal compartmental dissection must be met with a careful weighing of the risks and benefits to the patient. Perhaps the realistic goal of all reoperative surgery should not be to render the serum thyroglobulin level undetectable but rather to prevent local disease progression in critical areas of the neck. Long-term follow-up of these patients is warranted to determine the optimal surveillance and treatment paradigm.

Preoperative laryngoscopy should be performed before all reoperative procedures to determine the presence of recurrent laryngeal nerve (RLN) injury, which can help outline the approach to reoperative nodal dissection while minimizing the medicolegal ramifications of iatrogenic RLN injury [69,70]. Intraoperative RLN identification and dissection significantly reduce the risk of its injury and are superior to limited nerve exposure [46]. Recognition of the extralaryngeal branching of the RLN is also crucial during the operation. The motor fibres of RLN are located in the anterior branch while the posterior branch is only sensory in function. Therefore, great caution is required after the presumed identification of the RLN to ensure there is no unidentified anterior branch, which may lead to increased risk of postoperative nerve injury (Figure 8.5) [71]. The surgeon can expect to encounter difficulty in identifying and preserving the RLNs due to the fibrotic tissue that distorts the anatomy of the central neck area. Given the challenging nature of reoperative neck dissection, consideration of recurrent laryngeal nerve monitoring and special care to preserve the parathyroid vasculature are important.

(a) (b)

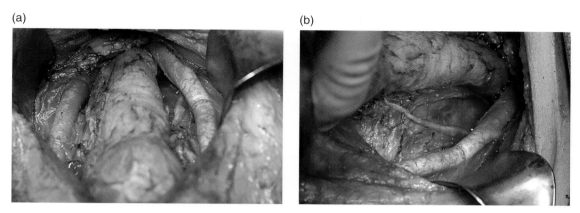

Figure 8.4 (a) Reoperative bilateral central compartment dissection of the neck nodal region. (b) Reoperative right central compartment dissection of the neck nodal region. The recurrent laryngeal nerve was dissected and preserved.

(a) (b)

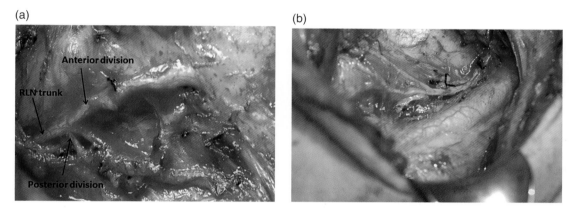

Figure 8.5 (a) Bifurcated recurrent laryngeal nerve (RLN) before entry into the larynx into anterior and posterior division. (b) Right RLN bifurcation into anterior and posterior division.

Complications

The most common complication associated with CND is hypoparathyroidism. Temporary hypoparathyroidism following CND occurs in 14–40% of cases [64,72–77]. This wide range of incidence can be partially attributed to the different normal reference levels and the definition of hypoparathyroidism. The high incidence of temporary hypoparathyroidism is likely due to the increased incidence of parathyroid reimplantation and inadvertent inclusion of parathyroid glands in the nodal dissection [40]. Though reports are mixed regarding the incidence of permanent hypoparathyroidism, a meta-analysis performed by Chisholm *et al.* [15] reported a 1.2% incidence as defined by the requirement for calcium

supplementation surpassing the 6–12 months period postoperatively. Other complications include injury to the recurrent laryngeal nerve or the external branch of the superior laryngeal nerve, which occurs in 1–2% of patients [64,72,73,78,79]. However, in experienced hands the addition of CND to total thyroidectomy for the treatment of thyroid cancer has not increased the nerve injury rates [64,72,73,80]. Therefore, the recent ATA recommendations for therapeutic or prophylactic CND should be interpreted in the light of available surgical expertise. Although this may increase the chance of future locoregional recurrence, overall this approach may be safer in less experienced surgical hands [5]. Sosa *et al.* [81] found that high-volume surgeons (defined as doing >100 cases = 5 years) had 75% fewer complications related to thyroid surgery than low-volume surgeons (4.3% versus 16.1%). However, there are no similar comparative studies done for outcomes related to CND. In cases of reoperative CND after either previous thyroidectomy or CND, reports have noted increased nerve injury rates up to 12% [78,79,82–84].

Conclusion

Central neck dissection for extensive thyroid cancer is a safe and effective procedure with low complication rates when performed by experienced surgeons. Therapeutic CND is recommended for all patients with clinically evident lymph node involvement. The precise role of prophylactic CND remains controversial; we suggest not performing prophylactic CND except in patients with large primary tumours. Functional compartmental *en bloc* neck dissection is favoured over 'berry picking'. Reoperative neck dissection for persistent/recurrent disease demands careful weighing of the risks and benefits to the patient due to the challenging nature of this procedure and increased risk of complications in the hands of inexperienced surgeons.

Disclosure

Conflict of interest: none. This research and work was fully supported by Tulane University and Tulane University Hospital. The authors have no financial interests in companies or other entities that have an interest in the information included in this chapter.

References

1 Siegel R, Ward E, Brawley O, Jemal A. Cancer statistics, 2011. The impact of eliminating socioeconomic and racial disparities on premature cancer deaths. CA Cancer J Clin 2011; 61(4): 212–36.

2 Boring CC, Squires TS, Tong T, Montgomery S. Cancer statistics, 1994. CA Cancer J Clin 1994; 44(1): 7–26.

3 Mazzaferri EL, Young RL. Papillary thyroid carcinoma: a 10 year follow-up report of the impact of therapy in 576 patients. Am J Med 1981; 70(3): 511–18.

4 Mazzaferri EL, Young RL, Oertel JE, Kemmerer WT, Page CP. Papillary thyroid carcinoma: the impact of therapy in 576 patients. Medicine (Baltimore) 1977; 56(3): 171–96.

5 Cooper DS, Doherty GM, Haugen BR, *et al.* Revised American Thyroid Association management guidelines for patients with thyroid nodules and differentiated thyroid cancer. Thyroid 2009; 19(11): 1167–214.

6 Grebe SK, Hay ID. Thyroid cancer nodal metastases: biologic significance and therapeutic considerations. Surg Oncol Clin North Am 1996; 5(1): 43–63.

7 Kouvaraki MA, Shapiro SE, Fornage BD, *et al.* Role of preoperative ultrasonography in the surgical management of patients with thyroid cancer. Surgery 2003; 134(6): 946–54; discussion 954–5.

8 Sivanandan R, Soo KC. Pattern of cervical lymph node metastases from papillary carcinoma of the thyroid. Br J Surg 2001; 88(9): 1241–4.

9 Kupferman ME, Patterson M, Mandel SJ, LiVolsi V, Weber RS. Patterns of lateral neck metastasis in papillary thyroid carcinoma. Arch Otolaryngol Head Neck Surg 2004; 130(7): 857–60.

10 Machens A, Hinze R, Thomusch O, Dralle H. Pattern of nodal metastasis for primary and reoperative thyroid cancer. World J Surg 2002; 26(1): 22–8.

11 Hamming JF, Roukema JA. Management of regional lymph nodes in papillary, follicular, and medullary thyroid cancer. In: Clark OH, Duh QY, Kebebew E (eds) Textbook of Endocrine Surgery, 2ndedn . Philadelphia: Saunders, 2005: 195–206.

12 Stojadinovic A, Ghossein RA, Hoos A, *et al.* Hurthle cell carcinoma: a critical histopathologic appraisal. J Clin Oncol 2001; 19(10): 2616–25.

13 Shindo M, Stern A. Total thyroidectomy with and without selective central compartment dissection: a comparison of complication rates. Arch Otolaryngol Head Neck Surg 2010; 136(6): 584–7.

14 White ML, Gauger PG, Doherty GM. Central lymph node dissection in differentiated thyroid cancer. World J Surg 2007; 31(5): 895–904.

15 Chisholm EJ, Kulinskaya E, Tolley NS. Systematic review and meta-analysis of the adverse effects of thyroidectomy combined with central neck dissection as compared with thyroidectomy alone. Laryngoscope 2009; 119(6): 1135–9.

16 Sippel RS, Chen H. Controversies in the surgical management of newly diagnosed and recurrent/residual thyroid cancer. Thyroid 2009; 19(12): 1373–80.

17 Cooper DS, Doherty GM, Haugen BR, *et al.* Management guidelines for patients with thyroid nodules and differentiated thyroid cancer. Thyroid 2006; 16(2): 109–42.

18 Arturi F, Russo D, Giuffrida D, *et al.* Early diagnosis by genetic analysis of differentiated thyroid cancer metastases in small lymph nodes. J Clin Endocrinol Metab 1997; 82(5): 1638–41.

19 Gimm O, Rath FW, Dralle H. Pattern of lymph node metastases in papillary thyroid carcinoma. Br J Surg 1998; 85(2): 252–4.

20 Machens A, Holzhausen HJ, Dralle H. Skip metastases in thyroid cancer leaping the central lymph node compartment. Arch Surg 2004; 139(1): 43–5.

21 Coatesworth AP, MacLennan K. Cervical metastasis in papillary carcinoma of the thyroid: a histopathological study. Int J Clin Pract 2002; 56(4): 241–2.

22 Ducci M, Appetecchia M, Marzetti M. Neck dissection for surgical treatment of lymphnode metastasis in papillary thyroid carcinoma. J Exp Clin Cancer Res 1997; 16(3): 333–5.

23 Gauger PG. Thyroid gland. In: Mulholland MW, Lillemoe KD, Doherty GM, et al. (eds) Greenfield's Surgery: Scientific Principles and Practice, 4th edn. Philadelphia: Lippincott Williams and Wilkins, 2006: 1289–309.

24 Noguchi M, Katev N, Miyazaki I. Controversies in the surgical management of differentiated thyroid carcinoma. Int Surg 1996; 81(2): 163–7.

25 Coburn MC, Wanebo HJ. Prognostic factors and management considerations in patients with cervical metastases of thyroid cancer. Am J Surg 1992; 164(6): 671–6.

26 Clark OH. Predictors of thyroid tumor aggressiveness. West J Med 1996; 165(3): 131–8.

27 Gilliland FD, Hunt WC, Morris DM, Key CR. Prognostic factors for thyroid carcinoma. A population-based study of 15,698 cases from the Surveillance, Epidemiology and End Results (SEER) program 1973–1991. Cancer 1997; 79(3): 564–73.

28 Mazzaferri EL, Jhiang SM. Long-term impact of initial surgical and medical therapy on papillary and follicular thyroid cancer. Am J Med 1994; 97(5): 418–28.

29 Tufano RP, Kandil E. Considerations for personalized surgery in patients with papillary thyroid cancer. Thyroid 2010; 20(7): 771–6.

30 Lundgren CI, Hall P, Dickman PW, Zedenius J. Clinically significant prognostic factors for differentiated thyroid carcinoma: a population-based, nested case–control study. Cancer 2006; 106(3): 524–31.

31 Tisell LE, Nilsson B, Molne J, et al. Improved survival of patients with papillary thyroid cancer after surgical microdissection. World J Surg 1996; 20(7): 854–9.

32 Carty SE, Cooper DS, Doherty GM, et al. Consensus statement on the terminology and classification of central neck dissection for thyroid cancer. Thyroid 2009; 19(11): 1153–8.

33 Stulak JM, Grant CS, Farley DR, et al. Value of preoperative ultrasonography in the surgical management of initial and reoperative papillary thyroid cancer. Arch Surg 2006; 141(5): 489–94; discussion 494–6.

34 Ahuja AT, Ying M. Sonographic evaluation of cervical lymph nodes. AJR 2005; 184(5): 1691–9.

35 Leboulleux S, Girard E, Rose M, et al. Ultrasound criteria of malignancy for cervical lymph nodes in patients followed up for differentiated thyroid cancer. J Clin Endocrinol Metab 2007; 92(9): 3590–4.

36 Snozek CL, Chambers EP, Reading CC, et al. Serum thyroglobulin, high-resolution ultrasound, and lymph node thyroglobulin in diagnosis of differentiated thyroid carcinoma nodal metastases. J Clin Endocrinol Metab 2007; 92(11): 4278–81.

37 Kresnik E, Gallowitsch HJ, Mikosch P, et al. Fluorine-18-fluorodeoxyglucose positron emission tomography in the preoperative assessment of thyroid nodules in an endemic goiter area. Surgery 2003; 133(3): 294–9.

38 Zbaren P, Becker M, Lang H. Pretherapeutic staging of hypopharyngeal carcinoma. Clinical findings, computed tomography, and magnetic resonance imaging compared with histopathologic evaluation. Arch Otolaryngol Head Neck Surg 1997; 123(9): 908–13.

39 Kim N, Lavertu P. Evaluation of a thyroid nodule. Otolaryngol Clin North Am 2003; 36(1): 17–33.

40 Hughes DT, Doherty GM. Central neck dissection for papillary thyroid cancer. Cancer Control 2011; 18(2): 83–8.

41 Roh JL, Park JY, Rha KS, Park CI. Is central neck dissection necessary for the treatment of lateral cervical nodal recurrence of papillary thyroid carcinoma? Head Neck. 2007; 29(10): 901–6.

42 Koo BS, Choi EC, Yoon YH, Kim DH, Kim EH, Lim YC. Predictive factors for ipsilateral or contralateral central lymph node metastasis in unilateral papillary thyroid carcinoma. Ann Surg 2009; 249(5): 840–4.

43 Son YI, Jeong HS, Baek CH, et al. Extent of prophylactic lymph node dissection in the central neck area of the patients with papillary thyroid carcinoma: comparison of limited versus comprehensive lymph node dissection in a 2-year safety study. Ann Surg Oncol 2008; 15(7): 2020–6.

44 Moo TA, Umunna B, Kato M, et al. Ipsilateral versus bilateral central neck lymph node dissection in papillary thyroid carcinoma. Ann Surg 2009; 250(3): 403–8.

45 Wada N, Duh QY, Sugino K, et al. Lymph node metastasis from 259 papillary thyroid microcarcinomas: frequency, pattern of occurrence and recurrence, and optimal strategy for neck dissection. Ann Surg 2003; 237(3): 399–407.

46 Farrag TY, Agrawal N, Sheth S, et al. Algorithm for safe and effective reoperative thyroid bed surgery for recurrent/persistent papillary thyroid carcinoma. Head Neck 2007; 29(12): 1069–74.

47 Kandil E, Friedlander P, Noureldine S, Islam T, Tufano RP. Impact of extensive neck dissection on survival from papillary thyroid cancer. ORL J Otorhinolaryngol Relat Spec 2011; 73(6): 330–5.

48 Quayle FJ, Moley JF. Medullary thyroid carcinoma: including MEN 2A and MEN 2B syndromes. J Surg Oncol 2005; 89(3): 122–9.

49 Ellenhorn JD, Shah JP, Brennan MF. Impact of therapeutic regional lymph node dissection for medullary carcinoma of

the thyroid gland. Surgery 1993; 114(6): 1078–81; discussion 1081–2.

50 Tisell LE, Hansson G, Jansson S, Salander H. Reoperation in the treatment of asymptomatic metastasizing medullary thyroid carcinoma. Surgery 1986; 99(1): 60–6.

51 You YN, Lakhani V, Wells SA Jr, Moley JF. Medullary thyroid cancer. Surg Oncol Clin North Am 2006; 15(3):639–60.

52 Kloos RT, Eng C, Evans DB, et al. Medullary thyroid cancer: management guidelines of the American Thyroid Association. Thyroid 2009; 19(6): 565–612.

53 Mazzaferri EL, Doherty GM, Steward DL. The pros and cons of prophylactic central compartment lymph node dissection for papillary thyroid carcinoma. Thyroid 2009; 19(7): 683–9.

54 Mazzaferri EL. What is the optimal initial treatment of low-risk papillary thyroid cancer (and why is it controversial)? Oncology (Williston Park) 2009; 23(7): 579–88.

55 Zetoune T, Keutgen X, Buitrago D, et al. Prophylactic central neck dissection and local recurrence in papillary thyroid cancer: a meta-analysis. Ann Surg Oncol 2010; 17(12): 3287–93.

56 Tuttle RM, Fagin JA. Can risk-adapted treatment recommendations replace the 'one size fits all' approach for early-stage thyroid cancer patients? Oncology (Williston Park) 2009; 23(7): 592, 600, 3.

57 Scheumann GF, Gimm O, Wegener G, Hundeshagen H, Dralle H. Prognostic significance and surgical management of locoregional lymph node metastases in papillary thyroid cancer. World J Surg 1994; 18(4): 559–67; discussion 567–8.

58 Sawka AM, Brierley JD, Tsang RW, et al. An updated systematic review and commentary examining the effectiveness of radioactive iodine remnant ablation in well-differentiated thyroid cancer. Endocrinol Metab Clin North Am 2008; 37(2): 457–80, x.

59 Ahn JE, Lee JH, Yi JS, et al. Diagnostic accuracy of CT and ultrasonography for evaluating metastatic cervical lymph nodes in patients with thyroid cancer. World J Surg 2008; 32(7): 1552–8.

60 Ito Y, Tomoda C, Uruno T, et al. Clinical significance of metastasis to the central compartment from papillary microcarcinoma of the thyroid. World J Surg 2006; 30(1): 91–9.

61 Moley JF, DeBenedetti MK. Patterns of nodal metastases in palpable medullary thyroid carcinoma: recommendations for extent of node dissection. Ann Surg 1999; 229(6): 880–7; discussion 887–8.

62 Bonnet S, Hartl D, Leboulleux S, et al. Prophylactic lymph node dissection for papillary thyroid cancer less than 2 cm: implications for radioiodine treatment. J Clin Endocrinol Metab 2009; 94(4): 1162–7.

63 Hughes DT, White ML, Miller BS, Gauger PG, Burney RE, Doherty GM. Influence of prophylactic central lymph node dissection on postoperative thyroglobulin levels and radioio-dine treatment in papillary thyroid cancer. Surgery 2010; 148(6): 1100–6; discussion 1006–7.

64 Sywak M, Cornford L, Roach P, Stalberg P, Sidhu S, Delbridge L. Routine ipsilateral level VI lymphadenectomy reduces postoperative thyroglobulin levels in papillary thyroid cancer. Surgery 2006; 140(6):1000–5; discussion 1005–7.

65 Mekel M, Nucera C, Hodin RA, Parangi S. Surgical implications of B-RafV600E mutation in fine-needle aspiration of thyroid nodules. Am J Surg 2010; 200(1): 136–43.

66 Sugitani I, Fujimoto Y, Yamada K, Yamamoto N. Prospective outcomes of selective lymph node dissection for papillary thyroid carcinoma based on preoperative ultrasonography. World J Surg 2008; 32(11): 2494–502.

67 Schuff KG, Weber SM, Givi B, Samuels MH, Andersen PE, Cohen JI. Efficacy of nodal dissection for treatment of persistent/recurrent papillary thyroid cancer. Laryngoscope 2008; 118(5): 768–75.

68 Clayman GL, Shellenberger TD, Ginsberg LE, et al. Approach and safety of comprehensive central compartment dissection in patients with recurrent papillary thyroid carcinoma. Head Neck 2009; 31(9): 1152–63.

69 Farrag TY, Samlan RA, Lin FR, Tufano RP. The utility of evaluating true vocal fold motion before thyroid surgery. Laryngoscope 2006: 116(2): 235–8.

70 Randolph GW. The importance of pre- and postoperative laryngeal examination for thyroid surgery. Thyroid 2010; 20(5): 453–8.

71 Kandil E, Abdel Khalek M, Aslam R, Friedlander P, Bellows CF, Slakey D. Recurrent laryngeal nerve: significance of the anterior extralaryngeal branch. Surgery 2011; 149(6): 820–4.

72 Palestini N, Borasi A, Cestino L, Freddi M, Odasso C, Robecchi A. Is central neck dissection a safe procedure in the treatment of papillary thyroid cancer? Our experience. Langenbecks Arch Surg 2008; 393(5): 693–8.

73 Henry JF, Gramatica L, Denizot A, Kvachenyuk A, Puccini M, Defechereux T. Morbidity of prophylactic lymph node dissection in the central neck area in patients with papillary thyroid carcinoma. Langenbecks Arch Surg 1998; 383(2): 167–9.

74 Roh JL, Park JY, Park CI. Total thyroidectomy plus neck dissection in differentiated papillary thyroid carcinoma patients: pattern of nodal metastasis, morbidity, recurrence, and postoperative levels of serum parathyroid hormone. Ann Surg 2007; 245(4): 604–10.

75 Steinmuller T, Klupp J, Wenking S, Neuhaus P. Complications associated with different surgical approaches to differentiated thyroid carcinoma. Langenbecks Arch Surg 1999; 384(1): 50–3.

76 Pereira JA, Jimeno J, Miquel J, et al. Nodal yield, morbidity, and recurrence after central neck dissection for papillary

thyroid carcinoma. Surgery 2005; 138(6): 1095–100, discussion 1100–1.

77 Gemsenjager E, Perren A, Seifert B, Schuler G, Schweizer I, Heitz PU. Lymph node surgery in papillary thyroid carcinoma. J Am Coll Surg 2003; 197(2): 182–90.

78 Kim MK, Mandel SH, Baloch Z, et al. Morbidity following central compartment reoperation for recurrent or persistent thyroid cancer. Arch Otolaryngol Head Neck Surg 2004; 130(10): 1214–16.

79 Moley JF, Lairmore TC, Doherty GM, Brunt LM, DeBenedetti MK. Preservation of the recurrent laryngeal nerves in thyroid and parathyroid reoperations. Surgery 1999; 126(4): 673–7; discussion 677–9.

80 Roh JL, Park JY, Park CI. Prevention of postoperative hypocalcemia with routine oral calcium and vitamin D supplements in patients with differentiated papillary thyroid carcinoma undergoing total thyroidectomy plus central neck dissection. Cancer 2009; 115(2): 251–8.

81 Sosa JA, Bowman HM, Tielsch JM, Powe NR, Gordon TA, Udelsman R. The importance of surgeon experience for clinical and economic outcomes from thyroidectomy. Ann Surg 1998; 228(3): 320–30.

82 Uruno T, Miyauchi A, Shimizu K, et al. Prognosis after reoperation for local recurrence of papillary thyroid carcinoma. Surg Today 2004; 34(11): 891–5.

83 Simon D, Goretzki PE, Witte J, Roher HD. Incidence of regional recurrence guiding radicality in differentiated thyroid carcinoma. World J Surg 1996; 20(7): 860–6; discussion 866.

84 Segal K, Friedental R, Lubin E, Shvero J, Sulkes J, Feinmesser R. Papillary carcinoma of the thyroid. Otolaryngol Head Neck Surg 1995; 113(4): 356–63.

Videoclip

This chapter contains the following videoclip. They can be accessed at: www.wiley.com/go/miccoli/thyroid

Video 8.1   Video-assisted central neck dissection. A thorough prophylactic central neck dissection can be performed with a minimally invasive approach (MIVAT).

CHAPTER 9

Extensive Surgery for Thyroid Cancer: Lateral Neck Dissection

Dana M. Hartl,[1] Haïtham Mirghani[1] and Daniel F. Brasnu[2]

[1]Department of Head and Neck Oncology, Institut Gustave Roussy, Villejuif, France

[2]Department of Otolaryngology Head Neck Surgery, University of Paris René Descartes and Georges Pompidou European Hospital, Paris, France

Introduction

Today, surgery remains the only treatment with curative intent for macroscopic lateral neck node metastases for differentiated and medullary thyroid cancer. With experience, lateral neck dissection can be routinely performed safely and effectively. Lateral neck dissection can mean many things, but the precise and currently accepted terminology should be understood and routinely employed. For thyroid cancer, therapeutic lateral neck dissection in the presence of known or suspected metastatic nodes is currently recommended, but prophylactic lateral neck dissection remains controversial for differentiated thyroid cancer and for some cases of medullary thyroid cancer. This chapter aims at clearly defining the different types of lateral neck dissections employed for thyroid cancer and their anatomical limits, indications and potential complications, with tips for rarer but typical locations to explore for 'hidden lymph nodes' and means to minimize morbidity.

Definitions

Historically, the first lateral neck dissections performed at the end of the 19th and beginning of the 20th centuries were *en bloc* resections of metastatic lateral neck nodes along with removal of the sternomastoid muscle, the spinal accessory nerve, the internal jugular vein and the submandibular gland [1]. In the 1950s, efficient and oncologically sound resection of metastatic nodes with preservation of these non-lymphatic structures was described, decreasing morbidity. Then in the 1960s, more limited neck dissections were described and prophylactic or elective lateral neck dissection, targeted at the groups of lymph nodes most likely to be diseased for a given tumour, became routine.

Compared to the earliest neck dissections or 'radical neck dissections' with removal of the sternomastoid muscle, the spinal accessory nerve and the internal jugular vein, the more limited dissections – 'functional', 'limited' or 'conservative' – are currently termed 'modified radical neck dissections', sparing one or more of the non-lymphatic structures [2,3]. The even more limited neck dissections are termed 'selective neck dissections'.

For more limited dissections, the neck nodes have been divided into groups or levels. Their designation by Roman numerals and letters by the American Head and Neck Society and the American Academy of Otolaryngology-Head and Neck Surgery (AAOHNS) is currently the most widely accepted nomenclature [1,4]. A neck dissection performed to remove known or highly suspected metastatic nodes is termed a 'therapeutic' neck dissection. That performed in the absence of known metastatic nodes is termed 'elective' or 'prophylactic' neck dissection [5].

Thyroid Surgery: Preventing and Managing Complications, First Edition. Edited by Paolo Miccoli, David J. Terris, Michele N. Minuto and Melanie W. Seybt.

© 2013 John Wiley & Sons, Ltd. Published 2013 by John Wiley & Sons, Ltd.

Neck dissection involves dissecting the non-lymphatic structures and removing, *en bloc*, the fatty, connective and lymphatic tissue (lymph nodes and lymphatic vessels) that surround these structures. This differs significantly from a lymphadenectomy (otherwise known as 'berry picking') in which only one or a few macroscopically involved nodes are removed. Lymphadenectomy is not recommended as the initial procedure for treatment of involved neck nodes, due to the co-existence of microscopically involved nodes with macroscopically involved nodes [6].

Indications

Differentiated thyroid cancer

For differentiated thyroid cancer (follicular and papillary carcinomas) with metastatic nodes in the lateral neck, a therapeutic neck dissection with 'functional compartmental *en bloc* neck dissection' is currently recommended [6]. For low-risk patients, metastatic neck nodes may not be related to survival. Nonetheless, one large retrospective database study of 9904 patients found that the presence of nodal metastases of papillary carcinoma was a significant risk factor for decreased overall survival (79% versus 82% at 14 years) [7]. Another study found that nodal metastasis of papillary thyroid carcinoma was a risk factor for increased mortality, but only for patients >45 years of age [8]. Finally, patients with over 10 metastatic nodes or more than three nodes with extracapsular spread carry a higher risk of neck recurrence [9].

Ultrasound characteristics of suspicious lymph nodes in differentiated thyroid cancer include a cystic appearance (with a sensitivity of 11% but a specificity of 100% in the study by Leboulleux *et al.*[10]), hyperechoic punctuations (or microcalcifications which have a sensitivity of 46% but a specificity of 100%), loss of the hyperechoic hilum (with a sensitivity of 100% but a specificity of 29%), and peripheral intranodal vascularization regardless of central vascularization (with a sensitivity and specificity of 86% and 82%, respectively). The loss of hilum in itself is non-specific, as are a round shape and hypoechogenicity. Confirmation of the metastatic nature of suspicious nodes should be attained preoperatively by ultrasound-guided fine needle aspiration cytological analysis and by measuring the thyroglobulin level in the needle washout fluid. Levels above 10 ng/mL are considered suspicious for malignancy [6,11–14].

For differentiated thyroid cancer, selective neck dissection with preservation of all of the non-lymphatic structures is generally feasible. There is currently no consensus and, generally low-level, contradictory evidence as to the optimal extent of therapeutic neck dissection, although complete resection of all macroscopic disease is the norm [15]. In the presence of large nodal metastases, the dissection may be particularly fastidious, requiring time and effort, but the functional outcome of preserving all of these structures largely compensates the surgeon's efforts. Extensive neck dissection for thyroid cancer can be safely performed with low recurrence rates [16].

Prophylactic lateral neck dissection, in the absence of known lateral metastases, is generally not recommended for differentiated thyroid cancer. Despite current recommendations, however, we have been performing prophylactic lateral neck dissection routinely for many years and have found that for patients with papillary carcinoma initially considered free of nodal metastases (T1–T3 cN0), up to 25% will have at least micrometastases in levels III and/or IV ipsilateral to the thyroid tumour [17]. Staging the neck using prophylactic lateral neck dissection (as well as prophylactic central neck dissection) can lead to lower doses of radioactive iodine for patients without occult metastases and higher doses of radioiodine and a more aggressive follow-up for patients found to have occult metastatic nodes [18,19]. Determining the impact of this approach on disease-free survival and quality of life will require further studies, however.

Medullary thyroid cancer

For medullary thyroid carcinoma, a therapeutic 'compartmental' or *en bloc* selective lateral neck dissection for patients with radiologically or clinically visible metastatic nodes and in the absence of widespread distant metastases is recommended [20]. Some, but not all, of these patients will experience a survival benefit. There is for now no predictive factor to preoperatively determine which of these patients will benefit from neck dissection. Patients with more than 10 metastatic nodes or involvement of more than two node levels will generally not achieve biological remission (normalization of calcitonin levels) even with extensive neck surgery [21–23]. There is no evidence in favour of isolated lymphadenectomy ('berry picking') of metastatic nodes for improving survival or quality of life in medullary thyroid cancer.

Prophlyactic lateral neck dissection for medullary thyroid cancer is advocated by some, when there is evidence of lymph node metastases in the central compartment (level VI), but this attitude is controversial in the absence of evidence showing improved survival [20]. The incidence of metastatic lateral nodes is significantly related to the number of metastatic nodes in the central compartment [24], and to the preoperative calcitonin levels [25]. One advantage of prophylactic lateral neck dissection in these cases may be a decrease in regional recurrence and local complications or pain that these recurrences may cause [21,26–30].

Basic technique: selective neck dissection levels III and IV ◉ (Videos 9.1, 9.2)

Patient position and skin incision

The basic technique, always performed under general anaesthesia, implies a patient in a supine position with neck extension. A neck roll may be used to extend the neck and pull the clavicles backward to maximally expose the regions of interest, especially the supraclavicular fossa. Care must be taken not to overextend the neck, which may cause prolonged postoperative neck pain. Care must also be taken to maintain the forearms supinated to prevent compression of the cubital nerve.

The skin incision is generally a low collar incision [31]. A level III and IV neck dissection can be performed through a Kocher-type incision, 5–7 cm long, the length being determined by the patient's morphology. Extension to levels I, II and V may require a lateral and superior extension of the incision or a second horizontal incision in the upper part of the neck (Figure 9.1).

Dissection of the anterior border and deep surface of the sternomastoid muscle

The external jugular vein has a variable position and may be preserved if it does not impede retraction of the sternomastoid muscle and access to the region, otherwise it should be sacrificed. The vascular pedicles to the sternomastoid muscle are coagulated (bipolar or monopolar cautery or other haemostatic devices) and divided. The dissection is terminated once the posterior border of the sternomastoid muscle is reached. Here, the fascia

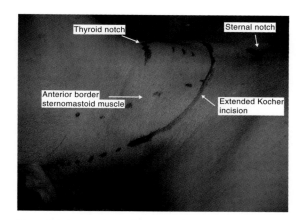

Figure 9.1 An extended Kocher incision for lateral neck dissection for thyroid cancer.

overlying the fatty and lymphatic tissue (middle cervical aponeurosis) is divided longitudinally, along the sternomastoid muscle. The omohyoid muscle may generally be preserved, with dissection of its lateral and deep surfaces (its vascular pedicle with a branch of the ansa hypoglossi generally needs electrocautery). This muscle can be retracted anteriorly or posteriorly, depending on the approach. In case of extensive or bulky disease, the omohyoid muscle may be sacrificed with no morbidity.

Anterior-to-posterior technique

This approach is particularly useful for performing a selective neck dissection of level III and/or IV via the Kocher incision. Visibility is improved if the surgeon stands on the opposite side of the neck dissection. The internal jugular vein is dissected in a subfascial plane (exposing the surface of the vein and its small collateral veins) from anterior to posterior and from the clavicle to the level of the cricoid cartilage for a level III and IV dissection. The fascia medial to the vein, starting at the lateral border of the sternohyoid muscle, should be removed or at least inspected for visible lymph nodes along the anterior surface of the vein. Care must be taken to preventively cauterize the small emissary veins often located at the lateral and deep aspects of the vein. The vein is then retraced medially, preferably with a blunt retractor (Figure 9.2a), taking care not to traumatize the vagus nerve that lies deep to the vein. The vagus nerve should be visualized, however, because it represents the deep and medial limit of the dissection which allows removal of any retrojugular nodes that may be present.

(a)

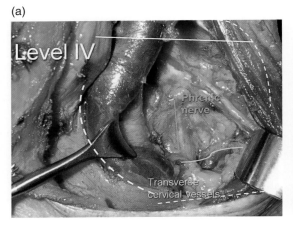

(b)

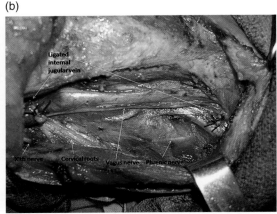

Figure 9.2 (a) Selective left level IV neck dissection; a blunt retractor on the internal jugular vein facilitates exposure. (b) Selective levels II-III-IV right neck dissection with resection of the internal jugular vein, necessary due to the invasion of the vascular wall by several metastatic nodes.

In differentiated thyroid cancer, metastatic nodes rarely invade the internal jugular vein or other structures. A meticulous dissection can thus generally free the vein from the nodes. In the rare cases where the wall of the vein is invaded, a small patch can be resected and repaired with a 6-0 prolene running suture. If more extensive invasion is found, the vein may have to be sacrificed. We generally ligate the vein with 2 ligatures superiorly and 2b ligatures inferiorly, using 0-0 vicryl or non-resorbable sutures (Figure 9.2b).

Lateral to the vagus nerve, the dissection plane is carried out horizontally, taking care to remain close to the fatty and lymphatic tissue, preserving the deep cervical fascia, and not to dissect too deeply toward the phrenic nerve at this level (Figure 9.3). The transverse cervical vessels are identified, preserved and dissected on their anterior surface. There is always a small branch of the artery that runs upward into the lymphatic tissue that should be cauterized before transection. The inferior border of the neck dissection is the superior border of the clavicle. The fatty/lymphatic tissue should be transected at this level, preferably with haemo- and lymphostasis with ligatures, clips or electric devices to avoid chyle leak. Large lymphatic vessels (or even the thoracic duct itself) may need to be ligated, especially in cases with low-lying large metastatic nodes in which dilation of the lymphatic vessels may be observed.

The dissection is then carried out from this level upward, remaining in close contact with the fatty/

lymphatic tissue and preserving the deep cervical fascia that overlies the phrenic nerve and the scalene muscles. Above the level of the omohyoid muscle, the lymphatic/fatty tissue should be dissected and explored for branches of the sensory cervical plexus running almost perpendicularly to the jugular vein. They should be preserved by dissecting their anterior aspect from the lymph nodes. The fat/lymphatics are transected at the level of the cricoid cartilage, the superior limit of level III.

Extension to level II

This dissection can be continued to include level II. This generally requires an extended skin incision. One continues the dissection along the lateral border of the sternohyoid muscle and then laterally, removing the fascia and nodes along the superior thyroid vascular pedicle. The dissection continues along the anterior aspect of the internal jugular vein and the facial vein, and then the medial and deep aspect of the internal jugular vein. The superior border of the level II dissection is the inferior border of the posterior belly of the digastric muscle which is dissected and retracted superiorly to improve visualization of the area (taking care not to excessively retract this area due to the proximity of the marginal mandibular branch of the facial nerve superficially and the hypoglossal nerve anteriorly).

Dissecting within the specimen is then recommended to find and preserve the branches of the cervical plexus

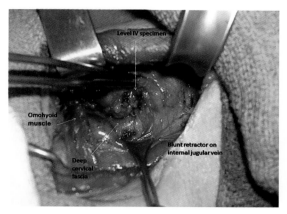

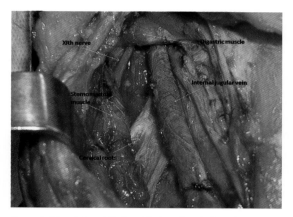

Figure 9.3 Left level IV selective neck dissection in an anterior-to-posterior direction. A blunt retractor retracts the internal jugular vein medially.

Figure 9.4 Levels II and III after right lateral neck dissection.

and the spinal accessory nerve. The spinal accessory nerve is found generally at the junction of the upper quarter-lower three-quarters of the sternomastoid muscle [32]. The dissection is carried out in the fatty tissue in an oblique axis along the supposed trajectory of the nerve (the nerve making an angle of approximately 45° with the superior quarter of the sternomastoid muscle). The nerve is then dissected either along its inferior border, for a neck dissection limited to level IIA, or on all sides, completely freeing it from the underlying tissue, in order to remove both levels IIA and IIB (Figure 9.4).

There is often an anastomosis between the third cervical root and the XIth nerve that should be preserved. The nerves are dissected along their anterior aspect, freeing the specimen. Dissection of level IIB requires completely freeing the spinal accessory nerve on all sides to remove the tissue situated cranially and posteriorly to the nerve, between the posterior belly of the digastric muscle, above, the sternomastoid muscle, laterally, and the medial scalene and levator scapulae muscles, posteriorly. Once the nerve is identified and dissected, the dissection frees the specimen from the deep cervical fascia. This deep dissection requires cauterization of the occipital artery that runs through this region.

Posterior-to-anterior technique

Once the fascia covering the fatty/lymphatic tissue is transected at the level of the posterior border of the sternomastoid muscle, the branches of the cervical plexus are found by dissecting the fatty/lymphatic tissue in a

direction that is perpendicular to the posterior border of the sternomastoid muscle. Once each branch is found, its anterior surface is dissected and the fatty/lymphatic tissue superficial to it is elevated. At the upper border of the clavicle, the tissue is transected, with ligatures, clips or electric haemostatic devices. The transverse cervical vessels are found at the deep aspect of the lymph nodes, and preserved, as above, with dissection of their anterior aspect, taking care to preserve the underlying deep cervical fascia, protecting the underlying phrenic nerve and scalenus muscles. Then the lateral aspect of the internal jugular vein is dissected and retracted medially and the vagus nerve visualized lying deep to the vein. The vagus nerve and the internal jugular vein are dissected subfascially from caudally to cranially, from the clavicle to a level corresponding to the cricoid cartilage (the superior boundary of level III), with electrocautery or ligation of any small emissary veins that may be present, especially at the posterior aspect of the vein. The surgical specimen can thus be freed from the vagus nerve and the internal jugular vein from down to up, and laterally to medially. We recommend dissecting the vagus nerve and the posterior aspect of the vein to ensure resection of metastatic nodes that frequently lie behind the vein. The dissection is continued medially, removing the fascia and nodes along the anterior aspect of the vein and those that may be found medial to the internal jugular vein, and superficial to the superior thyroid, lingual and facial veins. The lateral border of the sternohyoid muscle is the medial limit of the neck dissection.

In all cases, either the specimen is oriented with a diagram for pathological examination or the node levels are separated by the surgeon and sent for analysis in individual containers. Once the neck dissection completed, the regions not dissected (often levels V and I) should nonetheless be explored by palpation and dissected if macroscopically suspicious nodes are found.

One may need to dissect the neck structures in a different order than described here, especially in the presence of bulky metastatic nodes. In this case, the dissection is often carried out from the periphery to the centre, or, as a general rule 'from easy to difficult'.

In general, it is recommended to learn and master at least one of these approaches and to routinely use the same steps. The advantage of a routine is to gradually improve in terms of complications and length of time taken, and to be able to teach a logical, step-by-step procedure to junior surgeons. In the presence of large metastatic nodes, however, one may need to improvise and dissect the non-lymphatic structures described above in different ways, as the bulk of the disease may allow.

Complications

As for central neck dissection, for which the American Thyroid Association recommends surgical expertise [6], the outcomes of lateral neck dissection in terms of oncological resection and morbidity are improved when performed by high-volume surgeons [33]. The specific complications of lateral neck dissection are thoroughly discussed in Chapter 19 but a few limited indications need to be pointed out here.

General complications

Haematoma is an infrequent complication occurring soon after surgery, generally within the first 24 h. Drainage may require general anaesthesia, removal of the blood clots and haemostasis. Risk factors include untreated high blood pressure and heparin or vitamin K inhibitors, although low-dose aspirin has not been shown to increase haematoma formation. The presence of large metastatic nodes and extensive surgery may also increase the risk of haematoma formation. Local infection is also rare, and may be secondary to haematoma.

Children and adolescents, dark-skinned patients and patients with a history of keloids are at a higher risk for keloid scars and should be monitored in the weeks and months following surgery. In all patients, the scar should

not be exposed to sun or ultraviolet rays for 1 year, to avoid permanent pigmentation of the scar.

Specific complications

Chyle leak

Chyle leak is rare, occurring in approximately 1–4% of at-risk surgical cases. In the supraclavicular fossa on both sides, but particularly on the left behind and just lateral to the internal jugular vein, care should be taken to prevent this complication by systematically using ligatures or clips. Small lymphatics can be managed with electric haemostatic devices, however. In case of extensive nodal metastases, one can often observe a dilation of the lymphatic vessels. This should be managed with caution, using ligatures and clips more liberally.

Inadvertent damage to the thoracic duct or its branches on the left or, less frequently, of the great lymphatic vein on the right may be detected intraoperatively. Roh et al. reported a 5% incidence, all controlled intraoperatively [34].

The leak may not be apparent intraoperatively, with chyle appearing in the suction drains on postoperative day 1 or 2 (rarely later). The incidence reported by Roh et al. was 8%, with an almost equal incidence on the left and right sides. In most cases, conservative measures – diet modification, pressure dressing, drainage or repeated needle aspiration – are generally effective. Resolution may take 2–4 weeks, or more; however, diet modifications include a low-fat diet or total parenteral nutrition. There is low evidence in favour of any particular nutritional approach to chyle leak and currently no consensus. The nutritional status of the patient should be monitored carefully, however.

Spinal accessory nerve paresis or paralysis

Shoulder dysfunction and pain can be seen after dissection of the spinal accessory nerve, performed during dissection of levels II and V. Selective dissection of levels III and IV alone is not associated with shoulder dysfunction, and shoulder-related quality of life in this case has been shown to be no different from patients without any neck dissection.

There are few data on the incidence of permanent or temporary spinal accessory nerve impairment after later neck dissection specifically for differentiated thyroid carcinoma. Data from patients treated for squamous cell head and neck cancers meet with the further morbidity of radiation therapy. Data from the study by Capiello *et al.* of patients who underwent level II–IV neck dissection versus those with level II–V neck dissection without postoperative radiation therapy, after 1 year, showed a motor deficit in the shoulder in 5% of patients in the former group versus 15% in the latter group [35]. Upper limb strength impairment was 0% versus 20%. Pain was reported by 15% of the patients in both groups. Despite this, electromyographic abnormalities were found in the trapezius muscle in 20% and 85% of patients, respectively. Dissection of level V increases shoulder morbidity, but long-term subclinical impairment can be found even with dissection of level II.

Chronic pain in the shoulder may be due to spinal accessory nerve damage, but also to damage to the sensory cervical roots or to scarring. In the study by van Wilgen, only 51% of the patients complaining of shoulder pain an average of 3 years postoperatively had objective dysfunction of the spinal accessory nerve [36].

Preservation of the cervical roots has been shown to decrease the incidence of chronic pain and improve quality of life. Careful dissection and preservation of these nerves if possible can thus improve functional outcomes.

Anaesthesia, dysaesthesia, paraesthesia and pain

Temporary anaesthesia of the skin is common and generally subsides in 1–6 months. Anaesthesia of the earlobe is due to damage to or transection of the great auricular nerve (a branch of the cervical plexus crossing the upper one-third of the sternomastoid muscle). Loss of sensation is generally not permanent, but for now there is no means of predicting the quality of or the delay in recovery of sensation.

Other nerve injuries

The marginal mandibular branch of the facial nerve (cranial nerve VII) may be injured during lateral neck dissection, principally of level I and more rarely of level II, resulting in paralysis or paresis of the corresponding half of the lower lip (especially during talking and smiling). In level I dissection, extreme care should be taken to identify the nerve, avoiding extensive dissection of the nerve unless it is necessary. Generally, once the nerve is identified, the facial vessels can be divided below the level of the nerve, avoiding extensive nerve dissection. If dis-

section in this region is planned, facial nerve monitoring may be employed to ensure nerve identification. Injury to this nerve during level II dissection is most often due to the retractor retracting the posterior belly of the digastric muscle. These types of injuries most often result in neurapraxia, with spontaneous recovery of motion in several weeks or months. Physical therapy or other interventions have not been shown to hasten recovery of nerve function.

Injuries to the phrenic nerve, the vagus nerve, the hypoglossal nerve, the brachial plexus or the sympathetic plexus are rare, and will be treated in another section of this book.

Tips and tricks

How extensive should dissection be?

There is currently no consensus and, generally low-level, contradictory evidence as to the optimal extent of therapeutic neck dissection, although complete resection of all macroscopic disease is the norm [15]. Therapeutic neck dissection should be tailored to the extent of the disease, in order to remove all involved nodes and those that carry a high risk of involvement. Levels that are adjacent to a level with known metastases should generally be included in the dissection. Thus, a patient presenting with a known metastatic node in level III should undergo dissection of level III but also levels II and IV [37,38]. A complete selective submandibular neck dissection (IB) carries a significant risk of morbidity, especially for the marginal branch of the facial nerve, and to a lesser extent the lingual and hypoglossal nerves. This level is rarely involved by metastatic nodes. Routine dissection at this level is generally not performed and is only necessary if there are confirmed nodal metastases in that level. In many instances of limited metastatic involvement, the metastases and their surrounding fatty and lymphatic tissue can be removed with preservation of the gland and its vascularization [39].

Level II nodes

Level II is divided into IIA and IIB (see Figure 9.3). The risk of level II disease is considered to be higher for tumours involving the superior pole of the thyroid. These metastases arise from tumour cells drained by the lymphatics accompanying the superior thyroid vascular pedicle [40]. Koo *et al.* found that the presence of macro-scopic level III nodes was a risk factor for occult nodal metastases in level II [38]. They also found that extensive metastases in levels IIA, III and IV were predictive for metastases in level IIB. The incidence of metastatic nodes in level IIB is relatively rare, however, with reported rates ranging from approximately 3% to 5% [41,42].

Systematic clearing of level IIB in the absence of nodal metastases in IIA does not seem necessary, therefore. Sparing level IIB reduces the extent of dissection of the spinal accessory nerve and thus the risk of postoperative paresis and pain. However, sometimes nodal metastases are not apparent clinically at the time of operation and are only revealed after pathological analysis of the operating specimen. The intraoperative macroscopic evaluation of level IIA may thus not be reliable. Further studies of the necessary extent of lateral neck dissection to include level IIB are warranted.

Level V nodes

Level V nodes are very rarely involved in an isolated fashion, but are frequent if node levels III and IV are involved. In the study by Kupferman *et al.*, level V contained metastatic nodes in 53% of cases [43]. Patients with metastatic nodes in levels II, III and/or IV were significantly at risk of harbouring metastatic nodes in level V.

Level VA and B can be approached in two ways. The anterior approach passes between the branches of the sensory cervical plexus, medial to the sternomastoid muscle. The deep aspects of the nerve branches are dissected, then the posterior border of the sternomastoid muscle. Then the deep aspects of the medial and posterior scalene muscles are dissected, from anterior to posterior, preserving the deep cervical fascia. The dissection ends at the anterior border of the trapezius muscle, and removes all of the fatty and lymphatic tissue between the scalenes, the anterior border of the trapezius and the posterior border of the sternomastoid muscle. Care must be taken to identify and preserve the spinal accessory nerve at the posterior border of the sternomastoid muscle as it courses through the region to innervate the trapezius muscle.

The posterior approach passes laterally and posterior to the sternomastoid muscle, which implies elevating the posterior cutaneous flap from the lateral surface of the sternomastoid muscle all the way back to the anterior border of the trapezius muscle (Figure 9.5). The spinal accessory nerve is identified at the posterior border of the

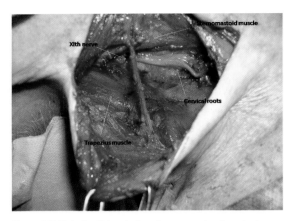

Figure 9.5 Right level V neck dissection, preserving the spinal accessory nerve (XIth nerve) and the lower sensory cervical roots.

sternomastoid muscle, generally at the junction of the upper two-thirds–lower one-third of the sternomastoid muscle where a posterior branch of the sensory cervical plexus crosses the posterior border of the muscle. The nerve is completely dissected and preserved. The sensory branches of the cervical roots should also be dissected on all sides and preserved, if tumour resection allows it. Then the posterior border of the sternomastoid muscle is dissected and reclined anteriorly. The lymphatic tissue is dissected off the medial and posterior scalene muscles from anterior to posterior, stopping at the anterior border of the trapezius muscle.

This dissection removes all of the tissue deep to the spinal accessory nerve. The lower limit of the dissection corresponds to the upper border of the clavicle As stated above, this more extensive dissection of the spinal accessory nerve increases the incidence of postoperative shoulder dysfunction and pain [35]. Preservation of the sensory cervical roots can improve outcomes, as can early rehabilitation with shoulder mobilization [44,45].

Level I nodes

Level I nodes – submental (IA) and submandibular (IB) – are also rarely involved by thyroid cancer, and generally not involved in the absence of adjacent macroscopic metastatic nodes. Complete selective neck dissection of these levels is not often necessary, unless macroscopic disease is present. The submental level (IA) is removed bilaterally due to the absence of an anatomical boundary between the left and right sides. Electrocautery can be used to dissect the anterior bellies of the digastric muscles. Then, starting at the level of the mandibular symphysis (preserving the periosteum), the tissue is removed from above to below, dissecting the anterior aspect of the mylohyoid muscle, which constitutes the deep boundary of the submental nodal level. The dissection continues down to the superior border of the hyoid bone, the inferior boundary. Dissection of level IA in itself carries very little morbidity.

A complete selective level IB neck dissection implies removal of the submandibular gland, as well as the lymphatic and fatty tissue in the submandibular region, between the lower border of the mandible, the mylohyoid muscle and mucosa of the floor of the mouth, the digastric and stylohyoid muscles. This is rarely necessary for thyroid carcinoma. The dissection requires identification and preservation of the marginal mandibular branch of the facial nerve, which, after raising the subplatysmal flap, is identified crossing the facial vein on its anterior surface. The facial vein and artery are generally ligated just below the nerve, although in some cases the anatomy of the artery is such that it may be preserved with ligation of its glandular branches. Then the dissection is carried out from anterior to posterior along the periosteum of the mandible, from the anterior belly of the digastric muscle, to the level of the stylohyoid muscle. Then the anterior belly of the digastric muscle is dissected from the lymphatic tissue. The underlying mylohyoid muscle is retracted anteriorly, after haemostasis of its vascular pedicle, and the lingual nerve and Wharton's duct are identified. Wharton's duct, the sublingual gland and the glandular branch of the lingual nerve are ligated (there is generally a small artery running along Wharton's duct at this level) and freed from the submandibular gland and tissue. The dissection then continues anterior to posterior along the superior border of the posterior belly of the digastric muscle, taking care to avoid trauma to the underlying hypoglossal nerve. The dissection terminates with ligation of the facial vein and artery at the level of the digastric muscle.

The potential complications of a complete submandibular neck dissection include paresis of the marginal mandibular branch of the facial nerve (with paralysis of the corresponding half of the lower lip), hemianaesthesia of the tongue and hemiparesis of the tongue. These complications are generally well tolerated and complete recovery of neurapraxia of these nerves generally occurs within several weeks or months. However, any neck asymmetry from removal of the gland will persist.

A compromise may also be reached to lower the morbidity of level IB dissection in the presence of small (1–2 cm) metastatic nodes without obvious invasion of the submandibular gland [39]. These nodes often lie anterior to the gland, and a limited dissection between the anterior belly of the digastric muscle, the mylohoid muscle, the gland and the lateral border of the vessels (avoiding the marginal mandibular branch of the facial nerve) may suffice to remove the metastatic nodes along with the surrounding fat and lymphatics. In other cases, the metastatic nodes lie posterior to the gland, and can be removed conservatively by dissecting the posterior border of the gland and the anterior border of the posterior belly of the digastric muscle, removing all of the adjacent fat and lymphatics.

What incision should I use?

Many types of neck incisions have been described for neck dissection. For thyroid cancer, the Kocher incision, more or less extended laterally and upward toward the mastoid process, optimizes exposure for complete neck dissection while minimizing aesthetic problems. The upward extension is less conspicuous if it is carried out about 2 cm (or more) posterior to the anterior border of the sternomastoid muscle. This curved and posterior incision also avoids a vertical incision in the neck which can become retracted and painful. Another option for thyroid cancer is to perform a double incision – a Kocher incision and a submandibular incision (described by MacFee) 4–5 cm below the mandible (Figure 9.6), run-

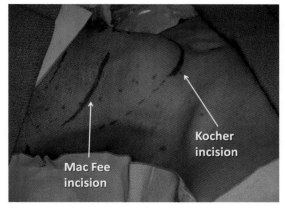

Figure 9.6 Example of a submandibular 'MacFee' incision for level II neck dissection.

ning along a line drawn from the mastoid process curving down to the level of the hyoid bone [44]. One must be particularly careful when using the double-incision strategy, however, due to reduced visibility under the intermediate skin flap, where metastatic nodes may be overlooked.

Where should I look for hidden lymph nodes?

There are several areas of predilection for metastatic nodes in thyroid cancer that are generally not addressed by standard selective lateral neck dissections.

• Below the clavicle, below the transverse cervical vascular pedicle above the subclavian artery and vein. These nodes are relatively frequent, and can be anterior (just below the inferior border of level IV) or posterior (below level VB). Palpation in these regions after complete neck dissection of levels IV and VB should be performed to rule out any forgotten metastatic nodes in this area. Care should be taken to avoid chyle or lymphatic leakage, with ligatures or clips, as stated above.

• Behind the sternoclavicular joint, in front of the common carotid artery. These nodes may be even lower, running along the route of the internal thoracic vessels, parallel to the lateral aspect of the sternum, down below the clavicle and to the level of the first or second rib. Metastatic nodes in this region are rare, and may be accessible by a cervical approach if the morphology of the patient is favourable (relatively thin, young patients with long necks, especially). Otherwise, resection of these metastatic nodes requires a sternotomy. If there are low-lying metastatic nodes in levels IV or VI, palpation behind the joint and sternum should be performed to rule out any forgotten nodes that still are often accessible from a cervical approach.

• Behind the common carotid artery. These metastases develop along the trajectory of the inferior thyroid artery (a region overlooked when performing a standard lateral neck dissection). These nodes can be resected from a lateral approach, from the central neck (the paratracheal region) or via a combined approach, especially for large metastases. The vagus nerve is particularly vulnerable when dissecting this area and special caution should be used. The sympathetic nerve is also located in this region, and trauma can lead to Horner's syndrome, which is generally regressive over several weeks or months.

• Medial to the common carotid artery at the level of the carotid bifurcation. These metastatic nodes develop along the route of the superior thyroid vascular pedicle. Nodes at this level can be adherent to the inferior constrictor muscle and removal may thus require careful dissection of the carotid bifurcation and the constrictor muscles. The origin of the superior thyroid artery is very close to the carotid bifurcation and careful ligation at this level (with oversewing using fine vascular sutures) is advisable, if necessary.

• Submandibular or submental nodes. As stated before, these are rare locations for metastases. They may be 'hiding' behind the facial vein. Palpation can generally find these nodes lying anteriorly or posteriorly to the submandibular gland. The route of spread to this region can be an upward spread from level II nodes or an upward spread from upper level VI or 'Delphian' (prelaryngeal) nodes, extending along the thyrohyoid muscle up to the level of the hyoid bone.

How to minimize complications?

Careful haemostasis during and after dissection is of course the general rule in surgery, as is an impeccable aseptic technique. A double aseptization of the skin may decrease postoperative infections, but prophylactic intra- or postoperative antibiotics do not [45,46]. Infection is a rare occurrence in lateral neck dissection (1–3%), but infection has been shown to be correlated with longer operative time [45,46].

Very careful lymphostasis is important. The left supraclavicular fossa is particularly at risk due to the presence of the thoracic duct and/or its branches, sometimes seen just behind the internal jugular vein. Large dilated lymphatics are often seen when large or numerous lymph node metastases are present. Ligatures or clips are our preferred choice for lymphostasis in these cases (most electric devices are not specifically designed for lymphatics). If the thoracic duct or large branches need to be transected in order to remove the lymph nodes, careful ligation is necessary. Biological adjuncts such as fibrin or cyanoacrylate glue or Tachosil® may also prevent lymphatic leakage and may be used prophylactically, once the ligaures or clips have ensured lymphostasis. A pressure dressing applied immediately postoperatively to the supraclavicular fossa may also minimize the leak. A suction drain should not be put directly in the supraclavicular fossa in this case.

The spinal accessory nerve is generally a 'robust' nerve and complete definitive paralysis is not common, even when the nerve is completely dissected, as for a level V dissection. However, care must be taken, because even transient paralysis or paresis and pain can be particularly handicapping. Bipolar (and not monopolar) cautery should be used around the nerve, but never too close to the nerve. The nerve itself should never be handled with forceps, but can be dissected and indirectly retracted by retracting the adjacent fascia or other tissues. As stated above, preservation of the sensory cervical roots should always be attempted.

Using Harmonic™ technology has been shown to decrease operating time for lateral neck dissections for thyroid cancer [47]. This is an advantage both for the patient, with potentially less blood loss and a lower risk of infection, and for the physician who can optimize operating room resources and potentially lower costs.

Finally, scar complications are minimized by careful skin closure, using resorbable sutures, fibrin glue and/or staples removed early. Patients should be advised to use UVA and B protective creams on the scar for 1 year. Prevention of keloid formation may be used for at-risk patients (young patients and dark-skinned patients): local cortisone creams or injections if an inflammatory scar develops, local application of silicone dressings, early referral to a specialized dermatologist or plastic surgeon.

Conclusion

With a precise knowledge of the anatomical boundaries and with experience, lateral neck dissection can be routinely performed safely and effectively. A meticulous technique is required to minimize morbidity. Knowledge of the paths of spread of lymphatic metastases of thyroid cancer is necessary to ensure complete surgical resection of macroscopic disease, a major prognostic factor in terms of recurrence and, in some cases, survival.

References

1 Ferlito A, Robbins KT, Shah JP, et al. Proposal for a rational classification of neck dissections. Head Neck 2011; 33(3): 445–50.

2 Robbins KT, Medina JE, Wolfe GT, Levine PA, Sessions RB, Pruet CW. Standardizing neck dissection terminology. Official report of the Academy's Committee for Head and Neck Surgery and Oncology. Arch Otolaryngol Head Neck Surg 1991; 117(6): 601–5.

3 Robbins KT. Classification of neck dissection: current concepts and future considerations. Otolaryngol Clin North Am 1998; 31(4): 639–55.

4 Robbins KT, Clayman G, Levine PA, et al. Neck dissection classification update: revisions proposed by the American Head and Neck Society and the American Academy of Otolaryngology-Head and Neck Surgery. Arch Otolaryngol Head Neck Surg 2002; 128(7): 751–8.

5 Ferlito A, Rinaldo A, Silver CE, et al. Elective and therapeutic selective neck dissection. Oral Oncol 2006; 42(1): 14–25.

6 Cooper DS, Doherty GM, Haugen BR, et al. Revised American Thyroid Association management guidelines for patients with thyroid nodules and differentiated thyroid cancer. Thyroid 2009; 19(11): 1167–214.

7 Podnos YD, Smith D, Wagman LD, Ellenhorn JD. The implication of lymph node metastasis on survival in patients with well-differentiated thyroid cancer. Am Surg 2005; 71(9): 731–4.

8 Zaydfudim V, Feurer ID, Griffin MR, Phay JE. The impact of lymph node involvement on survival in patients with papillary and follicular thyroid carcinoma. Surgery 2008; 144(6): 1070–7; discussion 1077–8.

9 Leboulleux S. Prognostic factors for persistent or recurrent disease of papillary thyroid carcinoma with neck lymph node metastases and/or tumor extension beyond the thyroid capsule at initial diagnosis. J Clin Endocrinol Metab 2005; 90(10): 5723–9.

10 Leboulleux S, Girard E, Rose M, et al. Ultrasound criteria of malignancy for cervical lymph nodes in patients followed up for differentiated thyroid cancer. J Clin Endocrinol Metab 2007; 92(9): 3590–4.

11 Frasoldati A, Pesenti M, Gallo M, Caroggio A, Salvo D, Valcavi R. Diagnosis of neck recurrences in patients with differentiated thyroid carcinoma. Cancer. 2003; 97(1): 90–6.

12 Boi F, Baghino G, Atzeni F, Lai ML, Faa G, Mariotti S. The diagnostic value for differentiated thyroid carcinoma metastases of thyroglobulin (Tg) measurement in wash-out fluid from fine-needle aspiration biopsy of neck lymph nodes is maintained in the presence of circulating anti-Tg antibodies. J Clin Endocrinol Metab 2006; 91(4): 1364–9.

13 Kim MJ, Kim EK, Kim BM, et al. Thyroglobulin measurement in fine-needle aspirate washouts: the criteria for neck node dissection for patients with thyroid cancer. Clin Endocrinol (Oxf) 2009; 70(1): 145–51.

14 Snozek CL, Chambers EP, Reading CC, et al. Serum thyroglobulin, high-resolution ultrasound, and lymph node thyroglobulin in diagnosis of differentiated thyroid

carcinoma nodal metastases. J Clin Endocrinol Metab 2007; 92(11): 4278–81.

15 Hasney CP, Amedee RG. What is the appropriate extent of lateral neck dissection in the treatment of metastatic well-differentiated thyroid carcinoma? Laryngoscope 2010; 120(9): 1716–17.

16 Grant CS, Stulak JM, Thompson GB, Richards ML, Reading CC, Hay ID. Risks and adequacy of an optimized surgical approach to the primary surgical management of papillary thyroid carcinoma treated during 1999–2006. World J Surg 2010; 34(6): 1239–46.

17 Hartl D, Leboulleux S, Al Ghuzlan A, et al. Optimization of staging of the neck with prophylactic central and lateral neck dissection for papillary thyroid carcinoma. Ann Surg 2012; 255(4): 777–83.

18 Hughes DT, White ML, Miller BS, Gauger PG, Burney RE, Doherty GM. Influence of prophylactic central lymph node dissection on postoperative thyroglobulin levels and radioiodine treatment in papillary thyroid cancer. Surgery 2010; 148(6): 1100–7.

19 Bonnet S, Hartl D, Leboulleux S, et al. Prophylactic lymph node dissection for papillary thyroid cancer less than 2 cm: implications for radioiodine treatment. J Clin Endocrinol Metab 2009; 94(4): 1162–7.

20 Kloos RT, Eng C, Evans DB, et al. Medullary thyroid cancer: management guidelines of the American Thyroid Association. Thyroid 2009; 19(6): 565–612.

21 Weber T, Schilling T, Frank-Raue K, et al. Impact of modified radical neck dissection on biochemical cure in medullary thyroid carcinomas. Surgery 2001; 130(6): 1044–9.

22 Scollo C, Baudin E, Travagli JP, et al. Rationale for central and bilateral lymph node dissection in sporadic and hereditary medullary thyroid cancer. J Clin Endocrinol Metab 2003; 88(5): 2070–5.

23 Machens A, Gimm O, Ukkat J, Hinze R, Schneyer U, Dralle H. Improved prediction of calcitonin normalization in medullary thyroid carcinoma patients by quantitative lymph node analysis. Cancer 2000; 88(8): 1909–15.

24 Machens A, Hauptmann S, Dralle H. Prediction of lateral lymph node metastases in medullary thyroid cancer. Br J Surg 2008; 95(5): 586–91.

25 Machens A, Dralle H. Biomarker-based risk stratification for previously untreated medullary thyroid cancer. J Clin Endocrinol Metab 2010; 95(6): 2655–63.

26 Dralle H, Damm I, Scheumann GF, et al. Compartment-oriented microdissection of regional lymph nodes in medullary thyroid carcinoma. Surg Today 1994; 24(2): 112–21.

27 Pelizzo MR, Boschin IM, Bernante P, et al. Natural history, diagnosis, treatment and outcome of medullary thyroid

cancer: 37 years experience on 157 patients. Eur J Surg Oncol 2007; 33(4): 493–7.

28 Machens A, Hinze R, Thomusch O, Dralle H. Pattern of nodal metastasis for primary and reoperative thyroid cancer. World J Surg 2002; 26(1): 22–8.

29 Quayle FJ, Benveniste R, DeBenedetti MK, Wells SA, Moley JF. Hereditary medullary thyroid carcinoma in patients greater than 50 years old. Surgery 2004; 136(6): 1116–21.

30 Quayle FJ, Moley JF. Medullary thyroid carcinoma: management of lymph node metastases. Curr Treat Options Oncol 2005; 6(4): 347–54.

31 Robbins KT, Oppenheimer RW. Incisions for neck dissection modifications: rationale for and application of nontrifurcate patterns. Laryngoscope 1994; 104(8 Pt 1): 1041–4.

32 Tatla T, Kanagalingam J, Majithia A, Clarke PM. Upper neck spinal accessory nerve identification during neck dissection. J Laryngol Otol 2005; 119(11): 906–8.

33 Morton RP, Gray L, Tandon DA, Izzard M, McIvor NP. Efficacy of neck dissection: are surgical volumes important? Laryngoscope 2009; 119(6): 1147–52.

34 Roh JL, Kim DH, Park CI. Prospective identification of chyle leakage in patients undergoing lateral neck dissection for metastatic thyroid cancer. Ann Surg Oncol 2008; 15(2): 424–9.

35 Cappiello J, Piazza C, Giudice M, de Maria G, Nicolai P. Shoulder disability after different selective neck dissections (levels II–IV versus levels II–V): a comparative study. Laryngoscope 2005; 115(2): 259–63.

36 Van Wilgen CP, Dijkstra PU, van der Laan BF, Plukker JT, Roodenburg JL. Shoulder complaints after neck dissection; is the spinal accessory nerve involved? Br J Oral Maxillofac Surg 2003; 41(1): 7–11.

37 Koo BS, Choi EC, Yoon YH, Kim DH, Kim EH, Lim YC. Predictive factors for ipsilateral or contralateral central lymph node metastasis in unilateral papillary thyroid carcinoma. Ann Surg 2009; 249(5): 840–4.

38 Koo BS, Seo ST, Lee GH, Kim JM, Choi EC, Lim YC. Prophylactic lymphadenectomy of neck level II in clinically node-positive papillary thyroid carcinoma. Ann Surg Oncol 2010; 17(6): 1637–41.

39 Takes RP, Robbins KT, Woolgar JA, et al. Questionable necessity to remove the submandibular gland in neck dissection. Head Neck 2011; 33(5): 743–5.

40 Qubain SW, Nakano S, Baba M, Takao S, Aikou T. Distribution of lymph node micrometastasis in pN0 well-differentiated thyroid carcinoma. Surgery 2002; 131(3): 249–56.

41 Vayisoglu Y, Ozcan C, Turkmenoglu O, et al. Level IIb lymph node metastasis in thyroid papillary carcinoma. Eur Arch Otorhinolaryngol 2010; 267(7): 1117–21.

42 Patron V, Bedfert C, Le Clech G, Aubry K, Jegoux F. Pattern of lateral neck metastases in N0 papillary thyroid carcinoma. BMC Cancer 2011; 11: 8.

43 Kupferman ME, Weinstock YE, Santillan AA, *et al.* Predictors of level V metastasis in well-differentiated thyroid cancer. Head Neck 2008; 30(11): 1469–74.

44 MacFee W. Transverse incisions for neck dissection. Ann Surg 1960; 151(2): 279–84.

45 Man LX, Beswick DM, Johnson JT. Antibiotic prophylaxis in uncontaminated neck dissection. Laryngoscope 2011; 121(7): 1473–7.

46 Johnson JT, Wagner RL. Infection following uncontaminated head and neck surgery. Arch Otolaryngol Head Neck Surg 1987; 113(4): 368–9.

47 Miccoli P, Materazzi G, Fregoli L, Panicucci E, Kunz-Martinez W, Berti P. Modified lateral neck lymphadenectomy: prospective randomized study comparing harmonic scalpel with clamp-and-tie technique. Otolaryngol Head Neck Surg 2009; 140(1): 61–4.

Videoclips

This chapter contains the following videoclips. They can be accessed at: www.wiley.com/go/miccoli/thyroid

Video 9.1   Left selective neck dissection levels III–IV.
Video 9.2   Modified right lateral neck dissection.

CHAPTER 10

Surgery for Retrosternal/Upper Mediastinal Thyroid/Parathyroid Disease

Jeffrey J. Houlton and David L. Steward
Department of Otolaryngology – Head and Neck Surgery, University of Cincinnati – Academic Health Center, Cincinnati, OH, USA

Introduction

Operations of the upper mediastinum offer a unique challenge to the endocrine surgeon, largely because limited access into the thoracic cavity challenges one of the most important tenets of surgical technique – maintain adequate exposure. This chapter reviews the surgical management of endocrine disorders of the upper mediastinum, including benign and malignant diseases of the thyroid and parathyroid glands.

Thyroid

Substernal goitre represents the most common thyroid disorder of the upper mediastinum. The frequency of substernal goitre excision, reported as a percentage of thyroidectomies performed, ranges from 2% to 19% [1]. This range lacks precision largely because there is no clear consensus in the literature for what constitutes a substernal goitre. The two most common definitions are any goitre that descends below the plane of the thoracic inlet, and any thyroid goitre/nodule in which the volume is more than 50% contained within the mediastinum [2–5]. Other less inclusive definitions include a goitre with extension to the aortic arch or a goitre in which the largest diameter resides within the chest [6,7]. However, the authors have found the most clinically relevant definition to include any goitre whose inferior extent cannot be delineated on thyroid ultrasound because of interference from the clavicles (with the patient's neck in an extended position). This definition includes goitres that have displayed the inclination for unopposed growth into the chest, and those for which ultrasonographic imaging is inadequate, necessitating evaluation by computed tomography (CT).

Anatomy

Substernal goitres are classified as either primary or secondary. A primary substernal goitre refers to a congenital/ectopic thyroid goitre that originates in the thoracic cavity and is in discontinuity with the cervical thyroid. Primary substernal goitres are rare, constituting 0.2–1% of all substernal goitres [8,9]. Secondary substernal goitres are acquired goitres that originate in the cervical thyroid. As they grow, their anterior extension becomes limited by the strap muscles and they slowly descend through the planes of the cervical fascia into the thoracic cavity. Most secondary goitres remain in continuity with the cervical thyroid but rarely, as they descend, their attachments atrophy and either become completely separated from the cervical thyroid or remain

Thyroid Surgery: Preventing and Managing Complications, First Edition. Edited by Paolo Miccoli, David J. Terris, Michele N. Minuto and Melanie W. Seybt.

attached by only a thin fibrous stalk. Clinically, the most important anatomical distinction between primary and secondary substernal goitres is their blood supply. Secondary substernal goitres receive their blood supply from cervical vessels, primarily the inferior thyroid artery, and maintain this cervical blood supply throughout their descent into the chest. By rule, primary substernal goitres receive their blood supply from an intrathoracic source [8,9]. As such, accessing and extirpating primary substernal goitres through a cervical approach is inadvisable, if not impossible.

Approximately 85% of secondary substernal goitres descend into the anterior mediastinum, in a pre- or para-tracheal position, anterior to the recurrent laryngeal nerves (RLN) [1,10–12]. More challenging are the 10–15% of secondary substernal goitres that descend into the posterior mediastinum, displacing the carotid and RLNs anteriorly [1,10–12]. This posterior location is problematic as it puts the RLN at higher risk of injury due to inadvertent traction or transection when this relationship is not fully appreciated [11–13]. Posterior exposure is also more challenging and can even prove limited with a midline sternotomy. Thoracotomy may be necessary for complete access [5,7,8,11–13].

Presentation/evaluation

Substernal goitres most commonly present in the fifth and sixth decades of life and are generally the result of slow-growing, inferiorly descending, multinodular goitres (MNG) [1,3–4]. However, they may be the result of thyroid carcinoma, large solitary adenomas or, much less frequently, chronic lymphocytic thyroiditis [3,14]. Presentation is variable and up to 40% of patients are asymptomatic on initial evaluation [5]. Asymptomatic substernal goitres may be discovered as part of the workup for cervical MNGs, or may be found incidentally on radiological studies. Alternatively, substernal goitres can produce compressive symptoms through impingement of essentially any structure that traverses the thoracic inlet, including the trachea, oesophagus or a cadre of neurovascular structures. Tracheal compression resulting in positional or exertional dyspnoea is the most commonly presenting compressive symptom, present in 30–90% of patients [3,5,13,15]. Patients with tracheal compression commonly report an inability to sleep supine, but also may manifest intermittent cough, airway obstruction or audible stridor. Dysphagia resulting from oesophageal

compression is reported frequently (15–60%). Hoarseness from stretching or compression of the RLN (1–3%) may be present and should raise concerns about displacement of the nerve or potential malignancy [5,16–19]. Superior vena cava syndrome, resulting from vascular compression, occurs up to 5% of the time and may occasionally be induced when the patient is asked to raise their arms above their head, a manoeuvre called Pemberton's sign [5,20]. Rarely substernal goitres have been reported to result in compression of the phrenic nerve, cervical sympathetic chain and brachial plexus [19,21,22].

Substernal goitres are often discovered on ultrasono-graphic imaging. However, CT is the radiographic study of choice to define the intrathoracic extent of the gland. A non-contrasted study is generally sufficient and will avoid inducing hyperthyroidism from an iodine bolus in patients with subclinical disease, present in up to 25% of patients with MNG [23]. As such, a thyroid function profile should be obtained with the initial workup. Evaluation with fine needle aspiration (FNA) may prove difficult as access is limited by the sternum/clavicles, and is generally unneces-sary as surgical excision is indicated even for benign disease. However, an FNA may be helpful in the setting of a large dominant nodule or if the mass exhibits rapid growth or suspicious radiographic features, and may be performed in flexion and extension or in sitting-up and supine positions. Flow-volume loops, advocated by some authors to objectively assess obstructive airway symptoms, are generally unnecessary as asymptomatic lesions still require excision [16]. Radionuclide studies may be helpful in the workup of an isolated mediastinal mass to evaluate potential thyroid origin, though this is a rare presentation in an endocrine surgery practice. Other mediastinal masses that mimic primary or detached secondary substernal goi-tre include neurogenic tumours, thymomas (Figure 10.1), bronchogenic/pericardial cysts, lymphomas and tera-tomas [24]. Lastly, laryngoscopy to evaluate vocal cord function is recommended for all patients with substernal goitres prior to undergoing surgery. The incidence of pre-operative RLN palsy for benign substernal goitres is 1–3% and is higher for patients with malignant disease [18,19].

Treatment of substernal goitres

In terms of treatment, the diagnosis of substernal goitre is itself an indication for surgical excision, which is recommended even for asymptomatic lesions, except in elderly or medically infirm patients. This approach is

(a)

(b)

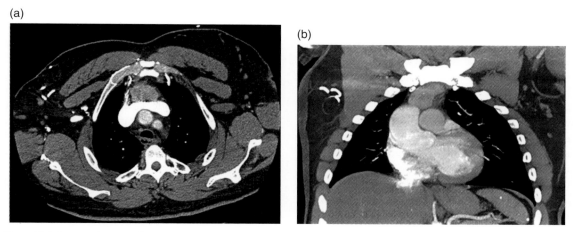

Figure 10.1 Contrasted computed tomography of the chest illustrating a partially enhancing upper mediastinal mass which extends to the level of the pulmonary artery and is separate from the cervical thyroid on axial (a) and coronal (b) views. The mass, originally thought to be consistent with a thymoma, was later found to be a detached secondary substernal goitre following sternotomy and excision by a thoracic surgeon.

justified for multiple reasons. First, the natural history of these lesions is persistent, albeit slow, growth into the chest once they have begun their descent. Even asymptomatic lesions are expected to become symptomatic and potentially life-threatening as time proceeds. As such, most patients presenting in their 50s and 60s are at their healthiest and most optimal age for surgery at presentation. Second, data suggest that substernal goitres have a low but not insignificant risk of carcinoma. In a large systematic review evaluating the risk of malignancy in patients presenting with substernal goitres, substernal goitres were found to herald malignancy in approximately 5–10% of patients [1]. This risk was not greater than that of cervical MNGs but once these lesions have begun their descent into the chest, serial surveillance, both cytologically and radiographically, becomes much more challenging. Lastly, as discussed below, medical alternatives to surgery have a very limited role in the management of substernal goitres.

Alternatives to surgery include observation, radioactive iodine (RAI) therapy and thyroid suppression with exogenous thyroid hormone. Observation is appropriate for patients who are poor surgical candidates, medically infirm or elderly patients who are asymptomatic and therefore unlikely to have their lifespan shortened by growth of a substernal goitre. A single treatment with radioactive iodine has been reported to reduce the volume of large compressive goitres by as

much as 30% [25,26]. However, RAI therapy has proven only moderately effective in relieving compressive symptoms and does not halt continued growth [25]. In addition, there is a theoretical concern that radiation thyroiditis may acutely worsen tracheal compression and lead to airway compromise. Radiation thyroiditis also has the potential to complicate future surgery by scarring tissue planes, an undesirable effect as transcervical substernal goitre excision relies heavily on smooth tissue planes for mobilization. While surgery is clearly the optimal therapy, RAI may be a reasonable option in the management of symptomatic elderly or infirm patients. Suppressive therapy with exogenous thyroid hormone is only minimally effective in reducing the size of substernal goitres [27]. In addition, suppressive therapy is not well tolerated in elderly or infirm patients, the exact population for whom a medical alternative to surgery would be beneficial [27]. As such, suppression with levothyroxine does not play a significant role in the management of substernal goitres.

Surgical management

The most important surgical consideration when excising substernal goitres is determining the likelihood of requiring a transthoracic approach. Almost always, substernal goitres can be mobilized from the chest through a cervical incision using gentle traction and blunt dissection and sternotomy is only very rarely required. Multiple retrospective studies, and several prospective case series, have attempted to determine the overall frequency of a thoracic approach for substernal goitre extirpation. Like most statistical analyses related to substernal goitres, however, the percentage of goitres which require a thoracic approach is largely dependent on how a substernal goitre is defined [1,5,6,10,11,16,17,28–30]. Netterville and associates defined a substernal goitre as a goitre with the majority of its volume residing within the chest, and reported requiring a thoracic approach in 15% of 150 patients undergoing excision [17]. In contrast, Cohen, using a similar definition, applied an extracervical approach in 4% of his 108-patient case series [5]. However, when a more inclusive definition of substernal goitre is used, such as any goitre that extends into the thoracic inlet, thoracic approach is required less than 2% of the time [1,28–30].

In order for substernal goitres to be mobilized transcervically, they must have smooth tissue planes that allow for easy blunt dissection, they must be small enough to fit through the thoracic inlet, and their bulk and blood supply must be accessible through the neck. Likewise, factors that limit a transcervical approach generally undermine one of these principles [1,4–13]. A 33-study systematic review by White et al. aimed to evaluate these factors [1]. They reported a significantly increased frequency of extracervical approach in the presence of an intrathoracic blood supply (primary substernal goitre), invasive malignancy, reoperation, substernal goitre extension past the aortic arch, and substernal goitre extension into the posterior mediastinum [1]. These factors are fairly intuitive and consistent with most other series, as invasive malignancies and reoperative goitres are frequently too 'sticky' to be bluntly mobilized, tumours that extend past the aortic arch may be too large to fit through the thoracic inlet, and substernal goitres with an intrathoracic blood supply or those that have significant posterior extension are difficult, if not impossible, to access through the neck [1,4–13].

In our personal experience, inferior extension below the aortic arch or into the posterior mediastinum warrants consultation with thoracic surgery but rarely requires a thoracic approach. In contrast, invasive malignancy with extrathyroidal extension into the mediastinum, primary substernal goitres or recurrent goitres generally do require a thoracic approach. Figure 10.2 illustrates a large right-sided substernal goitre that extends below the level of the aortic arch that was easily mobilized via a transcervical approach. In contrast, Figure 10.3 displays a malignant mediastinal goitre that invaded the serosa of the thoracic oesophagus and required a midline sternotomy for tumour excision.

Thoracic approaches for substernal thyroidectomy include the 'classic' midline sternotomy, mini-sternotomy or manubriotomy, and thoracotomy. In our experience, the mini-sternotomy almost always achieves adequate access to the upper mediastinum and is the least invasive of the three procedures. However, a complete midline sternotomy may be necessary for extremely large substernal goitres or malignancies. A thoracotomy is necessary for primary substernal goitres in the posterior mediastinum or for large or complex posterior descending secondary substernal goitres. It is possible to excise primary substernal goitres through an isolated thoracic procedure. However, a combined transcervical approach is necessary for all secondary substernal goitres, not only because most have a significant cervical component but also because their blood supply must be controlled through the neck.

Operative technique

The patient is positioned on top of a shoulder roll with the neck in extension to facilitate mobilization of the gland. Reverse Trendelenburg positioning will limit vascular engorgement and prove helpful during ligation of the superior pole vessels. A traditional low-collar incision is made in a horizontal neck crease. Subplatysmal skin flaps are raised superiorly and inferiorly in the plane of the superficial layer of the deep cervical fascia. The strap muscles are separated at the midline raphe down to their insertion at the manubrium. The sternothyroid muscle can be transected near its insertion on the thyroid cartilage to improve exposure superiorly and to improve mobility of large glands later on. The superior pole is isolated, the superior laryngeal nerve is identified and preserved, and the superior thyroid vasculature is ligated. The middle thyroid veins are isolated and divided.

At this juncture it is important to ensure that the RLN is not being displaced anteriorly by a posterior descending goitre. If a posterior goitre is suspected, the nerve can often be identified near its insertion point near the cricothyroid and inferior constrictor muscles posvterior to the superior pole. The exposed gland is placed under gentle traction with the Allis clamps. Alternatively, the gland may be retracted digitally by wrapping it in a moist

(a)

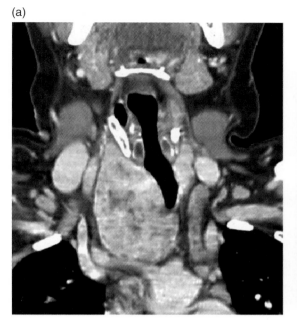

(b)

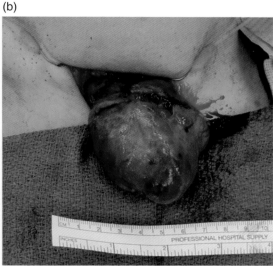

Figure 10.2 Contrasted coronal computed tomography (a) of a large right-sided substernal goitre extending to the level of the aortic arch. The accompanying intraoperative photo (b) illustrates uncomplicated mobilization from the chest.

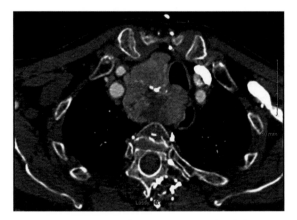

Figure 10.3 Contrasted axial computed tomography of a large invasive malignancy/mediastinal goitre involving the thoracic oesophagus. This lesion required midline sternotomy for resection.

sponge. Blunt dissection, in a plane posterior to the thyroid and the strap muscles, is employed to define the inferior extent of the goitre and an attempt is made to gently pull the goitre up and out of the chest. If the substernal goitre cannot be safely mobilized from the chest without tearing the gland, a sternotomy may be performed, though this is a rare occurrence. (Intracapsular morcellization has been advocated in the past for goitres that were too large to be mobilized through the thoracic inlet [7]. However, this technique is inadvisable due to risk of tumour spillage and, more importantly, because access for control of the expected haemorrhage is poor.) Following mobilization of the gland, the RLN and parathyroid glands are identified in the standard fashion (if not already delineated) and Berry's ligament is divided. Haemostasis is ensured and the wound is closed over a suction drain.

Surgery for malignant disease

Substernal goitre excisions for well-differentiated primary malignancies of the thyroid are similar to those for benign disease, though invasion of adjacent mediastinal structures more frequently necessitates sternotomy. As such, thoracic consultation is recommended for any patient with a cytologically malignant substernal goitre and when computed tomography does not reveal smooth tissue planes.

In terms of metastatic disease, the American Joint Committee on Cancer (AJCC) classifies metastatic disease of the superior mediastinum (level 7) as regional disease (N1b), not distant metastasis (M) [31]. This is consistent with anatomical evidence that reveals the superior mediastinal nodes to be in continuity with nodes of the central compartment [32]. However, few authors in the literature have formally advocated for superior mediastinal lymphadenectomy for grossly metastatic well-differentiated thyroid carcinoma of the upper mediastinum [32–34]. These several retrospective case series have generally described transcervical extirpation of gross mediastinal disease down to the level of the brachiocephalic vein/aortic arch without incurring significant morbidity (other than an increased incidence of hypocalcaemia) [32,33,35]. Yet neither the National Comprehensive Cancer Network (NCCN) nor the American Thyroid Association (ATA) makes formal recommendations for therapeutic superior mediastinal node dissection for grossly positive disease [36,37]. In addition, no studies have demonstrated a survival benefit of performing such an operation. As such, this practice has never been widely mandated, yet is generally performed to a variable degree as an extension of the central neck dissection.

We recommend performing superior mediastinal node dissection in continuity with central neck dissection for palpable metastatic disease, or disease larger than 1 cm, when it can be performed transcervically with low morbidity. This procedure is similar to the superior mediastinal dissection for recurrent or persistent hyperparathyroidism described below. Mediastinal lymphadenectomy that requires a sternotomy is generally not indicated even for persistent well-differentiated cancers that do not respond to RAI. Currently, no studies have justified the increased morbidity of sternotomy by any demonstrable survival benefit. Although it is conceivable that thoracic mediastinal dissection could be indicated on a palliative basis for disease causing significant airway compression, this is an uncommon scenario. There remains no defined role for extensive superior mediastinal node dissection on an elective basis (in the absence of gross disease), though we, like most authors, extend the central neck dissection to include substernal components to the level of the innominate artery.

Anaesthetic considerations

In our experience, even patients with large substernal goitres are almost always easily intubated transorally with a small-calibre endotracheal tube, quite anticlimactically.

However, anaesthetic induction should not be taken lightly and a dynamic collaboration with a trusted member of the anaesthetic team should be sought. Intubation can be complicated due to limited range of motion of the neck as well as the rare, but dreaded, inability to ventilate or intubate resulting from severe tracheal compression. In this situation, emergency tracheostomy is extremely difficult, as there is generally a significant cervical component to the goitre, and rigid bronchoscopy may be the most helpful means of securing an airway.

However, the best way of managing these airway emergencies is by avoiding them altogether. Patients with severe tracheal compression on CT scan, significant inspiratory stridor or severe supine dyspnoea should raise concerns about intubation difficulties. Awake flexible fibreoptic intubation is advocated in these higher risk cases so that spontaneous ventilation is maintained until the airway is secured without thoracic obstruction. If a more ominous airway situation is suspected, preparations for cardiopulmonary bypass can be considered prior to induction of anaesthesia. This can range from merely having femoro-femoral bypass available in an emergency to actually inserting arterial and venous catheters under local anaesthetic. These preparations are generally facilitated by the thoracic surgeon, who is undoubtedly involved in the care of any patient for whom bypass is being considered. Luckily, while it is important to consider these higher magnitude measures, they are rarely, if ever, needed [38].

Postoperative complications

Several studies indicate a higher overall morbidity/mortality, incidence of permanent hypoparathyroidism (0.5–5.8%) and incidence of RLN injury (0.9–14%) following substernal goitre excision compared to conventional thyroidectomy, though it is unclear how much sternotomy contributes to this morbidity [1,39]. The increased incidence of RLN injury is likely the result of anatomical distortion and it is critical to maintain a high suspicion that the nerve may be displaced anteriorly in order to avoid nerve injury.

Tracheomalacia, though difficult to define, is a unique complication of substernal goitre excision. When severe, it may require tracheostomy or tracheal resection, although in our experience the incidence of clinically significant tracheomalacia is quite infrequent. This is consistent with several series which report a low (0–5.8%)

incidence of tracheomalacia following substernal goitre excision, though tracheomalacia was reported as the most common indication for tracheostomy [1,40]. The risk of tracheomalacia was increased if the compressive goitre had been present for more than 5 years, was bilateral, caused significant tracheal compression or occurred in elderly patients [1,40].

Parathyroid

Over the last two decades the paradigm of parathyroid adenoma excision has shifted from routine four-gland exploration to the routine use of limited exploration for localized lesions. This shift is the result of significantly improved preoperative localization studies and the use of intraoperative parathyroid hormone (PTH) assays to confirm complete adenoma excision. However, even seemingly well-localized lesions can become fascinatingly challenging when ectopic adenomas, double adenomas, four-gland hyperplasia, supernumerary glands and false-positive localization studies are encountered. As such, each and every operation should be approached with the anticipation that a four-gland exploration, and potential superior mediastinal dissection, may be necessary.

Anatomical considerations

Ectopic parathyroid glands can be found superior to, inferior to, and along their embryological path of descent, from the angle of the mandible to the inferior pericardium, but are most commonly located within the anterior-superior mediastinum [41–43]. This mediastinal frequency is largely a contribution of the more commonly ectopic inferior glands, which arise within the thymus, perithymic tissue and thyrothymic ligament 5–7% of the time [41–43]. Inferior parathyroid glands, along with the thymus, are endodermal derivatives of the third pharyngeal pouch. These structures descend together from their peripharyngeal origin through the neck but separate as the inferior parathyroids halt at their orthotopic location, near the inferior pole of the thyroid, superficial to the RLN. Alternatively, inferior parathyroid glands may remain integrally involved with the thymus as it descends into the chest and become deeply embedded within the mediastinum or, more frequently, assume the aforementioned perithymic location. Similarly, supernumerary glands, which are present in up to 13% of patients, are located within the thymus two-thirds of the time [44].

The superior parathyroid glands are ectopically located within the posterior mediastinum 1% of the time [41,43]. The superior glands are endodermal derivatives of the fourth pharyngeal pouch. As such, they are located deep to the inferior glands and recurrent laryngeal nerve. This relationship is generally maintained even with ectopic glands. Superior glands are less variable in their location and less frequently ectopic compared to inferior glands, a feature generally attributed to their shorter descent during embryogenesis. Ectopic superior glands are most frequently retro-oesophageal, intrathyroidal, posterior mediastinal or located within the carotid sheath [41,42].

Indications for mediastinal dissection

Historically, before the widespread advent of preoperative localization, mediastinal dissection via sternotomy was indicated for any patient for whom a thorough cervical exploration for primary hyperparathyroidism was unrevealing or unsuccessful. This not infrequently included single-staged explorations of the neck followed by sternal splitting. Yet sternotomy failed to identify parathyroid pathology in at least 30% of patients [45]. Under the current paradigm, thoracic approaches for non-localized parathyroid disease are seldom employed and preoperative localization is considered mandatory prior to opting for sternotomy/deep mediastinal exploration. However, transcervical approaches to the superior mediastinum are still considered a mandatory tool in the endocrine surgeon's arsenal and are employed with relative frequency for parathyroid glands localized to the mediastinum or for 'missing' parathyroids.

Transcervical mediastinal dissection generally includes an anterior-superior dissection in combination with thymectomy. This approach is employed when an inferior parathyroid gland is 'missing' during exploration for an adenoma, when a subtotal parathyroidectomy (3½ gland excision) for hyperplasia fails to lower intraoperative PTH appropriately, and essentially any time primary hyperparathyroidism persists or recurs following four-gland exploration. Cervical thymectomy is also recommended for patients with MEN-1 and primary hyperparathyroidism given their propensity for hyperplasia and supernumerary glands. Posterior-superior mediastinal dissection is less frequently necessary and employed when an ectopic superior gland is missing or as a last step for a missing supernumerary gland. Mediastinal dissection is clearly indicated for disease that localizes to the mediastinum and, as discussed below, may infrequently require a thoracic approach.

Non-localized lesions

Our approach to localization starts with family history, biochemical workup and office ultrasound. If an obvious lesion exists on ultrasound and the diagnosis of primary hyperparathyroidism is confirmed, one-gland exploration is offered with possible conversion to bilateral exploration. If the ultrasound is equivocal or non-localizing, we then evaluate with sestamibi-single photon emission CT (SPECT) imaging. A dual-isotope sestamibi subtraction study can occasionally be useful for patients with cervical goitre but is of no additional value for mediastinal parathyroids unless a substernal goitre is present. If both the sestamibi imaging and the ultrasound are non-localizing, a situation that occurs around 10% of the time, four-gland exploration is offered [46]. We also reconfirm the biochemical workup to ensure that the diagnosis of primary hyperparathyroidism is correct. This should include an intact PTH assay, total calcium, serum albumin, vitamin D level and fractional excretion of calcium ratio or 24-h urine calcium collection to evaluate for familial hypocalciuric hypercalcaemia (FHH). We have found sestamibi-SPECT/CT fusion studies to be occasionally helpful for otherwise non-localizing lesions and most useful for evaluating mediastinal parathyroids. This is consistent with several studies that have shown SPECT/CT fusion to be a superior localization study compared to both sestamibi-SPECT and planar imaging [47–49]. SPECT/CT was also more sensitive and specific in localizing lesions of the mediastinum [47,49]. An obvious mediastinal parathyroid adenoma that was otherwise non-localizing is displayed in Figure 10.4. High-resolution CT, magnetic resonance imaging (MRI) and, rarely, selective venous sampling can also be used to evaluate the mediastinum.

Our general approach to four-gland exploration starts with unilateral dissection. If a suspicious lesion is not identified, the contralateral neck is explored. If all four glands are identified and not significantly abnormal, a decision is made whether four-gland hyperplasia is likely or whether a supernumerary adenoma exists. If hyperplasia is suspected, frozen sections are sent for pathological evaluation of hypercellularity. If a supernumerary adenoma is suspected then cervical thymectomy is performed. Mediastinal dissection is also performed as

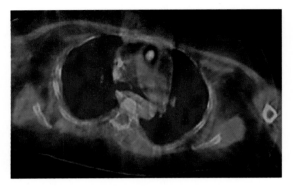

Figure 10.4 A sestamibi-SPECT/CT fusion study of an anterior mediastinal parathyroid adenoma which was otherwise non-localizing. This adenoma was resected via a transcervical approach.

a first step for a missing inferior gland. We find it far easier to evaluate the thymic contents by examining the specimen following anterior-superior mediastinal dissection, rather than exploring the thymic contents *in vivo*, unless the adenoma is readily apparent. If the anterior mediastinal dissection is unrewarding then our systematic exploration for a supernumerary adenoma continues to include the retro-oesophageal area, carotid sheath and posterior superior mediastinum. A hemithyroidectomy is not performed unless a suspicious lesion is present on office ultrasonography. Posterior mediastinal dissection is performed as the final step in exploration or when a superior parathyroid gland is missing. This includes exploring the mediastinal trachea and oesophagus as far as is feasible through the cervical incision.

Localized lesions

Parathyroid adenomas that localize to the superior mediastinum are most frequently accessed using a transcervical approach, as discussed below. However, up to 2% of all adenomas will require a thoracic approach. Several authors have cited anatomical landmarks which aid in determining the necessity for a thoracic approach, and have variably recommended that lesions located inferior to the manubrium, brachiocephalic vein or aortic arch be approached extracervically [50–53]. We have found glands located superior to the brachiocephalic vein to be easily accessible through a cervical approach. However, exposure inferior to the brachiocephalic vein is more difficult, although frequently dissection to the level of the aortic arch is possible utilizing anterior suspension, sternal or clavicular traction, and posterior displacement of the brachiocephalic vessels. If transcervical access is equivocal (i.e. if the adenoma is located below the brachiocephalic vein or if preoperative location is unclear) then we recommend approaching mediastinal exploration in a similar fashion to substernal goitre excision.

Access is first attempted via a cervical approach. If the adenoma is found to be too deep to expose, a mini-sternotomy is performed by a thoracic surgeon. If an adenoma is located within the aortic-pulmonary window or deep in the mediastinum, clearly sternotomy or thoracotomy is necessary and generally performed as an isolated thoracic approach. Classically, these deep mediastinal adenomas were accessed utilizing a median sternotomy; however, more recently video-assisted thoracoscopic (VATS) approaches have been used with a high rate of success [51–53]. VATS is performed with lower morbidity and is reported to be particularly useful for posterior adenomas located in the inferior mediastinum [51–53].

Anterior-superior mediastinal dissection

The patient is positioned in slight reverse-Trendelenburg and the neck is placed in extension. A Rultract Skyhook™ sternal retractor is set up for potential use following sterile draping. An incision is made within a horizontal skin crease superior to the sternal notch, unless a pre-existing incision exists. Superior and inferior subplatysmal skin flaps are raised in the plane of the superficial layer of the deep cervical fascia and distracted with a self-retaining retractor. The strap muscles are separated at the midline raphe down to the sternal notch and retracted laterally. The thymus is generally located just anterior to the brachiocephalic vessels. The thymic tissue is grasped with Allis clamps and traction is placed superomedially. Intrathymic parathyroid glands are fairly easily removed with blunt dissection following cervical delivery of the thymus. However, extrathymic, or unidentified, mediastinal parathyroid glands require a much more thorough dissection.

For thorough dissection, the carotid is traced to the brachiocephalic or subclavian artery and the RLNs are identified. Once the lateral dissection is finished, a thymectomy retractor may be used to facilitate inferior dissection. We prefer to use the Rultract Skyhook™ sternal retractor as described by Sukumar *et al.* and have found it

to be a helpful adjunct when avoiding sternotomy [54]. Inferior venous tributaries are ligated (we prefer to use the Harmonic Focus™) as they feed into the brachiocephalic vein and the thymus is bluntly separated from the innominate attachments. Using Allis clamps for superior traction, the specimen is separated from the pretracheal fascia with blunt dissection and the thyrothymic attachments are transected, if not previously released. The specimen is assessed and sent for pathological evaluation. The wound is closed in layers, typically without the use of a suction drain.

Posterior mediastinal dissection

If a localized adenoma exists in the posterior-superior mediastinum, a similar horizontal incision is made and the strap muscles are divided in the midline in the traditional central approach. Alternatively, a more lateral approach medial to the sternocleidomastoid muscle (SCM) and lateral to the strap muscles can be utilized. The lower SCM is skeletonized and the jugular vein and carotid artery are identified and retracted laterally. Blunt dissection proceeds dorsally to identify the trachea, RLN, oesophagus and prevertebral fascia. Army-Navy retractors are used to retract anteriorly along the trachea and oesophagus. No sharp dissection takes place and no vascular structures are ligated. The adenoma is palpated or identified visually and gently removed with an upward spreading motion using tonsil forceps. Superior traction with a Babcock forceps may be useful but disruption of the capsule should be avoided because of possible tumour spillage. Haemostasis is ensured and the wound is closed in layers, generally without the use of a suction drain.

Complications

Prevention of complications from superior mediastinal surgery necessitates thorough knowledge of the anatomy and embryology of the region, accurate preoperative imaging, and an emphasis on blunt dissection with appropriate traction/countertraction technique. Four-gland explorations result in higher rates of permanent hypocalcaemia compared to limited exploration. This is also true for bilateral explorations that include superior mediastinal dissection as glands are frequently devascularized during exploration and tracing of the RLN. Great care should be taken to preserve the vascular pedicle of the normal parathyroid glands. If a gland looks particularly dusky or if its blood supply becomes obviously violated, the gland should be auto-transplanted. The RLN is also at greater risk during mediastinal dissection as a longer section of the nerve is delineated.

Conclusion

Upper mediastinal surgery offers a unique challenge to the endocrine surgeon, largely because exposure through a cervical approach can prove difficult. Substernal goitres should be evaluated with CT and, when descent into the thoracic inlet is confirmed, surgical excision is appropriate. The vast majority of substernal goitres are easily excised via a transcervical approach. Substernal goitres that have an intrathoracic blood supply (primary substernal goitres), are invasively malignant, have been previously operated, extend past the aortic arch or reside within the posterior mediastinum are more likely to require a thoracic approach.

Operations performed for primary hyperparathyroidism, even for seemingly well-localized lesions, should be approached with the potential need for four-gland exploration, which may involve superior mediastinal dissection. Ectopic parathyroid glands are most frequently located in the thymus and perithymic tissue. Cervical thymectomy followed by evaluation of the specimen is far easier than *in vivo* exploration of the thymus if an adenoma is not readily visualized. Thoracic approaches to the mediastinum are rarely employed for non-localized parathyroid adenomas but may be necessary for localized lesions located inferior to the brachiocephalic vein if inaccessible through a cervical approach. SPECT/CT fusion is the most useful localization study for evaluating mediastinal adenomas.

Lastly, collaborative relationships with thoracic surgery must be stressed and are considered critical to successful endocrine surgery of the upper mediastinum.

References

1 White ML, Doherty GM, Gauger PG. Evidence-based surgical management of substernal goiter. World J Surg 2008; 32: 1285–300.

2 Hedayati N, McHenry CR. The clinical presentation and operative management of nodular and diffused substernal thyroid disease. Am J Surg 2002; 68: 245–52.

3 Allo MD, Thompson NW. Rationale for the operative management of substernal goiters. Surgery 1983; 94: 969–77.

4 Katlic MR, Wand C, Grillo HC. Substernal goiter. Ann Thorac Surg 1985; 39: 391–9.

5 Cohen JP. Substernal goiters and sternotomy. Laryngoscope 2009; 119: 683–8.

6 Vadasz P, Kotis L. Surgical aspects of 175 mediastinal goiters. Eur J Cardiothorac Surg 1998; 14: 393–7.

7 Lahey FH. Intrathoracic goiters. Surg Clin North Am 1945; 25: 609–18.

8 Foroulis CN, Rammos KS, Sileli MN, Papakonstantinou D. Primary intrathoracic goiter: a rare and potentially serious entity. Thyroid 2009; 19: 213–18.

9 Hall TS, Caslowitz P, Popper C. Substernal goiter versus intrathoracic aberrant thyroid: a critical difference. Ann Thorac Surg 1988; 46: 684–5.

10 Katlic MR, Grillo HC, Wang CA. Substernal goiter: analysis of 80 patients at Massachusetts General Hospital. Am J Surg 1985; 149: 283.

11 De Andrade MA. A review of 128 cases of posterior mediastinal goiter. World J Surg 1977; 1: 789–94.

12 Shahian DM, Rossi RL. Posterior mediastinal goiter. Chest 1988; 94: 599–602.

13 Landreneau RJ, Nawarawong W, Boley TM, Johnson JA, Curtis JJ. Intrathoracic goiter: approaching the posterior mediastinal mass. Ann Thorac Surg 1991; 52: 134–6.

14 Nervi M, Iacconi P, Spinelli C, Janni A, Miccoli P. Thyroid carcinoma in intrathoracic goiter. Langenbecks Arch Surg 1998; 383: 337–9.

15 Shaha AR, Burnett C, Alfonso A, Jaffe BM. Goiters and airway problems. Am J Surg 1989; 158: 378–81.

16 Shaha AR, Alfonso AE, Jaffe BM. Operative treatment of substernal goiters. Head Neck 1989; 11: 325–30.

17 Netterville JL, Coleman SC, Smith JC, Smith MM, Kay TA, Burkey BB. Management of substernal goiter. Laryngoscope 1998; 108: 1611–17.

18 Rowe-Jones JM, Rosswick RP, Leighton SE. Benign thyroid disease and vocal cord palsy. Ann Roy Coll Surg 1993; 75: 241–4.

19 Anders HJ. Compression syndromes caused by substernal goiters. Postgrad Med J 1998; 74: 327–9.

20 Lowry SR, Shinton RA, Jamieson G, Manche A. Benign multinodular goitre and reversible Horner's syndrome. BMJ 1988; 296: 529–30.

21 Manning PB, Thompson NW. Bilateral phrenic nerve palsy associated with benign goiter. Acta Chir Scand 1989; 155: 429–30.

22 Marcelino M, Nobre E, Conceicao J, et al. Superior vena cava syndrome and substernal goiter. Thyroid 2010; 20: 235–6.

23 Rieu M, Bekka S, Sambor B, Berrod JL, Fombeur JP. Prevalence of subclinical hyperthyroidism and relationship between thyroid hormonal status and thyroid ultrasono-

graphic parameters in patients with non-toxic nodular goiter. Clin Endocrinol 1993; 39: 67–71.

24 Blegvad S, Lippert H, Simper LB, Dybdahl H. Mediastinal tumours: a report of 129 cases. Scand J Thorac Cardiovasc Surg 1990; 24: 39.

25 Bonnema SJ, Knudsen DU, Bertelsen H, et al. Does radioiodine therapy have an equal effect on substernal and cervical goiters volumes? Evaluation by magnetic resonance imaging. Thyroid 2002; 12: 313–17.

26 Huysmans D, Hermus RM, Corstens F, Barentsz JO, Kloppengorg PW. Large, compressive goiters treated with radioiodine. Ann Intern Med 1994; 121: 757–62.

27 Shimaoka K, Sokal JE. Suppressive therapy of nontoxic goiter. Am J Med 1974; 57: 576.

28 Chauhan A, Serpell JW. Thyroidectomy is safe and effective for retrosternal goiter. ANZ J Surg 76: 238–42.

29 Hedayati N, McHenry CR. The clinical presentation and operative management of nodular and diffuse substernal thyroid disease. Am Surg 2002; 68: 245–51.

30 Hsu B, Reeve TS, Guinea AI et al. Recurrent substernal nodular goiter: incidence and management. Surgery 1996; 120: 1072–5.

31 Edge SB, Byrd DR, Compton CC, Fritz AG, Greene FL, Trotti A. AJCC Cancer Staging Manual, 6th edn . Berlin: Springer, 2010.

32 Khoo ML, Freeman JL. Transcervical superior mediastinal lymphadenectomy in the management of papillary thyroid carcinoma. Head Neck 2003; 25: 10–14.

33 Block MA, Miller JM, Horn RC. Significance of mediastinal lymph node metastases in carcinoma of the thyroid. Am J Surg 1972; 123: 702–5.

34 Zhang Q, Guo ZM, Fu JH, et al. Clinical evaluation of management of superior mediastinal metastasis from thyroid carcinoma with systemic superior mediastinal dissection via sternotomy approach: 12 cases report. Ai Zheng 2004; 23: 842–4.

35 Ducic Y, Oxford L. Transcervical elective superior mediastinal dissection for thyroid carcinoma. Am J Otolaryngol 2009; 30: 221–4.

36 NCCN. Clinical practice guidelines in oncology – thyroid carcinoma. Available at: www.nccn.org.

37 Cooper DS, Doherty GM, Haugen BR et al. Revised American Thyroid Association management guidelines for patients with thyroid nodules and differentiated thyroid cancer. Thyroid 2009; 19: 1167–214.

38 Gothard JWW. Anesthetic considerations for patients with anterior mediastinal masses. Anesthesiol Clin 2008; 26: 305–14.

39 Pieracci FM, Fahey TJ. Substernal thyroidectomy is associated with increased morbidity and mortality as compared with conventional cervical thyroidectomy. J Am Coll Surg 2007; 205: 1–7.

40 Shen WR, Kebebew E, Duh QY, Clark OH. Predictors of airway complications after thyroidectomy for substernal goiter. Arch Surg 2004; 139: 656–60.

41 Phitayakorn R, McHenry CR. Incidence and location of ectopic abnormal parathyroid glands. Am J Surg 2006; 191: 418–23.

42 Fancy T, Gallagher D, Hornig JD. Surgical anatomy of the thyroid and parathyroid glands. Otolaryngol Clin North Am 2010; 43: 221–7.

43 Akerstrom G, Malmaeus J, Bergstom R. Surgical anatomy of human parathyroid glands. Surgery 1984; 95: 14–21.

44 Wang C. The anatomic basis of parathyroid surgery. Ann Surg 1976; 183: 271–5.

45 Wang C, Gaz RD, Mondure AC. Mediastinal parathyroid exploration: a clinical and pathologic study of 47 cases. World J Surg 1986; 10: 687–95.

46 Siperstein A, Berber E, Barbosa GF, et al. Predicting the success of limited exploration for primary hyperparathyroidism using ultrasound, sestamibi, and intraoperative parathyroid horomone. Ann Surg 2008; 248: 420–8.

47 Akram K, Parker JA, Donohoe K, Kolodny G. Role of single photon emission computed tomography/computed tomography in localization of ectopic parathyroid adenoma: a pictorial case series and review of the current literature. Clin Nucl Med 2009; 34: 500–2.

48 Lavely WC, Goetze S, Friedman KP. Comparison of SPECT/CT, SPECT, and planar imaging with single- and dual-phase (99 m) Tc-sestamibi parathyroid scintigraphy. J Nucl Med 2007; 48: 1084–9.

49 Mullan BP. Nuclear medicine imaging of the parathyroid. Otolaryngol Clin North Am 2004: 37; 909–39.

50 Wells SA, Cooper JD. Closed mediastinal exploration in patients with persistent hyperparathyroidism. Ann Surg 1991; 214: 555–61.

51 Nwariaku FE, Snyder WH, Burkey SH, Watumull L, Mattews D. Inframanubrial parathyroid glands in patients with primary hyperparathyroidism: alternatives to sternotomy. World J Surg 2005; 29: 491–4.

52 Liu RC, Hill ME, Ryan JA. One-gland exploration for mediastinal parathyroid adenomas: cervical and thoracoscopic approaches. Am J Surg 2005; 189: 601–5.

53 Nilubol N, Beyer T, Prinz RA, Solorzano CC. Mediastinal hyperfunctioning parathyroids: incidence, evolving treatment, and outcome. Am J Surg 2007; 194: 53–6.

54 Sukumar MS, Komanapalli CB, Cohen JI. Minimally invasive management of the mediastinal parathyroid adenoma. Laryngoscope 2006; 116: 482–7.

CHAPTER 11

Reoperative Thyroid Surgery

N. Gopalakrishna Iyer[1] *and Ashok R. Shaha*[2]

[1] Department of Surgical Oncology, National Cancer Centre, Singapore
[2] Department of Surgery, Memorial Sloan-Kettering Cancer Center, New York, NY, USA

Introduction

One of the major challenges in thyroid surgery is in performing reoperative procedures in the neck. Apart from technical difficulties in operating in a hostile neck, the procedure can be further made difficult by the nature of the disease, previous surgical procedure (adequate versus inadequate) and other treatment modalities that may alter anatomy [1]. Complications are mainly related to the extent of recurrent disease, indications for reoperative surgery, proximity of recurrent disease to the recurrent laryngeal nerve and other important structures and adjuvant treatment modalities that have been used before [2]. In this regard, it is critical to avoid revision thyroid surgery as far as possible by performing the optimum surgical procedure during the initial thyroid surgery. Common indications for reoperative thyroid or neck surgery include (Box 11.1): inadequate primary surgery for benign or malignant disease, recurrent benign disease and recurrent malignant disease. This chapter will focus on the indications for reoperative surgery and technical considerations when reaccessing the neck.

Anatomical considerations

There are a number of anatomical considerations that should always be borne in mind when approaching the previously operated neck. Anatomical planes are usually less apparent, even more so if the patient has undergone prior treatment with external beam radiation or radioac-

> **Box 11.1 Indications for reoperative thyroid surgery**
>
> *Benign disease*
> Bleeding or haematoma
> Thyroid nodularity after initial thyroid lobectomy
> Recurrent thyroid nodularity after previous subtotal thyroidectomy for nodular goiter
> Recurrent Graves' disease after subtotal thyroidectomy
>
> *Recurrent or inadequately treated malignant pathology*
> Completion thyroidectomy after initial diagnosis of thyroid carcinoma and ipsilateral thyroid lobectomy
> Recurrent thyroid cancer in the thyroid bed
>
> *Reoperations for nodal disease*
> Lateral neck nodes (either clinically palpable or seen on ultrasound)
> Surgical exploration for persistent hypercalcitonaemia after initial surgery for medullary thyroid cancer

tive iodine. Some patients also undergo a more extensive fibrotic reaction than others, resulting in dissection through extensive scar tissue with adhesions between various structures in the neck. Important landmarks and vessels may be displaced by an absent thyroid gland. For example, the internal jugular vein or carotid artery may be in a more medial position. Similarly, the recurrent laryngeal nerve can be hitched up to the anterior surface of the thyroid. This is made worse if the tubercle of Zuckerkandl

---

Thyroid Surgery: Preventing and Managing Complications, First Edition. Edited by Paolo Miccoli, David J. Terris,
Michele N. Minuto and Melanie W. Seybt.
© 2013 John Wiley & Sons, Ltd. Published 2013 by John Wiley & Sons, Ltd.

is left behind during a subtotal thyroidectomy, which subsequently hypertrophies, pushing the nerve anteriorly. Reoperative surgery in this situation puts the nerve at much greater risk of injury that in the primary setting. The parathyroid glands may also be difficult to identify, but often fall laterally and hence may be safe during dissection.

Recurrent benign disease

Recurrent benign thyroid disease can usually be divided into those arising from inadequate surgery in the first instance and 'true recurrence'. A significant proportion of patients with recurrent benign disease likely had undergone partial or subtotal thyroidectomy procedures, which were common in the past. In patients with nodular goitre, recurrence in the contralateral lobe or in remnant thyroid tissue resulted in reoperative rates of up to 22% in some series, prompting prominent thyroid surgeons to favour total thyroidectomy in patients with multinodular goitres or Graves' disease [3]. In patients with recurrent hyperthyroidism from Graves' disease who had undergone a subtotal thyroidectomy, radioactive iodine ablation may be a safer option than reoperative surgery in most cases. In patients who have previously undergone a thyroid lobectomy presenting with contralateral recurrence, most of the issues associated with reoperative surgery can be avoided by not accessing the previously operated thyroid bed, and restricting the dissection to the side of the recurrence. Recurrent disease may also be confined to thyroid tissue left behind from inadequate clearance of the thyroid gland, and this includes the pyramidal lobe or thyrothymic tract. Recurrent disease in the pyramidal lobe can be removed easily, while recurrent retrosternal disease may be more difficult to remove, especially if it extends beyond the manubrio-sternal angle. The absence of a thyroid gland in the neck may potentially make it difficult to pull the gland out and deliver it into the neck, and the surgeon should be prepared to perform a sternotomy if necessary.

Recurrent malignant disease

While the incidence of differentiated thyroid cancer has increased, overall outcome remains excellent with disease-specific survival rates in the range 92–98% at 10 years and 84–94% at 40 years. The large majority of patients respond well to initial treatment with low risk for death and recurrence. Notwithstanding this, most series suggest that disease recurrence is seen in 10–30% of patients [4,5]. These rates are variable as they often depend on the definition of disease recurrence (thyroglobulinaemia versus structurally identifiable disease) or the distinction between persistent and recurrent disease. The rate of recurrence also depends on the histological subtype: well-differentiated, papillary or minimally invasive follicular thyroid cancers have lower recurrence rates (5–20%), compared to patients with widely invasive follicular or Hurthle cell carcinomas or aggressive variants of papillary carcinoma such as tall cell or insular carcinomas where recurrence rates are 25–73% [6–9].

Recurrence can be defined merely by increasing thyroglobulin levels (hyperthyroglobulinaemia) with no defined disease identifiable or structural disease seen on imaging. Structural disease recurrence can be broadly classified as local, regional or distant metastases. Cervical nodal metastasis in the lateral compartment is the most common presentation, representing 85% of cases, followed by local recurrence in the thyroid bed (including central compartment and superior mediastinal disease), seen in 32% of recurrent thyroid cancers [10]. Distant metastases represent 12% of all recurrences and tend to be discovered most frequently in the lung (50%), followed by bone (25%), lungs and bone (20%) and other sites (5%) [11–13].

Investigations and evaluation

The role of investigative modalities is to define the recurrent disease, identify any variations in anatomy due to previous surgery and identify any complications from previous surgery.
- *Ultrasound.* High-resolution imaging of the neck can be achieved with visualization of the thyroid bed and lateral neck compartments. Ultrasound-guided fine needle aspiration (FNA) biopsy is a useful adjunct to confirm or refute recurrent malignant disease, if applicable.
- *Cross-sectional imaging – computed tomography (CT) scans or magnetic resonance imaging (MRI).* Cross-sectional imaging is important to evaluate either bulky or large-volume recurrences or in situations where the anatomy may be altered [14]. This is also important if recurrence extends down to the mediastinum.

• *Fibreoptic laryngoscopy.* The vocal cords should be evaluated in all patients with recurrent disease where surgical exploration is contemplated (even in patients with normal voice) [1,15]. Pre-existing vocal cord paralysis may influence surgical decision with regard to clearing the contralateral paratracheal region and intraoperative nerve monitoring.

• *Positron emission tomography (PET) scan.* Routine use is not indicated in the long-term follow-up of patients. Scenarios where it may be useful include patients with rising thyroglobulin levels and no disease seen on ultrasound or RAI scans and those with metastatic disease. The extent of fluorodeoxyglucose (FDG) avidity and standard uptake values are also important prognostic markers in patients with both locoregional recurrence and distant metastatic disease [16].

Surgical principles

General

Patient safety is always paramount when contemplating reoperative surgery to the neck, and there are a number of considerations to keep in mind. First and foremost, the indications for surgery need to be carefully considered. In benign disease, reoperative surgery should be limited in patients who are symptomatic or toxic or those with potentially malignant disease. For patient who have recurrent Graves' disease, due consideration should be given to RAI ablation, to avoid surgery, Similarly, in patients with equivocal FNA results of a follicular lesion, a watchful waiting approach may be indicated when operating in a previously dissected thyroid bed. Even for likely tumour recurrence, the American Thyroid Association (ATA) suggests a more conservative approach as the detection of small, subcentimetre nodules in the thyroid bed and/or small lymph node metastases with borderline thyroglobulin (Tg) levels is becoming a common clinical dilemma [17]. Given the indolent nature of these low-volume lesions, there is questionable value in risking such patients to the surgical complications. The general philosophy is to reassess these patients with serial Tg levels and repeat ultrasound at 6–12-month intervals [1,18]. If there is no progression in size of the subcentimetre nodules or Tg levels, these patients may be safely observed without any intervention.

Certainly the best scenario for reoperative surgery is when the surgeon has performed the first procedure himself or herself. Otherwise, the surgeon should make every attempt to obtain the operative notes of the primary procedure, or communicate with the first surgeon as to the procedure itself, particularly the status of the recurrent laryngeal nerve, parathyroid gland and any variations in anatomy noted during the first procedure. A helpful adjunct in the reoperative setting is the use of nerve monitoring systems to permit easier identification of the recurrent laryngeal nerve, and to avoid nerve injury, but these are no substitutes for actual identification, dissection and tracing the nerve completely.

Local/thyroid bed disease

Recurrent disease (benign or malignant) in the central compartment or thyroid bed tends to be more difficult to manage, due to scarring from the previous dissection in the area, RAI therapy or external beam irradiation [19]. Moreover, if recurrent malignant disease is found to be locally invasive, a more aggressive approach may be needed [20,21]. This may require radical resection of the recurrent laryngeal nerve, trachea, cricotracheal complex, oesophageal musculature, larynx (laryngectomy) and/or pharynx (pharyngolaryngectomy). In contrast, contraindications to surgical extirpation should always be borne in mind and excluded when considering radical procedures. These include patient factors that preclude surgical intervention, extensive tumour invasion involving the prevertebral musculature and carotid encasement. In addition, there is little value in extensive surgery if there is clear evidence of transformation to undifferentiated or anaplastic cancer.

Technical considerations

There are several issues to consider when planning or executing reoperative surgery in the central compartment. In most cases, the surgical incision can be placed over the previous scar; this may require some extension if better exposure is required. The key component of reoperative surgery in the central compartment is vigilance to prevent injury to the recurrent laryngeal nerve. Nerve monitoring is an important and useful adjunct in identifying and preserving the recurrent laryngeal nerve [2,22]. But whether it is available or not, it is important to approach the central compartment with care, dissect bluntly, cut only structures that are well identified and attempt to identify the nerve before any major surgery is done.

It is important to understand the surgical anatomy of the nerve in a postthyroidectomy patient. On the right side, it often assumes an oblique path to reach the tracheo-oesophageal groove, while it tends to be more longitudinal on the left. It may be hitched up to the anterolateral edge of the trachea, or may be displaced laterally from previous surgery. Sometimes, a retrograde approach may be required to identify the nerve in the region of Berry's ligament, just inferior to the cricothyroid muscle. However, one has to bear in mind that the nerve may be bifid, and this approach may risk inadvertent injury to one of the branches. One option when dealing with unilateral disease recurrence is to avoid dissecting the contralateral paratracheal region and avoid the risk of injuring the contralateral nerve altogether. A further issue to consider is the persistence or recurrence of nodal disease along the trachea into the superior mediastinum. Long-standing disease may be associated with neovascularization from the innominate vessels, and care should be taken to dissect this out of the mediastinum. The Harmonic® scalpel (Harmonic Technology, Ethicon Endosurgery) is a useful tool to perform this dissection with adequate haemostasis, but the surgeon should always be aware of the location of the innominate vein and artery when performing this manoeuvre. Adherent or extensive disease in this region may necessitate a median sternotomy or clamshell approach to allow a formal nodal dissection of all mediastinal compartments, and a thoracic surgeon should be involved in this setting.

Lateral neck disease from thyroid cancer

Lateral compartment nodal metastases represent the most common site of recurrent malignant disease, and can be easily managed with an appropriate neck dissection, with minimal morbidity. In some cases, patients may develop recurrent neck disease after a prior lateral neck dissection. In this situation, reoperative neck surgery is technically more challenging, and should be performed by surgeons familiar with reoperative surgery in a hostile neck [2].

There are a number of pitfalls to reoperative surgery in the neck apart from the usual complications which patients should be made aware of. First is the possibility that the abnormal node may not be found during reoperative surgery, especially if the node is small. Second, re-do neck dissections may not clear all nodal tissue and patients may develop further lymphadenopathy in the future. Similarly, thyroglobulin levels may not normalize if there is residual microscopic disease, and in these circumstances patients may not achieve biochemical cure [1].

Alternative strategies to eradicate nodal metastases in the hostile neck include the use of radiofrequency ablation (RFA) or percutaneous injection of ethanol under ultrasound guidance, directly ablating the abnormal lymph node [23,24]. While the results of these studies appear to be promising for both techniques, patient numbers are small with limited follow-up data.

Technical considerations

The aim when dealing with lateral neck disease is to perform an appropriate clearance of the neck, which usually comprises a selective neck dissection clearing levels IIA–III and IV. Clearance of levels I, IIB and V should only be considered if there is nodal disease in these regions. In patients who have not undergone surgery in the lateral neck, this procedure is not technically challenging as it usually involves a virgin field. Nevertheless, there are a few considerations to bear in mind. The dissection can often be completed with an extension of the thyroidectomy incision horizontally across a lower neck skin crease. Unless the neck is long and there is high level II disease, it is unnecessary to extend the incision upwards to the mastoid in a 'hockey stick' manner. The latter often results in an unsightly scar from the vertical component of the incision, which can also be symptomatic.

During the dissection, it is important to preserve most of the neck structures, including the sternocleidomastoid muscle, internal jugular vein (IJV), accessory, phrenic and vagus nerve and cervical plexus branches. If the nodes are adherent to the IJV, they can usually be shaved off easily or removed with a cuff of the vein, which can then be repaired primarily. Care should be taken when dissecting nodes in the lower level IV region, especially on the left side, where all soft tissue should be carefully divided and ligated to prevent chyle leaks from the thoracic duct. This can be facilitated by using the Harmonic® scalpel when dissecting level IV tissue off from behind the clavicle. Similarly, there are often diseased level IV nodes found in the plane between the IJV and carotid artery or posterior to the carotid artery. These need to be

---

Box 11.2 Complications of neck dissection during reoperative surgery

Hypoparathyroidism:
- transient
- permanent

Chyle leak/chyloma

Bleeding and haematoma

Seroma

Wound infection

Nerve injuries:
- accessory nerve
- hypoglossal nerve
- ramus mandibularis
- vagus nerve
- sympathetic chain (Horner's syndrome)
- brachial plexus
- phrenic nerve
- cutaneous cervical plexus

---

carefully dissected and removed without injury to the vagus nerve and sympathetic trunk. Failure to do so may result in vocal cord palsy or Horner's syndrome (Box 11.2).

Re-do neck dissections in previously operated necks are more difficult and need experience to deal with. These can usually be done with an incision placed in the previous scar. Dissection should proceed cautiously as the IJV or carotid artery may be hitched up and appear soon after the platysma is divided, or be injured when raising the platysmal flap. One technique to facilitate raising the flap is to use blunt dissection to displace the soft tissue and demonstrate the flap clearly. It is often difficult to remove nodal disease from underlying structures, and it may be necessary to take a more radical approach and remove adherent structures such as the muscle, nerve or vein, even though one may be tempted to shave the nodes off. These are decisions that have to be made intraoperatively by an experienced surgeon.

Surgery for distant metastases from thyroid cancer

Surgery for distant metastases may be required to palliate symptoms (e.g. bone metastases), where serious complications are expected (e.g. intracranial haemorrhage, spinal compression, etc.) or to improve quality of life. There is no established role for metastatectomy in a curative setting as solitary or limited distant metastasis amenable to curative resection is an uncommon situation. However, there are good retrospective data to suggest that in these rare situations, complete metastatectomy may be associated with improved survival for localized distant disease, particularly for non-RAI-avid disease [25–27].

Surgical complications

Details on surgical complications and strategies to avoid them will be discussed in subsequent chapters (see Box 11.2). However, it is important to note that complications are more likely during reoperative procedures, with overall transient complication rates reported at 8% and a permanent morbidity rate of 3.8% [28]. With regard to specific complications compared to primary surgery, reoperative dissection of the thyroid bed results in higher rates of permanent recurrent laryngeal nerve palsy (3.4% versus 1.1%) and hypoparathyroidism (3.9% versus 1.2%) [29].

Conclusion

Reoperative thyroid surgery can comprise complex procedures with increased risk for the patient. These procedures should only be undertaken by surgeons with adequate training and experience to deal with the issues therein, and not by the occasional thyroid surgeon. Where possible, a more conservative or non-surgical approach may be preferred. Existing adjuncts may help in the procedure, but ultimately surgeon knowledge of neck anatomy and variations in an operated neck is the most useful guide to safe surgery. Patient safety is paramount and surgical decisions need to balance adequate oncological clearance with surgical risks.

References

1 Shaha AR. Revision thyroid surgery – technical considerations. Otolaryngol Clin North Am 2008; 41: 1169–83, x.

2 Iyer NG, Shaha AR. Complications of thyroid surgery: prevention and management. Minerva Chir 2010; 65: 71–82.

3 Reeve TS, Delbridge L, Brady P, Crummer P, Smyth C. Secondary thyroidectomy: a twenty-year experience. World J Surg 1988; 12: 449–53.

4 Hay ID, Thompson GB, Grant CS, *et al.* Papillary thyroid carcinoma managed at the Mayo Clinic during six decades (1940–1999): temporal trends in initial therapy and long-term outcome in 2444 consecutively treated patients. World J Surg 2002; 26: 879–85.

5 Shah JP, Loree TR, Dharker D, Strong EW, Begg C, Vlamis V. Prognostic factors in differentiated carcinoma of the thyroid gland. Am J Surg 1992; 164: 658–61.

6 Rossi RL, Cady B, Silverman ML, Wool MS, Horner TA. Current results of conservative surgery for differentiated thyroid carcinoma. World J Surg 1986; 10: 612–22.

7 Sanders LE, Cady B. Differentiated thyroid cancer: reexamination of risk groups and outcome of treatment. Arch Surg 1998; 133: 419–25.

8 Sanders LE, Silverman M. Follicular and Hurthle cell carcinoma: predicting outcome and directing therapy. Surgery 1998; 124: 967–74.

9 Stojadinovic A, Ghossein RA, Hoos A, *et al.* Hurthle cell carcinoma: a critical histopathologic appraisal. J Clin Oncol 2001; 19: 2616–25.

10 Schlumberger MJ. Papillary and follicular thyroid carcinoma. N Engl J Med 1998; 338: 297–306.

11 Durante C, Haddy N, Baudin E, *et al.* Long-term outcome of 444 patients with distant metastases from papillary and follicular thyroid carcinoma: benefits and limits of radioiodine therapy. J Clin Endocrinol Metab 2006; 91: 2892–9.

12 Dinneen SF, Valimaki MJ, Bergstralh EJ, Goellner JR, Gorman CA, Hay ID. Distant metastases in papillary thyroid carcinoma: 100 cases observed at one institution during 5 decades. J Clin Endocrinol Metab 1995; 80: 2041–5.

13 Casara D, Rubello D, Saladini G, *et al.* Different features of pulmonary metastases in differentiated thyroid cancer: natural history and multivariate statistical analysis of prognostic variables. J Nucl Med 1993; 34: 1626–31.

14 Aygun N. Imaging of recurrent thyroid cancer. Otolaryngol Clin North Am 2008; 41: 1095–106, viii.

15 Randolph GW, Kamani D. The importance of preoperative laryngoscopy in patients undergoing thyroidectomy: voice, vocal cord function, and the preoperative detection of invasive thyroid malignancy. Surgery 2006; 139: 357–62.

16 Robbins RJ, Wan Q, Grewal RK, *et al.* Real-time prognosis for metastatic thyroid carcinoma based on 2-[18 F]fluoro-2-deoxy-D-glucose positron emission tomography scanning. J Clin Endocrinol Metab 2006; 91: 498–505.

17 Cooper DS, Doherty GM, Haugen BR, *et al.* Revised American Thyroid Association management guidelines for patients with thyroid nodules and differentiated thyroid cancer. Thyroid 2009; 19: 1167–214.

18 Tuttle RM, Leboeuf R, Shaha AR. Medical management of thyroid cancer: a risk adapted approach. J Surg Oncol 2008; 97: 712–16.

19 Richer SL, Wenig BL. Changes in surgical anatomy following thyroidectomy. Otolaryngol Clin North Am 2008; 41: 1069–78, vii.

20 Patel KN, Shaha AR. Locally advanced thyroid cancer. Curr Opin Otolaryngol Head Neck Surg 2005; 13: 112–16.

21 Price DL, Wong RJ, Randolph GW. Invasive thyroid cancer: management of the trachea and esophagus. Otolaryngol Clin North Am 2008; 41: 1155–68, ix–x.

22 Shindo M, Chheda NN. Incidence of vocal cord paralysis with and without recurrent laryngeal nerve monitoring during thyroidectomy. Arch Otolaryngol Head Neck Surg 2007; 133: 481–5.

23 Dupuy DE, Monchik JM, Decrea C, Pisharodi L. Radiofrequency ablation of regional recurrence from well-differentiated thyroid malignancy. Surgery 2001; 130: 971–7.

24 Lewis BD, Hay ID, Charboneau JW, McIver B, Reading CC, Goellner JR. Percutaneous ethanol injection for treatment of cervical lymph node metastases in patients with papillary thyroid carcinoma. AJR 2002; 178: 699–704.

25 Shoup M, Stojadinovic A, Nissan A, *et al.* Prognostic indicators of outcomes in patients with distant metastases from differentiated thyroid carcinoma. J Am Coll Surg 2003; 197: 191–7.

26 Stojadinovic A, Shoup M, Ghossein RA, *et al.* The role of operations for distantly metastatic well-differentiated thyroid carcinoma. Surgery 2002; 131: 636–43.

27 Lee J, Soh EY. Differentiated thyroid carcinoma presenting with distant metastasis at initial diagnosis: clinical outcomes and prognostic factors. Ann Surg 2010; 251: 114–19.

28 Lefevre JH, Tresallet C, Leenhardt L, Jublanc C, Chigot JP, Menegaux F. Reoperative surgery for thyroid disease. Langenbecks Arch Surg 2007; 392: 685–91.

29 Menegaux F, Turpin G, Dahman M, *et al.* Secondary thyroidectomy in patients with prior thyroid surgery for benign disease: a study of 203 cases. Surgery 1999; 126: 479–83.

CHAPTER 12

How to Use Energy Devices and their Potential Hazards

Paolo Miccoli[1] and Michele N. Minuto[2]
[1] Department of Surgery, University of Pisa, Pisa, Italy
[2] Department of Surgical Sciences (DISC), University of Genoa, Genoa, Italy

Introduction

For many years it was advocated that the most viable cauterization system for thyroid vessels was the bipolar electrocautery, because it allowed concentration of all the electrical energy and consequent high temperatures in a single limited point, thus reducing heat transmission to critical structures. Cauterization was reserved only for very small vessels, and the clamp and tie technique was by far the most common way to divide the main pedicles of the thyroid gland. In the last decade, however, the introduction of other haemostatic systems, already available in abdominal surgery, proved to be potentially very useful also in neck surgery and in particular for thyroid surgery. This new class of instruments is generally better known as 'energy devices', since they all utilize different forms of energy, not necessarily and not simply just the heat produced by electricity but also radiofrequency or ultrasound. Although they all generate a significant elevation of temperature in the tissues [1], the temperatures reached by these instruments are never as high as those of standard monopolar electrocautery.

The most modern instruments used to determine haemostasis and division of the vessels might be divided into two main classes:

- radiofrequency based
- Harmonic® technology (Ethicon Endo-Surgery Inc.).

Radiofrequency (see Video 12.1, 12.2)

In this system there is a quick on-and-off energy delivery, defined as 'pulsing'; during energy turn-off, the system assesses the state of the tissue and can vary its output according to the received feedback. A positive side-effect of the power interruption is that the tissue cools for a short time, reducing the overall temperature. The feedback is based on tissue resistance to the power flow and to its impedance; this latter is the signal which allows the system to stop the power supply since desiccation has been reached. The most recent platform utilizes a non-pulsing energy delivery (fusion algorithms technology). The adjustments made by the generator during the fusion cycle are controlled through the tissue reaction in real time. This allows the operator to eliminate the energy pulsing and then to accelerate the process of fusion – the shorter interval of energy application supposedly reduces the thermal spread. In a recent paper investigating lateral thermal spread following *ex vivo* application of four commonly utilized energy devices (monopolar cauthery, bipolar diathermy, ultrasonic scissors and radiofrequency), the latter (Ligasure™, Covidien; Figure 12.1) developed a temperature at the tip of the instrument of 44.2 °C [2,3], following a 5-sec application at the highest power setting. In the same study, temperature at the Ligasure™ tip

Thyroid Surgery: Preventing and Managing Complications, First Edition. Edited by Paolo Miccoli, David J. Terris,
Michele N. Minuto and Melanie W. Seybt.
© 2013 John Wiley & Sons, Ltd. Published 2013 by John Wiley & Sons, Ltd.

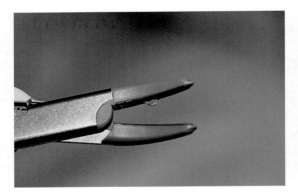

Figure 12.1 Ligasure Small Jaw™: the new generation allows tissues to be cut by means of the little blade inside the sheaths.

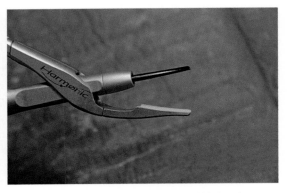

Figure 12.2 Harmonic Focus®: the white-coated blade is the one considered 'inactive', whereas the opposite blade is the 'active' one (it reaches the hottest temperatures).

after use for 15 sec on porcine muscle remained above 42°C for 15 sec.

👁 Harmonic® technology (Video 12.3)

This system can be defined as ultrasonic since it uses a blade moving at 'ultrasonic' speed. In this device electric energy is transformed into mechanical vibration: one of the two shears vibrates at 55,000 Hz per second, while the other shear is completely inactive. The transformation from one to the other form of energy is produced by a transducer which electrically activates two dishes of pie-zoelectric ceramics that make the active shear vibrate (Figure 12.2). Several effects are obtained by this ultra-sonic movement:

- rapid vaporization occurring at a much lower tempera-ture than usual due to the pressure exerted on vessels by the two-shears grip
- protein coaptation
- rupture of hydrogen bonds and protein denaturation

The coapted proteins and the wall of the vessel, folding along its layers due to the water vaporization, form a seal that closes the vessels to a diameter of 7 mm.

These effects can be obtained at a temperature between 50° and 100° but generally satisfactory coagulation and division of the structures can be obtained at a temperature of 60°. In contrast, electrocautery can reach temperatures as high as 400°. In spite of this significant difference, the surgeon should refrain from being too confident and remain aware that even relatively 'low' temperatures can

damage critical structures such as the recurrent nerve or the external branch of the superior laryngeal nerve and even the blood supply to the parathyroid glands. Furthermore, the tip of the instrument can reach higher temperatures and this is probably responsible for some of the tracheal injuries described in the literature. An impor-tant advantage of this technology is that the two shears are made of different materials and act in different ways: one is the active blade which is metallic and moves at ultra-sonic speed, the other is totally inactive and is made of Teflon. It is intuitive that the latter never reaches high temperatures. If the surgeon bears this simple difference in mind, most of the possible damage to tissues can be avoided, by simply manoeuvring the device in order to minimize the proximity of the metallic shear to the critical structures, in particular the nerves whose myelin coat is notoriously very sensitive to heat (Figure 12.3).

Another claimed advantage is that no electricity passes through the patient during its utilization. It is not clear, though, whether this avoids the general risks arising from the use of electrical energy in the human body. However, patients with pacemakers can draw an important benefit from the use of this technology. In fact, traditional surgi-cal diathermy (monopolar) may inhibit or trigger a pace-maker in demand mode, damage the pacing system or cause it to go into its automatic safety reversion mode, and can also cause thermal damage to the heart through the lead electrode. There are several reports of safely con-ducted operations using ultrasonic devices, therefore avoiding monopolar electrocautery, especially when the site of surgery (e.g. upper abdomen for a cholecystectomy,

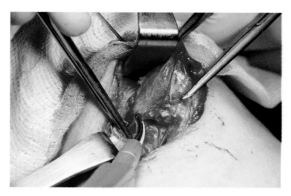

Figure 12.3 Intraoperative application of the Harmonic Focus®: notice that the 'inactive' blade of the instrument is oriented toward the more delicate structures (the inferior laryngeal nerve on the right of the shears, in this case), to avoid excessive heating.

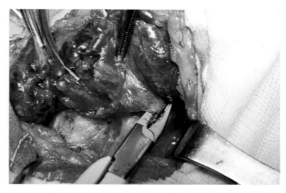

Figure 12.4 Intraoperative application of the Ligasure Small Jaw™: notice the inferior laryngeal nerve on the left side of the instrument.

breast surgery) was close to the pacemaker [4,5]. Moreover, in the near future, when magnetic resonance imaging might be necessary during an operation, such as in the case of 'automatic robotic surgery', the possibility of using an instrument able to obtain haemostasis with no electricity passing through the body might become of paramount importance.

The most important difference between radiofrequency and ultrasonic technology is that radiofrequency instruments can only induce haemostasis but not the contemporary division of structures; this potential drawback in the last generation of devices has been partially solved by introducing a subtle blade inside one of the shears that severs the vessel at the end of coagulation. However, this change implies larger shears which of course are less delicate when using the instrument for dissection (Figure 12.4).

To avoid any possible damage from heat transmission, a surgeon approaching this technology for the first time should be led by an experienced operator for at least 20 interventions.

A further issue never stressed in literature is represented by the risks arising from incorrect sterilization of such disposable instruments. It is well known that in some surgical settings, they are utilized several times after gas sterilization. On this point, the manufacturers are very strict and they carefully warn surgeons that, as in any delicate technology, this attitude might seriously jeopardize the instrument function. It is, for example, quite obvious that cleaning the shears with a brush may

significantly affect the overlapping of the two shears. In contrast, an over-delicate cleaning of the instrument might leave microscopic debris or blood clots which can compromise the sterilization itself. Finally, incorrect use would raise important legal issues in cases of unexpected complications.

Evidence from the literature

Although it has been claimed that these instruments might produce a better outcome in terms of complications in thyroid surgery, the only real advantage clearly demonstrated in the literature is the reduction in operative time (Table 12.1). On this issue the different authors are basically unanimous, although with different results. The results in the literature must obviously be interpreted according to other factors, such as the experience of the surgeon both in conventional surgery and in the use of devices of this kind.

The issue of the reduction in operative time involves an aspect that is becoming more and more important [6]: the possibility of reducing costs that could help to offset the increased expense deriving from the use of these emerging technologies. In fact, the cost of one of these disposable instruments is generally never lower than $500 and thus its use must also be evaluated on an economical basis. If the cost of the operating room per hour was carefully analysed, it would be obvious that time saving which allows performance of an extra operation will produce increased income for the hospital. If one considers that

Table 12.1 Summary of publications evaluating the operative time of thyroidectomies performed using any energy device.

Author	Number of patients	Operative time using energy devices (min)	Operative time using knot-tying technique (min)
Siperstein *et al.* 2002 [7]	86/85	132±39	161±42
Voutilainen *et al.* 2000 [8]	19/17	99.1±26.7	134.9±49.4
Manouras *et al.* 2005 [9]	94/90	87.30±21.30	101.60±34.20
Saint Marc *et al.* 2007 [10]	100/100	42.50±11.20	48.90±6.80
Cipolla *et al.* 2008 [11]	53/52	104.00±12.70	110.00±15.60
Foreman *et al.* 2009 [12]	106/77	82.80	94.09
Hallgrimsson *et al.* 2008 [13]	27/24	121 (84–213)	172 (66–268)

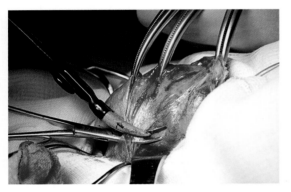

Figure 12.5 Intraoperative application of a reusable radiofrequency-based instrument: the BiClamp® (ERBE Elektromedizin GmbH).

using a single instrument instead of threads and possibly clips is a further reduction of the costs of a procedure, it is reasonable to conclude that these new technologies do not necessarily represent an unjustified extension of the expenses. Moreover, both ultrasound-based and radiofrequency systems can be available as reusable instruments (Figure 12.5): shears can be resterilized, even though only for a limited number of cases. Unfortunately, the ergonomy of these devices is quite poor.

As mentioned above, no evidence exists in the literature that the complications peculiar to thyroid and, to a lesser extent, parathyroid surgery have been reduced by the introduction of this class of haemostatic instruments. In particular, the recurrent nerve palsy rate has remained the same in all papers comparing energy devices with conventional clamp and tie techniques. In spite of two sporadic reports in which a reduction of postoperative hypoparathyroidism was present, though not reaching statistical evidence, this result has not been confirmed in larger series.

TIPS AND TRICKS

- A wet 'peanut' on the nerve when using energy in its vicinity can significantly lower the temperature.

- The relationship between tension, pressure, time of application and haemostasis should always be present in the surgeon's mind. If the maximum haemostasis is desired, tissues should be kept quite loose with limited pressure on them.

- The position of the inactive blade in relation to the critical structures is important to reduce the risks of heat transmission (see Figure 12.3).

- It is essential to keep the tip of the instrument in view in any phase of the application (the tip is the hottest part of the instrument!)

- The last generation of tools, which now have significantly improved ergonomy, can also be used during dissection. A major caveat is the temperature of the shears: they take a short while to become cold after coagulation and before using them to dissect ('residual heat'). Remember that aluminium, for example, cools more quickly than other metals.

- Immediately after use, do not put the instrument on the patient's dressing: it might burn it and damage the patient's body.

- Energy devices and the Harmonic® in particular are protein advantageous since the mechanism of coagulation passes through a protein coaptation; for this reason the vessel should always be grasped between the two shears with a 'generous' amount of surrounding connective tissue.

- The Harmonic® is characterized by early failure, if any; once the coagulation has been obtained, no late failures are to be expected.

It must be borne in mind that overconfident use of these instruments might jeopardize the nervous structures to the point of serious damage. In fact, these are far from being 'cold' instruments: for this reason, meticulous attention must be paid to the critical distance between the shears (in particular the 'active' shear) and the nerve. Manufacturers often give optimistic instructions in terms of the extent of heat transmission, but these should be taken into account in a very critical way. There are other parameters to evaluate besides merely distance, in particular the timing and level of power delivery. Several thermographic and histological studies have precisely determined the safe distance between the instrument and the nerve. It would be advisable for endocrine and neck surgeons to critically appraise the literature about this issue and compare data with their own experience.

References

1 Sutton PA, Awad S, Perkins AC, Lobo DN. Comparison of lateral thermal spread using monopolar and bipolar diathermy, the Harmonic Scalpel and the Ligasure. Br J Surg 2010; 97(3): 428–33.

2 Cakabay B, Sevinç MM, Gömceli I, Yenidogan E, Ulkü A, Koç S. LigaSure versus clamp-and-tie in thyroidectomy: a single-center experience. Adv Ther 2009; 26(11): 1035–41.

3 Oussoultzoglou E, Panaro F, Rosso E, et al. Use of BiClamp decreased the severity of hypocalcemia after total thyroidectomy compared with LigaSure: a prospective study. World J Surg 2008 32(9): 1968–73.

4 Nandalan SP, Vanner RG. Use of the harmonic scalpel in a patient with a permanent pacemaker. Anaesthesia 2004; 59(6): 621.

5 Epstein M, Mayer J Jr, Duncan B. Use of an ultrasonic scalpel as an alternative to electrocautery in patients with pacemakers. Ann Surg 1998; 65: 1802–4.

6 Sebag F, Fortanier C, Ippolito G, Lagier A, Auquier P, Henry JF. Harmonic scalpel in multinodular goiter surgery: impact on surgery and cost analysis. J Laparoendosc Adv Surg Tech A 2009; 19(2): 171–4.

7 Siperstein AE, Berber E, Morkoyun E. The use of the harmonic scalpel vs conventional knot tying for vessel ligation in thyroid surgery. Arch Surg 2002; 137(2): 137–42.

8 Voutilainen PE, Haglund CH. Ultrasonically activated shears in thyroidectomies: a randomized trial. Ann Surg 2000; 231(3): 322–8.

9 Manouras A, Lagoudianakis EE, Antonakis PT, Filippakis GM, Markogiannakis H, Kekis PB. Electrothermal bipolar vessel sealing system is a safe and time-saving alternative to classic suture ligation in total thyroidectomy. Head Neck 2005; 27(11): 959–62.

10 Saint Marc O, Cogliandolo A, Piquard A, Famà F, Pidoto RR. LigaSure vs clamp-and-tie technique to achieve hemostasis in total thyroidectomy for benign multinodular goiter: a prospective randomized study. Arch Surg 2007; 142(2): 150–6; discussion 157.

11 Cipolla C, Graceffa G, Sandonato L, Fricano S, Vieni S, Latteri MA. LigaSure in total thyroidectomy. Surg Today 2008; 38(6): 495–8.

12 Foreman E, Aspinall S, Bliss RD, Lennard TW. The use of the harmonic scalpel in thyroidectomy: 'beyond the learning curve'. Ann R Coll Surg Engl 2009; 91(3): 214–16.

13 Hallgrimsson P, Lovén L, Westerdahl J, Bergenfelz A. Use of the harmonic scalpel versus conventional haemostatic techniques in patients with Grave disease undergoing total thyroidectomy: a prospective randomised controlled trial. Langenbecks Arch Surg 2008; 393(5): 675–80.

Videoclips

This chapter contains the following videoclips. They can be accessed at: www.wiley.com/go/miccoli/thyroid

Video 12.1   Total lobectomy with the Ligasure Small Jaw™. The Ligasure Small Jaw™ uses radiofrequency energy, controlled through a feedback system based on tissue resistance to the power flow and to its impedance.

Video 12.2   Total thyroidectomy with radiofrequency-based technology. The Ligasure™ allows a delicate and safe dissection with minimal thermal spread at the tip of the instrument (above 42°C in animal tests).

Video 12.3   Total thyroidectomy with the Harmonic Focus®. The Harmonic Focus® transforms electric energy into mechanical vibration, allowing the coagulation and section of vessels to a diameter of 7 mm.

PART III

Intraoperative Complications: The 'Classic' Issues

CHAPTER 13
The Recurrent Laryngeal Nerve

David Goldenberg¹ and Gregory W. Randolph²

¹ Division of Otolaryngology – Head and Neck Surgery, Pennsylvania State University, Milton S. Hershey Medical Center, Hershey, PA, USA
² Massachusetts Eye and Ear Infirmary, and Endocrine Surgical Service, Massachusetts General Hospital, and Department of Otolaryngology Head and Neck Surgery, Harvard Medical School, Boston, MA, USA

Introduction

The recurrent laryngeal nerve (RLN) was first identified and named by Galen in the second century. Galan found that vagal sectioning in a pig resulted in aphonia. Until this time, speech was thought to be controlled by the heart [1]. In the seventh century, Paulus Aeginata suggested that the RLN could be avoided during surgical treatment of the thyroid. Vesalius, in the 16th century, provided anatomical drawings of the RLN and superior laryngeal nerve (SLN) distribution. In the late 1800s Billroth ceased performing thyroidectomies as a result of haemorrhage and postoperative sepsis. Wolfler later reviewed 44 of Billroth's patients operated on over 5 years and noted a 29.5% RLN paralysis rate.

SURGICAL ANATOMY

Recurrent laryngeal nerve microanatomy

The vagus nerve was described in modern form first by Willis in the 1600s [2]. The cervical branches of the vagus encountered during thyroid surgery include the SLN, both internal and external branches, and the RLN. The SLN's *internal branch* brings general visceral afferents to the lower pharynx, supraglottic larynx, vocal cords, and base of tongue, and brings special visceral afferents to the epiglottic taste buds. The SLN's *external*

branch brings branchial efferents to the cricothyroid muscle and inferior constrictor. The internal branch of the SLN may also provide motor contributions to the posterior cricoarytenoid muscle and intra-arytenoid muscle, and the external branch of the SLN may provide limited motor input to the anterior thyroarytenoid muscle. The RLN contains branchial efferents to the inferior constrictor, cricopharyngeus, all laryngeal intrinsic muscles except the cricothyroid muscle, general visceral afferents from the larynx (vocal cords and below), upper oesophagus and trachea [3]. RLN branches also convey sympathetic and parasympathetic branches to the lower pharynx, larynx, trachea and upper oesophagus. Apart from the larynx and pharynx, the vagus provides afferent and parasympathetic innervation to the heart, oesophagus, stomach, intestines, liver, spleen and kidneys.

Recurrent laryngeal nerve gross surgical anatomy

The right vagus runs from the posterior aspect of the jugular vein in the neck base to cross anterior to the first part of the subclavian artery. The RLN branches and courses up and behind the subclavian artery (fourth branchial arch), running medially along the pleura and cranially behind the common carotid artery into the right thoracic inlet in the base of the neck. The left vagus courses from the carotid sheath in the left neck base anterior to the aortic arch (sixth arch, ligamentum arteriosus). The RLN branch curves up under the aortic

Thyroid Surgery: Preventing and Managing Complications, First Edition. Edited by Paolo Miccoli, David J. Terris, Michele N. Minuto and Melanie W. Seybt.

arch just lateral to the obliterated ductus arteriosus. Because of its course around the right subclavian artery, the right RLN enters the neck base at the thoracic inlet more laterally than the left recurrent does [4]. The right RLN then ascends the neck, entering the thoracic inlet,

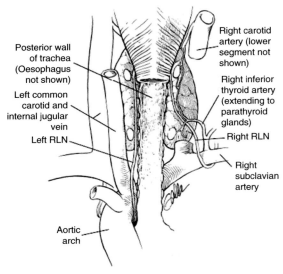

Figure 13.1 Differences in RLN course on the right and left side. Reproduced from Randolph [22] with permission from Elsevier.

emerging from under the common carotid artery, travelling from lateral to medial as it travels superiorly, ultimately crossing the inferior thyroid artery. It assumes a paratracheal position in the last centimetre of its course as it approaches the lowest edge of the inferior constrictor (Figure 13.1). At this point, it travels under the inferior-most fibres of the inferior constrictor the cricopharyngeus muscle, extending deep to the inferior constrictor and up behind the cricothyroid articulation to enter the larynx (Figure 13.2). In approximately 30% of cases the RLN actually penetrates the lowest fibres of the inferior constrictor on its way to the larynx [5].

The point of disappearance of the RLN under the lowest fibres of the inferior constrictor will, in this chapter, be termed the 'laryngeal entry point' and represents the distal-most exposure of the RLN in the thyroid surgical field. The left RLN emerges from underneath the aortic arch and enters the thoracic inlet in a more paratracheal position and extends upward in or near the tracheo-oesophageal groove, ultimately crossing the distal branches of the left inferior thyroid artery. The left RLN extends underneath the inferior fibres of the inferior constrictor and up behind the cricothyroid cartilaginous articulation to enter the larynx. For the last centimetre or so before laryngeal entry, the RLN travels close to the lateral border of the trachea.

Figure 13.2 Side view of the larynx, showing the ligament of Berry and laryngeal entry point relative to palpable landmark of inferior thyroid cartilage cornu. Reproduced from Randolph [22] with permission from Elsevier.

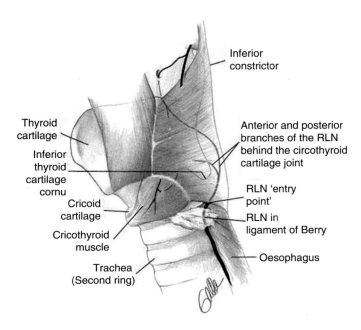

The length of the RLN from vagal takeoff to laryngeal entry point is 8.5 cm on the right and 10 cm on the left. The RLN diameter averages approximately 2 mm, ranging from 1 to 3 mm [6].

Non-recurrent recurrent laryngeal nerve

The non-recurrent RLN occurs in 0.5–1% of cases and is associated with a right subclavian artery takeoff from the distal aortic arch [7]. The right subclavian in these cases follows a retro-oesophageal course to the right or, less commonly, between the oesophagus and the trachea [7]. The non-recurrent RLN derives from the vagus as a direct medial branch in the neck and extends, depending upon its level of takeoff from the vagus, with a downward looping course from behind the carotid artery to the laryngeal entry point. The takeoff of the nonrecurrent RLN from the vagus may occur as high as the thyroid superior pole or as low as the inferior thyroid artery. The non-recurrent nerve may be very closely related to the inferior thyroid artery. It may be bifid or have multiple branches in 18–40% of cases [8]. A non-recurrent RLN is shown in Figure 13.3.

Rates of iatrogenic recurrent laryngeal nerve damage

Permanent RLN paralysis rates have been reported in the 1–2% range in experienced hands. The rates of RLN paralysis after thyroidectomy in many studies are likely under-estimated. Probably the important reason underlying RLN paralysis underestimation is that not all patients undergo postoperative laryngeal examination. In some practices, only patients who are significantly and persistently symptomatic have their larynxes inspected. Second, most injuries are not detected intraoperatively by the surgeon. Lo, for example, found that surgeons had recognized intraoperative injury in only 1% of cases when, in fact, surgical injury had occurred in nearly 7% of patients [9].

Lastly, those thyroid surgery groups with unfavourable data are less likely to report their findings. With symptomatic assessment of vocal cord function, a human tendency exists to 'identify success and ignore failure' [9]. All patients should have preoperative and postoperative laryngeal examination if we are to appreciate the true rate at which RLN injury occurs. Although the rate of RLN paralysis with thyroidectomy in expert hands may be low, many current reports document rates in the 6–8% range, with some reports of up to 23% [10,11].

The rates of RLN paralysis during thyroid surgery are greater in cases associated with:
* lack of RLN identification during surgery
* bilateral surgery
* surgery for cancer
* surgery associated with significant lymph node resection
* surgery for Graves' disease or thyroiditis
* revision surgery
* surgery associated with substernal goitre
* surgery associated with longer operating room times or greater blood loss
* patients brought back to surgery because of bleeding.

A recent study by Abadin *et al.* showed that RLN injuries comprised 46% of all sources of thyroid surgery malpractice litigation between 1989 and 2009 [12]. Lydiatt stated that in unilateral RLN injury lawsuits, four out of six (67%) were settled in favour of plaintiffs and lack of informed consent was alleged in seven of nine (78%) cases [12].

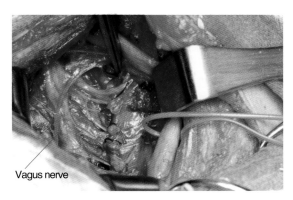

Vagus nerve

Figure 13.3 Intraoperative view of a non-recurrent RLN with one main branch arising from the vagus, and multiple minor branches.

Visualization and approach to the recurrent laryngeal nerve during surgery

The surgeon should endeavour to identify the RLN in all cases of thyroidectomy. Lahey and Crile were both early advocates for finding the RLN during every thyroidectomy. Most studies prove that RLN visual identification during thyroidectomy is associated with lower rates of postoperative RLN paralysis.

General identification principles

An important rule that we follow is that no structure is cut until the RLN is identified visually and electrically. If this single rule is strictly adhered to, RLN injury, and certainly transection injury, should be rare. To identify the RLN, a bloodless field is essential. In cases of goitrous enlargement of the gland, the strap muscles can be retracted, but they should be transected without hesitation if additional exposure is needed. As the strap muscles are retracted laterally, so the thyroid and laryngotracheal complex should be retracted as one unit medially to open up the lateral thyroid region. Care should be taken as excessive retraction on the thyroid can lead to nerve traction injury. The distal course of the RLN may extend ventrally and follow a course along the upper cervical trachea obliquely upward out of the tracheo-oesophageal groove as the thyroid lobe is retracted. As the thyroid is dissected and freed from its cervical attachments, it is progressively pulled medially and the airway itself is to some degree displaced upwardly and rotated through this retraction. This distal upward course of the RLN may become accentuated through these manoeuvres and result in injury, especially during subtotal lobectomy, which may not involve visualization of the last centimetre or so of the RLN's course [4]. A nerve in this circumstance may be injured through placement of clamps or suturing of the thyroid remnant. Once total lobectomy is complete, blood often oozes from the ligament of Berry area. To control bleeding, patience is recommended, rather than indiscriminate cautery or clamping.

A neurosurgical pledget, used to brush the area with a suction tip to allow full view of the RLN and the bleeding sites, with careful discrete bipolar cautery or specific clamping of the identified small bleeder, is best. Minimal oozing can be controlled with Surgicel.

The surgical approach to finding the RLN during may vary depending on the type of case. The approach to the nerve can be empirically divided into three specific approaches. Keep in mind that a nerve identified through any technique is a nerve well identified. Nonetheless, three separate approaches to nerve identification can be helpful during thyroidectomy.

Inferior approach to the recurrent laryngeal nerve

The inferior approach was introduced by Sedgwick and described by Lore. In this approach, the RLN is identified toward the thoracic inlet laterally for the right RLN and typically more medially in the tracheo-oesophageal groove on the left. This technique uses the RLN triangle [13] which, as described by Lore, has its apex inferior in the thoracic inlet. The medial wall is formed by the trachea, the lateral wall by the medial edge of the retracted strap muscles, and the superior base by the lower edge of the retracted thyroid's inferior pole. The RLN is found in a loose areolar bed and typically exists proximal to the inferior thyroid artery crossing point and proximal to any extralaryngeal nerve branching. This can be helpful in the setting of revision surgery, where the nerve can be found in an undissected region caudal to the previous surgery scar. The disadvantage of this approach is that it involves dissection of a relatively long segment of RLN toward the laryngeal inlet. One must be cautious, in this long cranial-caudal length of RLN dissection, that the inferior parathyroid gland is not devascularized. One must also consider in this approach on the right the potential for a non-recurrent right RLN (Figure 13.4a).

Superior approach to the recurrent laryngeal nerve

In the superior approach, the RLN is found at the laryngeal entry point just above the ligament of Berry. The advantage of this approach is that the RLN's entry to the larynx represents its most constant position in the neck. The larynx may be deviated or rotated, but the nerve will always relate to the lateral cricoid and enter at the cricoid's inferior edge. This approach is especially useful for large cervical or substernal goitres, where the nerve cannot be found inferiorly or laterally. The inferior cornu of the thyroid cartilage may be palpated to approximate the location of the nerve in this region. The nerve is also more easily located in this area once one is oriented to the anterior arch of the cricoid anteriorly. Once this region is identified, nerve stimulation can be helpful to focus the dissection. Once the nerve is identified in this area, it can be dissected retrograde and reflected off the undersurface of the thyroid lobe. The disadvantage of this approach is that the ligament of Berry is fibrous and well vascularized. The superior pole also must be taken down first so the external branch of the superior laryngeal nerve and the superior parathyroid gland can be identified

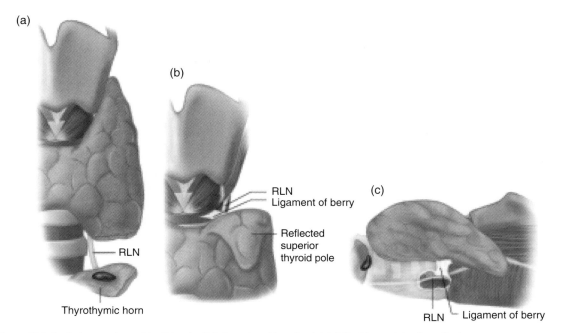

(a)

(b)

(c)

RLN
Ligament of berry

Reflected
superior
thyroid pole

RLN

Thyrothymic horn

RLN — Ligament of berry

Figure 13.4 Surgical approaches to identifying the RLN. Reproduced from Randolph [23] with permission from Elsevier.

and avoided. This approach may be more technically challenging with a large superior pole. However, this is a very useful and reliable method for nerve identification when other approaches fail or in the setting of a non-recurrent RLN (Figure 13.4b).

Lateral approach to the recurrent laryngeal nerve

The lateral approach is the most commonly used method (Figure 13.4c), in which the RLN is found laterally at the midpole level with medial thyroid lobe retraction. This is applicable to many routine cases.In this approach, the tubercle of Zuckerkandl can be used as a landmark for finding the RLN. The tubercle is almost always medial to and overlying the RLN.

The advantage of the lateral approach is that it limits the length of RLN dissection. It does, however, dissect the RLN over the region where thyroid tissue is brought close to the nerve, just at and below the ligament of Berry.

This is not a suitable approach for large cervical or substernal goitres or if there is extensive scar from previous surgery. It is also notable that because the nerve is identified quite distally in its course, extralaryngeal branching may occur at this level; caution must be exercised to recognize all branches that may occur in this distal segment of the RLN's course. One must be especially cautious regarding finding a posterior branch and mistaking this as the entire nerve trunk which could place an existing anterior branch at risk during the final portion of ligament of Berry dissection.

Landmarks for locating the recurrent laryngeal nerve

The laryngeal entry point

This represents the most constant position of the RLN in the neck. Regardless of goitrous displacement or non-recurrence of the RLN, the nerve will always be found here. Finding the nerve at the laryngeal entry point can be difficult despite its anatomical constancy, because of the adjacent tough, fibrous and well-vascularized ligament of Berry. The nerve may be behind or within the ligament and may have thyroid tissue very closely associated with it in this region. The RLN's laryngeal entry point is approximately 1 cm below and just anterior to the thyroid cartilage's inferior horn, which can be easily palpated (see Figure 13.2).

Ligament of Berry

The fibrous ligament of Berry anchors the thyroid to the laryngotracheal complex, and is also known as the posterior suspensory ligament of the thyroid. The ligament of Berry can be regarded as a condensation of the thyroid capsule, arising from the posterolateral aspect of the cricoid, first, second and, occasionally, third tracheal rings, and extends to the corresponding deep surface of the medial aspect of the bilateral thyroid lobes. The ligament of Berry is separate and distinct from the significantly less robust anterior suspensory ligament, which arises from the midline and paramidline upper cervical trachea to extend to the corresponding deep surface of the thyroid isthmus. The ligament of Berry is both dense and well vascularized, deriving a branch along its inferior edge from the inferior thyroid artery. This artery is well known to thyroid surgeons and can result in troublesome haemorrhage during the final phase of dissection. The ligament can be very closely associated with adjacent thyroid tissue that, to a varying degree, can infuse the substance of the ligament of Berry, and in so doing, approximate the RLN. The RLN often crosses deep to the ligament of Berry; Berlin found that in 30% of cases the RLN coursed through the ligament itself.

Tubercle of Zuckerkandl

The tubercle of Zuckerkandl is an anatomical structure first described by Madelung in 1867, and later by the Viennese anatomist Emil Zuckerkandl, in 1902. The tubercle of Zuckerkandl is believed to represent the remnants of the lateral thyroid processes and includes the ultimobranchial bodies and C cells. These bilateral structures arise as a proliferation of pharyngeal endoderm from the ventral portion of the fourth pharyngeal pouch and the vestigial fifth pouch. The tubercle of Zuckerkandl is described as being nearly always superficial to the recurrent laryngeal nerve, so serving as an accurate landmark for its identification in thyroid surgery [14,15].

Recurrent laryngeal nerve and inferior thyroid artery

The inferior thyroid artery (ITA) derives as an upwardly directed branch of the thyrocervical trunk and extends under the carotid artery into the central neck. It loops downward more medially, extending to the thyroid at the midpolar level of the thyroid. The RLN and the inferior thyroid artery have a variable relationship. The RLN may be deep or superficial, or may ramify branches of the artery. The basic relationship, however, is that the artery and nerve intersect. Hollingshead has described the RLN as being deep to the inferior thyroid artery in about 50% of cases, running between the inferior thyroid artery branches in 25% of cases, and running anterior to the inferior thyroid artery in 25% of cases. Given the varying course of the inferior thyroid artery, coupled with the potential for its absence and parallel course to the RLN, the RLN/ITA crossing point is a variable and thus poor landmark for routine RLN identification [16] (see Video 13.1).

Damage to the recurrent laryngeal nerve

Mechanisms of iatrogenic RLN injury include mechanical, thermal or vascular factors. Focal demyelination after minimal injury of the RLN (e.g. compression) leads to a temporary blockage of nerve conduction (neurapraxia) that generally recovers completely and spontaneously after 6–8 weeks. More severe trauma to the RLN (e.g. crush, stretch or ischaemic injuries) can damage the myelin sheath (axonotmesis) which can still recover spontaneously but leads to muscular contractions that are of poor quality and thus the voice is affected. More violent trauma to the RLN (e.g. laceration or severe crush or stretch injuries) leads to interruption of the endoneurial, perineurial and/or epineurial sheaths (neurotmesis), which is followed by incomplete or absent nerve regrowth.

Voice changes after recurrent laryngeal nerve injury

Paralytic dysphonia and dysphagia after RLN injury may cause significant morbidity and may be profound enough to necessitate change in vocation [17]. Any disruption in the luminal surface of the vocal cord results in a disruption of this process and a coarse change to the character of the voice, generically called *hoarseness*. The change to the voice resulting from vocal cord paralysis is more accurately termed *breathiness* and represents a weakened voice due to relative glottis incompetence during phonation due to the lateral resting position typical for most paralysed vocal cords. The degree of breathiness relates to the degree to which the affected fold is laterally displaced and the resulting degree to which the two folds fail to meet during phonation.

On fibreoptic laryngoscopy, the vocal fold usually remains in the paramedian position initially. This and postintubation oedema often allow for a fairly normal voice and voice changes may not present definitively for days to weeks. With time, the paralysed vocal fold will atrophy, causing the voice to worsen. The glottal air leak during phonation causes a breathy-rough voice and possible hoarseness. Laryngeal examination reveals an immobile fold that appears bowed/atrophic and laterally displaced. This lateral vocal fold displacement leads to a glottis gap resulting in air escape during phonation (breathy voice) and possibly allowing aspiration of saliva or ingested fluids. Some patients with long-standing unilateral vocal fold paralysis may have minimal vocal complaints. However, most patients with unilateral laryngeal paralysis do have some vocal impairment, ranging from mild vocal fatigue to severe hoarseness. In some cases, the glottis is incompetent; the patient is aphonic and aspirates during swallowing.

Although voice and swallowing can be significantly affected by unilateral laryngeal paralysis, the glottic airway is generally not obstructed in the adult. In bilateral paralysis, the airway is always impaired to some degree. Acute bilateral paralysis usually results in acute and severe upper airway obstruction, requiring emergency tracheotomy or intubation. Other patients may have a marginal but adequate airway initially, with increasing obstruction over time. In bilateral paralysis, vocal symptoms nearly always take a back seat to respiratory problems. Symptoms virtually always change over time, because of recovery of motion on the paralysed side, development of contralateral compensatory function, or shifting of vocal fold position toward the midline.

Intraoperative neural electrophysiological monitoring of the recurrent laryngeal nerve

Recurrent laryngeal nerve monitoring represents an adjunct to, and extension of, routine visual identification of the nerve during surgery. Electrical identification of the RLN, analogous to facial nerve monitoring during parotid surgery, reinforces but does not substitute for its visual identification, and provides the surgeon with a new functional dimension of surgical anatomy. Electrical confirmation complements the visual impression and avoids visual false positives. RLN monitoring during thyroidectomy has three specific functions: to facilitate neural identification, to aid in neural dissection, and to prognosticate regarding postoperative neural function. Although monitoring is very helpful in terms of neural identification and is a tremendous adjunct in neural dissection during thyroidectomy, the principal benefit of RLN monitoring is intraoperative prediction of postoperative function.

Once the RLN has been successfully identified with the use of the various stimulation and recording methods previously described, continuous electromyographic (EMG) monitoring is performed with the goal of maintaining the neural integrity of the nerve during the resection. Direct observation of a nerve does not assess function and cannot evaluate nerve injury. Because neural monitoring represents a new technique, it has been the subject of great controversy. Intraoperative neural monitoring has been evaluated by many through the limited lens of studies looking at the rates of paralysis with or without monitoring. The vast majority of these studies are insufficiently powered and deny the many categories of benefit that typically become apparent to a surgeon through routine application of neural monitoring only after several months.

Proving the benefit of intraoperative neural monitoring is difficult. Eisele notes that to show a reduction in RLN paralysis rates from 2% to 1% per nerves at risk, a study group of approximately 1000 patients (assuming $\alpha = 0.05$, power 0.8, 1 tailed t-test) would be necessary [18]. Although it is difficult to prove benefit, many series show excellent results associated with neural monitoring [19].

Normative values for the pre- and postresection minimum thresholds of the RLN have been established. A 2003 study from the University of Michigan described their experience with postcricoid surface electrodes during thyroidectomy and parathyroidectomy surgery. This study involved 53 patients with 81 total at-risk RLNs and resulted in a single case of transient vocal fold paresis and a single case of permanent paresis. They reported an average preresection threshold current of 0.57 mA ($\pm$ 0.48 mA) and an average postresection threshold current of 0.42 mA ($\pm$ 0.55 mA).

Choby *et al.* performed a study on a larger patient population (80 patients) and more at-risk nerves (111 RLNs), and showed consistent and reproducible minimum thresholds of RLN stimulation. This study establishes normal RLN threshold levels for average preresection (0.50 mA; range 0–1.3 mA), postresection (0.47 mA; range 0.2–1 mA), and difference in pre- and postresection minimum threshold levels (–0.03 mA; range –0.9 to –0.6 mA) [20].

There are several methods of evaluating EMG potentials from stimulation of the RLN. Recording techniques can use either surface or needle electrodes. A fibreoptic laryngoscope or laryngeal mask anaesthesia is sometimes used for visual inspection of the vocal folds on stimulation of the RLN. Surgeons may use laryngeal palpation techniques to detect muscular activity during nerve stimulation.

A pair of subdermal electrodes or fine-hooked wire electrodes can be inserted directly into the vocal folds using simultaneous direct laryngoscopy. Alternatively, needle electrodes may be inserted through the cricothyroid membrane into the vocal muscle. Needle electrodes are not without disadvantages. Placement of endolaryngeal needle electrodes can be quite challenging and requires a skilled surgeon. Inserted needles are susceptible to dislocation of the electrodes during muscle contraction. Some have pointed out that the risk of using needle electrodes includes electrode displacement resulting in vocal cord haematomas, lacerations, needle breakage and possible inadvertent rupture of the endotracheal tube balloon.

Surface electrodes have gained widespread use in the field of intraoperative monitoring for recording laryngeal muscles. Two types of surface electrodes are commonly used: postcricoid surface electrodes and intralaryngeal surface electrodes that are integrated into the endotracheal tube. These ready-made endotracheal tubes are considerably more expensive than standard endotracheal tubes. An alternative is to attach sticky surface electrodes directly onto a standard endotracheal tube. One of the concerns regarding the use of surface electrodes (whether integrated or attached) is the possibility of tube migration during surgery, which significantly reduces the sensitivity of the surface electrodes because placement is no longer optimal [21]. Laryngeal palpation on stimulation of the RLN can be used for gross assessment of muscular response. This technique involves palpation of the posterior cricoarytenoid muscle contraction in response to RLN stimulation. Randolph *et al.* concluded that laryngeal palpation was as sensitive as the EMG assessment using surface or hooked wire electrodes [16].

References

1 Dedo HH. The paralyzed larynx: an electromyographic study in dogs and humans. Laryngoscope 1970; 80(10): 1455–517.

2 Steinberg JL, Khane GJ, Fernandes CM, Nel JP. Anatomy of the recurrent laryngeal nerve: a redescription. J Laryngol Otol 1986; 100(8): 919–27.

3 Brok HA, Copper MP, Stroeve RJ, Ongerboer de Visser BW, Venker-van Haagen AJ, Schouwenburg PF. Evidence for recurrent laryngeal nerve contribution in motor innervation of the human cricopharyngeal muscle. Laryngoscope 1999; 109(5): 705–8.

4 Hunt PS, Poole M, Reeve TS. A reappraisal of the surgical anatomy of the thyroid and parathyroid glands. Br J Surg 1968; 55(1): 63–6.

5 Wafae N, Vieira MC, Vorobieff A. The recurrent laryngeal nerve in relation to the inferior constrictor muscle of the pharynx. Laryngoscope 1991; 101(10): 1091–3.

6 Sepulveda A, Sastre N, Chousleb A. Topographic anatomy of the recurrent laryngeal nerve. J Reconstr Microsurg 1996; 12(1): 5–10.

7 Henry JF, Audiffret J, Denizot A, Plan M. The nonrecurrent inferior laryngeal nerve: review of 33 cases, including two on the left side. Surgery 1988; 104(6): 977–84.

8 Watanabe A, Kawabori S, Osanai H, Taniguchi M, Hosokawa M. Preoperative computed tomography diagnosis of non-recurrent inferior laryngeal nerve. Laryngoscope 2001; 111(10): 1756–9.

9 Lo CY, Kwok KF, Yuen PW. A prospective evaluation of recurrent laryngeal nerve paralysis during thyroidectomy. Arch Surg 2000; 135(2): 204–7.

10 Wagner HE, Seiler C. Recurrent laryngeal nerve palsy after thyroid gland surgery. Br J Surg 1994; 81(2): 226–8.

11 Foster RS Jr. Morbidity and mortality after thyroidectomy. Surg Gynecol Obstet 1978; 146(3): 423–9.

12 Abadin SS, Kaplan EL, Angelos P. Malpractice litigation after thyroid surgery: the role of recurrent laryngeal nerve injuries, 1989–2009. Surgery 2010; 148(4): 718–22; discussion 722–3.

13 Lore JM Jr, Kim DJ, Elias S. Preservation of the laryngeal nerves during total thyroid lobectomy. Ann Otol Rhinol Laryngol 1977; 86(6 Pt 1): 777–88.

14 Sheahan P, Murphy MS. Thyroid tubercle of Zuckerkandl: importance in thyroid surgery. Laryngoscope 2011; 121(11): 2335–7.

15 Pelizzo MR, Toniato A, Gemo G. Zuckerkandl's tuberculum: an arrow pointing to the recurrent laryngeal nerve (constant anatomical landmark). J Am Coll Surg 1998; 187(3): 333–6.

16 Randolph GW, Kobler JB, Wilkins J. Recurrent laryngeal nerve identification and assessment during thyroid surgery: laryngeal palpation. World J Surg 2004; 28(8): 755–60.

17 Moley JF, Lairmore TC, Doherty GM, Brunt LM, DeBenedetti MK. Preservation of the recurrent laryngeal nerves in thyroid and parathyroid reoperations. Surgery 1999; 126(4): 673–7; discussion 677–9.

18 Eisele DW. Intraoperative electrophysiologic monitoring of the recurrent laryngeal nerve. Laryngoscope 1996; 106(4): 443–9.

19 Timon CI, Rafferty M. Nerve monitoring in thyroid surgery: is it worthwhile? Clin Otolaryngol Allied Sci 1999; 24(6): 487–90.

20 Choby G, Hollenbeak CS, Johnson S, Goldenberg D. Surface electrode recurrent laryngeal nerve monitoring during thyroid surgery: normative values. J Clin Neurophysiol 2010; 27(1): 34–7.

21 Johnson S, Goldenberg D. Intraoperative monitoring of the recurrent laryngeal nerve during revision thyroid surgery. Otolaryngol Clin North Am 2008; 41(6): 1147–54, ix.

22 Randolph GW (ed). Surgery of the Thyroid and Parathyroid Glands. Philadelphia: Saunders/Elsevier, 2003.

23 Randolph GW. Surgical anatomy, intraoperative neural monitoring, and operative management of the RLN and SLN. In: Duh QY, Clark OH, Kebebew E (eds) Atlas of Endocrine Surgical Techniques. Surgical Techniques Atlas Series. Philadelphia: Saunders, 2010.

Videoclips

This chapter contains the following videoclips. They can be accessed at: www.wiley.com/go/miccoli/thyroid

Video 13.1 Unusual presentations of inferior laryngeal nerves. The inferior laryngeal nerve (ILN) can assume unusual positions because of their relationships with thyroid/parathyroid nodule(s) and rare anatomical conditions (non-recurrent -ILN).

CHAPTER 14

The Superior Laryngeal Nerve

Tammy M. Holm[1] and Sara I. Pai[2]

[1] Department of General Surgery, Brigham and Women's Hospital, and Harvard Medical School, Boston, MA, USA
[2] Departments of Otolaryngology – Head and Neck Surgery and Oncology, Johns Hopkins School of Medicine, Baltimore, MD, USA

Introduction

Identification with preservation of the superior laryngeal nerve (SLN) has become one of the refinements of thyroid surgery over the past 150 years. Historically, little attention has been paid to the functional importance of the SLN as it has been overshadowed by the often devastating complications associated with injury to the recurrent laryngeal nerve (RLN). Perspectives on the significance of SLN injury began shifting in the mid 1930s when a leading opera singer, Amelita Galli-Curci, underwent surgery to remove a large goitre. Postoperatively, Galli-Curci's diminished vocal range and poor vocal endurance were attributed to injury of the SLN during her thyroidectomy. Recent analysis of the events surrounding Galli-Curci's vocal decline suggest that SLN injury was, in fact, not a likely contributing factor [1]. Nonetheless, the media attention surrounding Galli-Curci's surgery highlighted the importance of SLN preservation among both the general public and greater surgical community.

Anatomy and physiology

The SLN originates as a branch of the vagus nerve (cranial nerve X) arising from the middle of the nodose ganglion with contributions from the superior cervical sympathetic ganglion. The SLN descends posteromedial to the internal carotid artery, bifurcating into two main branches, an external branch (EBSLN) and an internal branch (IBSLN), as it crosses posterior to the external carotid artery (Figure 14.1).

The IBSLN is the larger of the two and classically pierces the thyrohyoid membrane superior to the superior laryngeal artery before dividing into the superior, middle and inferior branches. The inferior branch also communicates with the recurrent laryngeal nerve via the ansa of Galen. The IBSLN consists of primarily sensory and autonomic nerves supplying the mucosal lining of the supraglottis and glottis. The superior branch of the IBSLN provides sensation to the lingual surface of the epiglottis and the lateral glosso-epiglottic fossae. The middle branch of the IBSLN innervates the aryepiglottic fold, true vocal folds, vestibular (false vocal) folds and the posterior aspect of the arytenoids. The inferior branch supplies the interarytenoid muscle. There is also a connecting branch uniting the IBSLN and EBSLN *vis-á-vis* the foramen thyroideum which is found in 4–30% of cases [2]. The sensory function of the IBSLN is responsible for the laryngeal cough reflex serving to protect patients from aspiration. Fortunately, the anatomical course of the IBSLN, namely superior and deep to the operative field, largely protects it from injury during thyroidectomy.

The EBSLN descends posterior to the sternothyroid muscle together with the superior thyroid artery (STA). It courses superficial to the inferior constrictor, piercing it just lateral to the inferior horn of the thyroid cartilage terminating in the cricothyroid (CT) muscle . The EBSLN is primarily motor in function. It enters the CT muscle as either a single trunk, which further divides to supply each

Thyroid Surgery: Preventing and Managing Complications, First Edition. Edited by Paolo Miccoli, David J. Terris, Michele N. Minuto and Melanie W. Seybt.

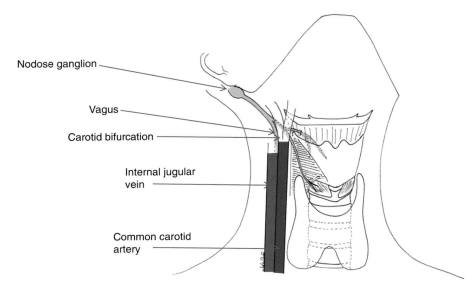

Nodose ganglion

Vagus

Carotid bifurcation

Internal jugular
vein

Common carotid
artery

Figure 14.1 Superior laryngeal nerve anatomy. The superior laryngeal nerve (SLN) originates from cranial nerve X at the nodose ganglion, descending posteromedial to the internal carotid artery and bifurcating as it crosses posterior to the external carotid artery. The internal branch penetrates the thyrohyoid membrane while the external branch continues with the superior thyroid vessels before terminating in the cricothyroid muscle. Nerve, yellow; internal jugular vein, blue; carotid artery, red.

of the three bellies of the CT muscle, or as multiple branches. The CT muscle provides vocal strength and duration, particularly at higher pitches. Contraction of the CT pivots the inferior cornu of the thyroid cartilage posteriorly upon the cricoid cartilage, thereby stretching the vocal cords (Figure 14.2). Interestingly, recent cadaveric studies have identified communicating nerves between the EBSLN and the recurrent laryngeal nerve, thus suggesting significant innervation to laryngeal muscles other than the CT [3]. Specifically, the EBSLN has been shown to give off motor branches to the ipsilateral thyroarytenoid muscle and sensory branches to the subglottic mucosa and the area surrounding the cricoarytenoid joint [4]. This connection, referred to as the 'human communicating nerve' or the 'CT connection branch', has been identified in 44–85% of larynges studied [2,3,5]. These communicating nerves may explain the residual vocal cord innervation observed in some cases following injury to the RLN.

Anatomical variation

The origin of the EBSLN is typically described by its relationship to either the superior thyroid artery or the superior pole of the thyroid. Unfortunately, these landmarks themselves often vary according to neck length, thyroid size and ethnicity. Further contributing factors to the challenge of EBSLN identification and preservation is the observation that the course of the nerve may be asymmetrical 15–25% of the time within the same patient [6,7]. Multiple classification systems have been developed to identify more consistent surgical landmarks for EBSLN identification and/or preservation.

Cernea classified the course of the EBSLN into three groups based on the position of the nerve relative to the superior thyroid pole [8] (Figure 14.3). In type 1 variants (23%), the EBSLN crosses the superior thyroid vessels one or more centimeters above the horizontal plane at the superior border of the superior thyroid pole. In type 2a variants (15%), the nerve crosses less than 1 cm above the upper border of the superior thyroid pole while in type 2b variants (54%), the nerve crosses behind and below the upper border. Type 2b variants are more common in large goitres. The type 2 variants are most vulnerable to iatrogenic injury in thyroidectomy. Kierner and colleagues developed a slightly different classification system with four variants [9]. Types 1, 2 and 3 coincide with Cernea types 1, 2a and 2b, respectively. However, they describe an

Figure 14.2 Cricothyroid contraction. As the cricothyroid muscle contracts, the thyroid cartilage tilts inferiorly, shifting the cricoid cartilage posteriorly and thereby stretching the vocal cords. Vocal cords, red.

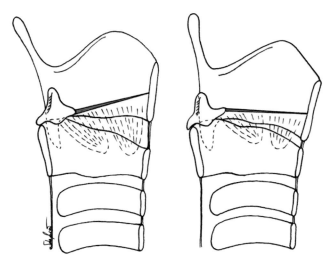

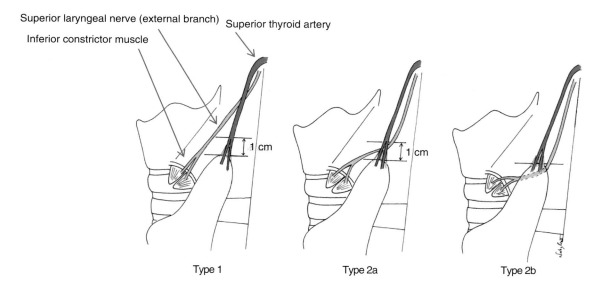

Superior laryngeal nerve (external branch) Superior thyroid artery

Inferior constrictor muscle

1 cm

1 cm

Type 1   Type 2a   Type 2b

Figure 14.3 Classification of the EBSLN – Cernea classification. The EBSLN is classified relative to the superior thyroid pole. In the type 1 variant, the EBSLN crosses the superior thyroid vessels at least 1 cm (*double arrows*) above the superior border of the thyroid pole. In the type 2a variant, the EBSLN crosses less than 1 cm above the superior border of the thyroid (*double arrows*). In type 2b variants, the nerve crosses behind and below the superior pole of the thyroid (*dotted lines*) thereby placing it at increased risk of inadvertent damage during dissection of the superior pole. EBSLN, yellow; superior thyroid artery, red.

incidence of 42% type 1, 30% type 2 and 14% type 3. Type 4 variants (14%) occur when the nerve crosses the STA immediately above the upper pole of the thyroid gland [6].

More recently, Friedman and colleagues developed a classification system to describe the intraoperative iden-tification of the EBSLN as it courses to the CT muscle [10]. They describe variations of the EBSLN relative to the inferior constrictor (Figure 14.4). In type 1 variants, the EBSLN descends with the superior thyroid vessels, either superficial or lateral to the inferior constrictor,

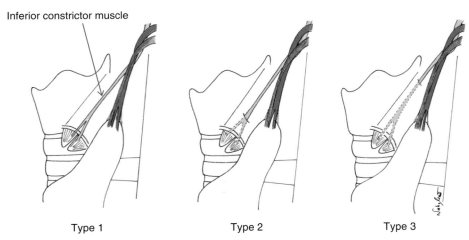

Type 1   Type 2   Type 3

Figure 14.4 Classification of the EBSLN – Friedman classification. The EBSLN is classified relative to the inferior constrictor. In type 1 variants, the EBSLN travels with the superior thyroid vessels superficial or lateral to the inferior constrictor. In type 2 variants, the EBSLN pierces the inferior constrictor just above the inferolateral edge of the thyroid cartilage (*dotted lines*). In type 3 variants, the EBSLN pierces the inferior constrictor early in its descent (*dotted lines*), travelling deep to the muscle prior to entering the cricothyroid.

until it terminates in the CT. In type 2 variants, the EBSLN penetrates the inferior constrictor 1 cm above the inferolateral edge of the thyroid cartilage. Finally, in type 3 variants, the EBSLN penetrates the superior aspect of the inferior constrictor and then continues deep to the muscle before piercing the CT.

Nerve monitoring

As the clinical significance of EBSLN function becomes more apparent, preservation has become paramount to achieving excellent surgical outcomes. Visual identification of the EBSLN is challenging on two fronts. First, it is a small-calibre nerve not easily visualized or palpated. Second, recent technical innovations including minimally invasive, mini-incision and video-assisted (MIVAT) thyroidectomy restrict the operative field, thereby limiting the surgeon's ability to visualize the nerve successfully. Neuromonitoring provides an adjunct to direct visualization for safe and effective identification.

Intraoperative neuromonitoring is a widely utilized technique for identification of the recurrent laryngeal nerves. Traditionally, an endotracheal tube is outfitted with electrodes which allow for direct contact with the vocal cords during surgery. Stimulation of the RLN results in an audible signal and/or electromyograph (EMG) wave. In a similar fashion, electrodes may be placed directly within the CT muscle and stimulation of the EBSLN will result in an audible signal and visible muscle contraction.

A recent prospective study of 10 patients undergoing minimally invasive thyroidectomy found that the EBSLN could be preserved in 100% of cases [11]. Bipolar electrodes were placed directly within the CT muscle and the EBSLN was identified by direct stimulation of the nerve. If the nerve could not be visualized, the stimulation probe was applied to the vessels entering the superior thyroid pole to rule out inadvertent entrapment of the EBSLN. The Voice Handicap Index-10 (VHI-10), a validated tool for patient self-appraisal of voice handicap severity, was used to assess evidence of nerve injury. All patients experienced preserved VHI-10 handicap scores 3 weeks after surgery. This study led to a prospective trial of 47 patients randomized to nerve monitoring or no nerve monitoring during thyroidectomy under local/regional anaesthesia with intravenous sedation [12]. Nerve monitoring was found to improve visualization of the EBSLN and resulted in better VHI-10 scores in patients who underwent nerve monitoring compared to those who did not. These studies are limited by their reliance on subjective patient functional assessment and lack videostroboscopy or flexible fiberoptic laryngoscopy confirmation of pre- and postoperative CT function.

Surgical approach

The close association of the EBSLN with the STA makes it quite vulnerable to injury during thyroid surgery. Surgical principles dictate preservation of anatomical structures through direct visualization of the nerve, as opposed to avoiding the course of the nerve. Cernea and others report a lower incidence of postoperative CT dysfunction in cases where the EBSLN is directly identified compared to when it is not [8]. In a separate randomized prospective study of 59 patients, the rate of EBSLN injury in dissections where the nerve was not identified was almost twice that of dissections where the EBSLN was identified – 14% versus 8% [13]. However, these studies did not account for surgical strategies to avoid EBSLN injury, i.e. ligation of the STA vessels directly on the thyroid gland. One randomized prospective study of 289 patients undergoing thyroidectomy found that ligation of STA branches close to the thyroid gland successfully avoids EBSLN injury as effectively as ligation of the STA after identification of EBSLN [14].

Some surgeons recommend the use of a nerve stimulator together with transection of the sternothyroid muscle at its attachment to the thyroid cartilage [10]. Using this technique, successful identification and preservation of the EBSLN were reported up to 85% of the time. Pagedar & Freeman modified this approach by foregoing the nerve stimulator and transecting the sternothyroid muscle at its midpoint [15]. The lateral surface of the CT and the EBSLN is exposed by bluntly dissecting superiorly into the avascular space between the larynx and superior thyroid pole. This technique allowed for successful EBSLN identification and preservation 98% of the time. However, these techniques are becoming less favored with the current trend towards smaller incisions.

There is some debate as to whether visualization of the nerve alone is sufficient to confirm EBSLN identification. In a study aiming to map the compound muscle action potential of the CT muscle using EMG, the gold standard for nerve identification, Selvan and colleagues found that 'nerves' visually identified by the surgeon were not often

verified by EMG and were in fact tendinous or thin, non-neural fibres within the region [16]. This would suggest that the addition of the nerve stimulator could be useful both for verifying visual EBSLN identification and for ruling out entrapment of the nerve while ligating the vessels at the superior pole [11,12,17]. While the small size and variable anatomical course may lead to difficulty in nerve visualization and identification, the nerve stimulator, when appropriately used, can provide some reassurance to surgeons that they are not going to transect the EBSLN. This approach is particularly useful in mini-incision thyroidectomy where the surgical field is limited.

Preservation of the EBSLN remains a challenge with the introduction of video-assisted and robotic thyroidectomy. Early studies in MIVAT suggest improved identification given the magnification introduced by the endoscope. Berti and colleagues report 'incidentally' identifying the EBSLN in 195 out of 300 VAT cases [18]. A recent prospective, randomized case–control study of 72 patients evaluated the role of intraoperative neuromonitoring in EBSLN identification during MIVAT and found that EBSLN was identified in 84% in the neuromonitoring group versus 42% in the non-monitored cohort [19].

Injury

Symptoms of CT muscle paralysis resulting from EBSLN injury include hoarseness, decreased vocal range, particularly with high pitches, decreased voice projection and voice fatigue. Symptoms of clinical injury may be directly assessed via indirect laryngoscopy, laryngeal EMG or fiberoptic stroboscopic laryngoscopy. The reported incidence of injury varies widely, with more recent reports suggesting a rate of approximately 2–28% [17,20,21]. Overall, increased injury has been associated with failure to identify the EBSLN intraoperatively.

While the course of the IBSLN largely protects it from injury during thyroidectomy, some patients will report increased dysphagia, coughing and swallowing difficulties consistent with IBSLN injury postoperatively. Clinical assessment is achieved via laryngopharyngeal sensory testing where pooling of secretions and loss of sensation to endoscope touch are evaluated. A recent prospective study found that pre- and postoperative laryngopharyngeal sensory testing failed to reveal sensory changes following thyroidectomy despite subjective patient complaints of postoperative dysphagia and globus sensation [22].

Rehabilitation

Patients suffering from SLN injury are best managed with aggressive speech therapy with a focus on isolated CT muscle strength training [23]. Voice rehabilitation is the mainstay of therapy, improving frequency range, projection and vocal control [24]. Unlike recurrent laryngeal nerve injury, surgical intervention with vocal fold injection, medialization or nerve grafting is rarely pursued in SLN injury.

Conclusion

"Can the thyroid in the state of enlargement be removed? Should the surgeon be so foolhardy to undertake it, every stroke of the knife will be followed by a torrent of blood and lucky it would be for him if his victim lived long enough for him to finish his horrid butchery. No honest and sensible surgeon would ever engage in it." (Samuel Gross MD, 1848)

We have made remarkable advancements in thyroid surgery over the past 150 years. The field is moving toward perfecting an operation once considered life-threatening, with smaller incisions, shorter hospital stays, preservation of both the recurrent and superior laryngeal nerves as well as parathyroid function. Innovations in video-assisted and robotic surgery have led to improved field visualization despite smaller and more cosmetically appealing incisions. Neuromonitoring serves as an important adjunct to the abbreviated operative field allowing for confirmation of nerve identification and thus improved preservation. While our approach to thyroidectomy continues to advance rapidly, the elegance of thyroid surgery continues to rest in the details: precise identification and preservation of important structures within the multilayered, complex anatomical network of the human neck.

References

1 Crookes PF, Recabaren JA. Injury to the superior laryngeal branch of the vagus during thyroidectomy: lesson or myth? Ann Surg 2001; 233(4): 588–93.

2 Sanudo JR, Maranillo E, Leon X, Mirapeix RM, Orus C, Quer M. An anatomical study of anastomoses between the laryngeal nerves. Laryngoscope 1999; 109(6): 983–7.

3 Wu BL, Sanders I, Mu L, Biller HF. The human communicating nerve. An extension of the external superior laryngeal nerve that innervates the vocal cord. Arch Otolaryngol Head Neck Surg 1994; 120(12): 1321–8.

4 Mu L, Sanders I. The human cricothyroid muscle: three muscle bellies and their innervation patterns. J Voice 2009; 23(1): 21–8.

5 Maranillo E, Leon X, Ibanez M, Orus C, Quer M, Sanudo JR. Variability of the nerve supply patterns of the human posterior cricoarytenoid muscle. Laryngoscope 2003; 113(4): 602–6.

6 Poyraz M, Calguner E. Bilateral investigation of the anatomical relationships of the external branch of the superior laryngeal nerve and superior thyroid artery, and also the recurrent laryngeal nerve and inferior thyroid artery. Okajimas Folia Anat Jpn 2001; 78(2–3): 65–74.

7 Mishra AK, Temadari H, Singh N, Mishra SK, Agarwal A. The external laryngeal nerve in thyroid surgery: the 'no more neglected' nerve. Indian J Med Sci 2007; 61(1): 3–8.

8 Cernea CR, Ferraz AR, Nishio S, Dutra A Jr, Hojaij FC, dos Santos LR. Surgical anatomy of the external branch of the superior laryngeal nerve. Head Neck 1992; 14(5): 380–3.

9 Kierner AC, Aigner M, Burian M. The external branch of the superior laryngeal nerve: its topographical anatomy as related to surgery of the neck. Arch Otolaryngol Head Neck Surg 1998; 124(3): 301–3.

10 Friedman M, LoSavio P, Ibrahim H. Superior laryngeal nerve identification and preservation in thyroidectomy. Arch Otolaryngol Head Neck Surg 2002; 128(3): 296–303.

11 Inabnet WB, Murry T, Dhiman S, Aviv J, Lifante JC. Neuromonitoring of the external branch of the superior laryngeal nerve during minimally invasive thyroid surgery under local anesthesia: a prospective study of 10 patients. Laryngoscope 2009; 119(3): 597–601.

12 Lifante JC, McGill J, Murry T, Aviv JE, Inabnet WB 3rd. A prospective, randomized trial of nerve monitoring of the external branch of the superior laryngeal nerve during thyroidectomy under local/regional anesthesia and IV sedation. Surgery 2009; 146(6): 1167–73.

13 Hurtado-Lopez LM, Pacheco-Alvarez MI, Montes-Castillo Mde L, Zaldivar-Ramirez FR. Importance of the intraoperative identification of the external branch of the superior laryngeal nerve during thyroidectomy: electromyographic evaluation. Thyroid 2005; 15(5): 449–54.

14 Bellantone R, Boscherini M, Lombardi CP, *et al.* Is the identification of the external branch of the superior laryngeal nerve mandatory in thyroid operation? Results of a prospective randomized study. Surgery 2001; 130(6): 1055–9.

15 Pagedar NA, Freeman JL. Identification of the external branch of the superior laryngeal nerve during thyroidectomy. Arch Otolaryngol Head Neck Surg 2009; 135(4): 360–2.

16 Selvan B, Babu S, Paul MJ, Abraham D, Samuel P, Nair A. Mapping the compound muscle action potentials of cricothyroid muscle using electromyography in thyroid operations: a novel method to clinically type the external branch of the superior laryngeal nerve. Ann Surg 2009; 250(2): 293–300.

17 Jonas J, Bahr R. Neuromonitoring of the external branch of the superior laryngeal nerve during thyroid surgery. Am J Surg 2000; 179(3): 234–6.

18 Berti P, Materazzi G, Conte M, Galleri D, Miccoli P. Visualization of the external branch of the superior laryngeal nerve during video-assisted thyroidectomy. J Am Coll Surg 2002; 195(4): 573–4.

19 Dionigi G, Boni L, Rovera F, Bacuzzi A, Dionigi R. Neuromonitoring and video-assisted thyroidectomy: a pro-spective, randomized case–control evaluation. Surg Endosc 2009; 23(5): 996–1003.

20 Aluffi P, Policarpo M, Cherovac C, Olina M, Dosdegani R, Pia F. Post-thyroidectomy superior laryngeal nerve injury. Eur Arch Otorhinolaryngol 2001; 258(9): 451–4.

21 Teitelbaum BJ, Wenig BL. Superior laryngeal nerve injury from thyroid surgery. Head Neck 1995; 17(1): 36–40.

22 Wasserman JM, Sundaram K, Alfonso AE, Rosenfeld RM, Har-El G. Determination of the function of the internal branch of the superior laryngeal nerve after thyroidectomy. Head Neck 2008; 30(1): 21–7.

23 Eckley CA, Sataloff RT, Hawkshaw M, Spiegel JR, Mandel S. Voice range in superior laryngeal nerve paresis and paralysis. J Voice 1998; 12(3): 340–8.

24 Dursun G, Sataloff RT, Spiegel JR, Mandel S, Heuer RJ, Rosen DC. Superior laryngeal nerve paresis and paralysis. J Voice 1996; 10(2): 206–11.

CHAPTER 15

The Parathyroid Glands in Thyroid Surgery

Maisie Shindo

Department of Otolaryngology, Oregon Health and Science University, Portland, OR, USA

Introduction

Parathyroid glands were first discovered in the Indian rhinoceros, and they are the last major organ to be discovered in humans [1]. They secrete parathyroid hormone (PTH), an 84-amino acid peptide, which induces the release of calcium from bone, increases renal calcium reabsorption in the renal tubules, and stimulates the conversion of the inactive form of vitamin D (25-hydroxyvitamin D) to its bioactive form, 1,25-dihydroxyvitamin D ($1,25(OH)_2$-D) in the kidney. The latter in turn increases intestinal absorption of calcium. Damage to parathyroid glands results in hypoparathyroidism, which reduces renal calcium reabsorption as well as formation of $1,25(OH)_2$-D. Both effects result in reduced serum calcium.

Parathyroid preservation during thyroidectomy

The most common complication of total thyroidectomy is hypocalcaemia. The incidence of hypocalcaemia following total thyroidectomy can be as high as 50%. In general, this is a transient problem and in the hands of experienced surgeons, the risk of permanent hypocalcaemia is 1%. Understanding the locations and vascular anatomy of these glands is critical to parathyroid preservation during thyroidectomy.

Anatomy

Each human typically has four parathyroid glands, two superior and two inferior. The inferior parathyroid glands are derived from the third pharyngeal pouch and descend caudally with the thyroid and thymus. The superior parathyroid glands are derived from the fourth pharyngeal pouch, attach to the posterior surface of the superior or midportion thyroid and migrate caudally with it. This pattern of migration explains the variability in the locations of the parathyroid glands, resulting in many possible locations of ectopic or supernumerary parathyroid glands. The limited course of the superior glands leads to less variability in location compared with the inferior gland. The inferior parathyroid glands can typically be found anterior to a plane drawn through the recurrent laryngeal nerve. They can be found just inferior, lateral or posterior to the inferior pole of the thyroid (Figure 15.1) though they can be quite variable in location. The superior parathyroid glands are less variable in location, the vast majority of them typically located near the cricothyroid joint, just superior to where the recurrent laryngeal nerve enters the larynx (Figure 15.2). The blood supply to the parathyroid glands is primarily from the inferior thyroid artery, and in some there is contribution from the superior thyroid artery (Figure 15.3). Each gland typically weighs 35–40 mg, measures 3–8 mm in each dimension and can vary in colour from light yellow to reddish brown.

Thyroid Surgery: Preventing and Managing Complications, First Edition. Edited by Paolo Miccoli, David J. Terris,
Michele N. Minuto and Melanie W. Seybt.
© 2013 John Wiley & Sons, Ltd. Published 2013 by John Wiley & Sons, Ltd.

(a)

(b)

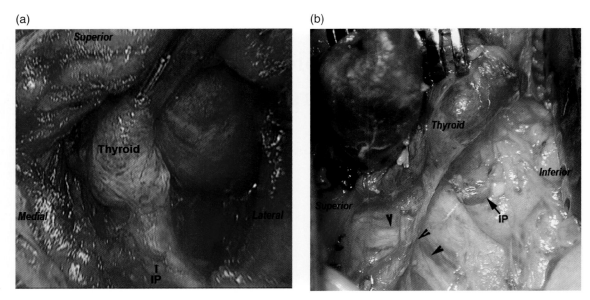

Figure 15.1 Typical locations for inferior parathyroid gland. (a) Left inferior parathyroid (IP) at the tip of the lower pole of thyroid. (b) Right inferior parathyroid (IP) posterior to the inferior pole of the thyroid. Arrowheads, recurrent laryngeal nerve.

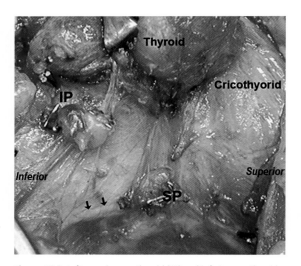

Figure 15.2 Left superior parathyroid (SP) and inferior parathyroid (IP). Arrows, recurrent laryngeal nerve.

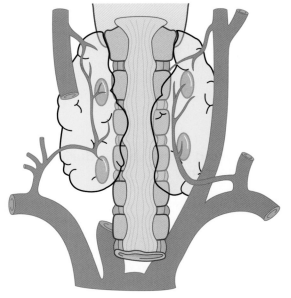

Figure 15.3 Parathyroid blood supply.

Parathyroid preservation

One of the greatest challenges during thyroid surgery is to identify the parathyroid glands and meticulously preserve them with their blood supply. During thyroidectomy, dissection should be kept along the thyroid capsule to minimize inadvertent removal or devascularization of the parathyroid glands. Meticulous atraumatic gentle handling of the parathyroid gland and its blood supply is critical to its survival. The parathyroid gland should be gently dissected off the thyroid capsule. It is not uncommon to encounter small vessels between the parathyroid

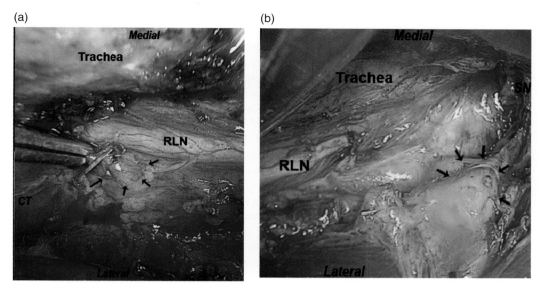

Figure 15.4 Right paratracheal compartment after total thyroidectomy and paratracheal node dissection. (a) Preservation of superior parathyroid (SP; CT, cricothyroid) and (b) arrows point to preserved inferior parathyroid. RLN, recurrent laryngeal nerve.

and thyroid capsule. These vessels should be controlled without injuring the parathyroid gland, and cautery should be avoided on the gland. If it is necessary to divide these vessels near the parathyroid gland, haemoclips or fine tip bipolar should be used, keeping the bipolar tip at least 2–3 mm away from the parathyroid. When performing *en bloc* central compartment dissection, every attempt should be made to identify and preserve the superior parathyroid glands (Figure 15.4a), since the inferior ones are often embedded in the paratracheal contents and removed with the specimen. If the inferior gland is found during the thyroidectomy, its vascular pedicle should be identified, which typically courses lateral to the gland. Once the parathyroid gland is successfully peeled off the thyroid capsule, it should be reflected laterally or inferiorly on its pedicle and carefully preserved prior to completing the paratracheal compartment dissection (Figure 15.4b).

Autotransplantation

Parathyroid glands can be adherent to or embedded within the thyroid capsule and be inadvertently removed during thyroidectomy. When performing compartment-oriented central neck dissection for malignancy, the inferior parathyroid glands, and at times the more caudally lying superior glands, may be removed with the specimen.

Therefore the specimen should be inspected for parathyroid gland(s) prior to passing it off the field. Pederson *et al.* described the use of γ-probe and sestamibi injection to help differentiate parathyroid from other tissues during thyroidectomy and central neck dissection [2]. Another similar study by Grubbs and colleagues concluded that it can be helpful to determine the radioactive count if measured *ex vivo* in the central compartment dissection specimen for identifying parathyroid glands but not in the thyroid specimen [3]. Any parathyroid gland found should be removed for reimplantation. Prior to reimplantation, a small portion of the tissue may be biopsied and sent for frozen section confirmation of parathyroid tissue, as the parathyroid gland can be visually challenging to differentiate from fat or lymph nodes. Once histologically confirmed, the parathyroid tissue should be cut into 1×1×3 mm pieces and reimplanted into intramuscular pocket(s) in the sternocleidomastoid muscle. The reimplanted site(s) should be marked with a haemoclip and or permanent coloured suture (Figure 15.5).

Risk of postoperative hypocalcaemia

Potential causes of postoperative hypocalcaemia after total thyroidectomy include injury and devascularization

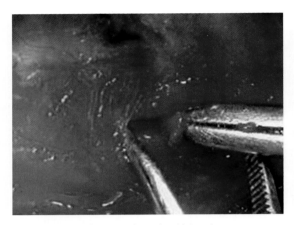

Figure 15.5 Reimplantation of parathyroid tissue into sternocleidomastoid muscle.

of the parathyroid glands, inadvertent removal of parathyroid glands, and calciuretic effect of intravenous fluid. Extent of surgery has an impact on the risk of hypocalcaemia. Several earlier studies have reported high incidences of postoperative transient hypocalcaemia, as high as 70%, with total thyroidectomy and central compartment lymph node dissection, and permanent hypocalcaemia ranging from 1% to 15% [4–8]. These statistics were primarily based on comprehensive bilateral paratracheal node dissection. In analysing the incidence of hypocalcaemia from bilateral versus unilateral central compartment lymph node dissection, it appears that the risk from bilateral dissection is higher than that of unilateral dissection [6, 9–11]. Another study also showed that adding unilateral or selective central neck dissection to total thyroidectomy does not increase the risk of postoperative hypocalcaemia [12]. With regard to correlating the thyroid pathology with postoperative hypocalcaemia, total thyroidectomy for large compressive goitres, substernal goitres and for chronic hyperthyroidism due to Graves' disease has been shown to be associated with increased risk of postoperative hypocalcaemia [13–16]. Females also appear to be more likely than males to develop hypocalcaemia following total thyroidectomy [6,15].

Postoperative management of hypocalcaemia

Patients admitted for observation should be assessed for symptoms and signs of hypocalcaemia. Classic symptoms of hypocalcaemia are neuromuscular excitability in the

form of muscle twitching, spasms, tingling and numbness. In severe cases carpopedal spasm can develop and progress to tetany and seizures. Severe hypocalcaemia can also cause cardiac dysrhythmias. In patients without overt signs, underlying neuromuscular excitability can become evident with provocation. One test is eliciting a Chvostek's sign where tapping the preauricular region over the facial nerve induces facial muscle twitching. Approximately 10% of normal people have a positive Chvostek's sign; conversely, patients with hypoparathyroidism and biochemically confirmed hypocalcaemia may not demonstrate a Chvostek's sign [17]. Another test is inflation of a blood pressure cuff to induce hypoxia in muscles, which can precipitate carpopedal spasm (Trousseau's sign). Trousseau's sign is relatively specific for hypocalcaemia – 94% of hypocalcaemic patients display a positive sign, compared with 1% of normocalcaemic people [17]. A calcium level may be checked the next morning, and two sequential calcium levels should be drawn 6–8 h apart the next day since the calcium may not drop until well beyond 24 h after surgery. Patients can be discharged if the sequential calcium levels are stable or demonstrate an upward trend.

Normal range for plasma calcium in most laboratories is 8.5–10.2 mg/dL (or 2.2–2.5 mmol/L). Since most of the body's plasma calcium is bound to albumin, a decrease in plasma albumin will lower the plasma calcium level even though the free calcium remains the same. Therefore if the albumin level is low, the plasma calcium should be corrected such that 0.8 should be added to the total calcium for every drop in albumin of 1.0. When in doubt, it can be helpful to obtain a free calcium level by measuring ionized calcium. Normal range for ionized calcium in most labs is 1.12–1.32. Calcium levels also inversely correlate with pH such that alkalosis lowers the ionized calcium and acidosis elevates it. Therefore a hypocalcaemic patient who hyperventilates can develop respiratory alkalosis, thus lowering the free calcium and aggravating paraesthesias and possibly inducing tetany.

Surgeons and endocrinologists employ a variety of different postoperative regimens for treatment of hypocalcaemia. While there is no consensus on this issue, there are some general principles that can guide medical management of hypocalcaemic patients after thyroidectomy. Should symptoms develop or serum calcium values corrected for albumin drop below 8.0 mg/dL, oral calcium carbonate should be initiated at a dose of 1.5–4 g/day.

Patients with severe hypocalcaemia, i.e. less than 7.0 mg/dL, or symptoms such as cramps and tetany, require replacement with intravenous calcium. These patients should be monitored on telemetry since they can also develop electrocardiogram (ECG) changes, such as prolonged QT interval. Calcium gluconate is preferred over calcium chloride for intravenous administration, as the latter is associated with increased risk of tissue necrosis. If only the chloride form is available and must be used, it should be administered via a central venous line. The initial dose for infusion is 1 g (93 mg of elemental calcium) to 2 g diluted in 250 cc of dextrose solution given over 10–20 min. If the calcium persistently remains below 7 mg/dL, a continuous intravenous infusion should be initiated. Continuous infusion is typically given as 10 g/L solution infused at a rate of 1–3 mg of elemental calcium/kg/h. It is also important to administer vitamin D, as it is the mainstay in the treatment of hypoparathyroidism. A variety of vitamin D preparations are available, including ergocalciferol (vitamin D_2), cholecalciferol (vitamin D_3) and calcitriol, which is the biologically active form of vitamin D (1,25-dihydroxyvitamin-D_3). Calcitriol should be used instead of the inactive forms (D_2, D_3), since there is a lack of parathyroid hormone to convert the inactive form to the active form. The typical dose of calcitriol is 0.25–0.5 μg.

Three major trends in postoperative calcium management have emerged in recent years moving toward early discharge. The idea is to predict who is at risk of developing hypoparathyroidism and treat early so that hypocalcaemia is not prolonged. One is to measure serum calcium and phosphate levels before and after surgery. However, there is very little consensus about when and how often those levels should be measured. Sam and colleagues analysed changes in phosphate levels between the night of surgery and the following morning in 111 patients who underwent total thyroidectomy and found that all those who became hypocalcaemic had an overnight rise in serum phosphate to >1.44 mmol/L [18].

Another approach is routine empiric supplementation of calcium with or without calcitriol (vitamin D) and discharging the patient the following day if the calcium is normal. Routine use of oral calcium supplements has been shown to reduce the incidence and severity of post-thyroidectomy hypocalcaemia and facilitate early discharge [19,20]. If this approach is to be taken, the patient should be educated on signs and symptoms of hypocalcaemia and may be instructed to go for a calcium check the following morning.

A third method that has been proposed in recent years is using intraoperative rapid PTH, drawn some time between right after skin closure to 6 h after, for predicting the risk of hypocalcaemia. Laboratories measure intact parathyroid hormone levels using immunoassays. The assay technique was then modified to obtain a PTH level rapidly during parathyroid surgery to determine success. The application of this intraoperative rapid PTH (IOPTH) was then expanded to thyroidectomy patients for predicting postoperative hypocalcaemia. Noordzig pooled results of post-thyroidectomy PTH measurements in 457 patients from nine studies and found that the immediate postoperative PTH was <10 pg/dL in those who became hypocalcaemic [21]. Numerous studies have published similar findings. The absolute value of immediate postoperative PTH level at which the patient is at risk of becoming hypocalcaemic ranged from 8 to 16 pg/dL or 1.7–3.7 pmol/L [22–30]. Some have also advocated using percent drop from preoperative level as a predictor. However, there is a great deal of variability in the results of these studies, the percent drop from preoperative level that predicts postoperative hypocalcaemia ranging from 30% to 70% [22,23,27]. Post-thyroidectomy PTH levels predict hypocalcaemia but lack 100% accuracy. Progressive and severe hypocalcaemia is unlikely in the setting of a normal PTH level and hence PTH can be cautiously used to facilitate discharge within 24 h for these patients. In addition, PTH levels can be used to implement early treatment with calcium and/or vitamin D supplements to reduce the incidence and severity of hypocalcaemia [31–33].

There is no uniform concrete algorithm for checking and managing postoperative calcium. If postoperative IOPTH is below normal range (i.e. less than 5 pg/dL), calcium supplements should be initiated, and two sequential calcium levels should be drawn 6–8 h apart the next day since the calcium may not drop until well beyond 24 h after surgery. The preferred type and dose of supplements vary; most start with calcium carbonate 1000–2000 mg every 8 h. Calcitriol 0.25–0.5 μg daily may also be administered in these patients. The patient can be discharged if sequential calcium levels demonstrate an upward trend. If postoperative IOPTH is above 10 pg/dL and the morning calcium is within normal range, the patient can be discharged. In these patients if the corrected calcium is at the lower range of normal, it is not unreasonable to send them home with oral calcium and have them recheck a level as an outpatient the next day. If the postoperative IOPTH is between 5 and 10 pg/dL and the morning calcium level is below normal range, oral calcium supplementation should be started if the patient is not already on calcium. The calcium level should be rechecked in 6 h and monitored as described above. If the calcium is extremely low, i.e. less than 7 mg/dL, or the patient experiences symptoms of neuromuscular excitability, intravenous calcium gluconate should be administered as outlined above.

Permanent hypoparathyroidism

Permanent hypoparathyroidism is treated with long-term calcium and calcitriol replacement. A new promising treatment modality for hypoparathyroidism is administration of recombinant human I-34 PTH (terapeptide) [34,35]. In a 3-year study in 12 children, subcutaneous PTH(I-34) was compared with calcium and calcitriol treatment, and the authors concluded that PTH(1-34) therapy is safe and effective [34]. Whether this represents the treatment of choice in adults with hypoparathyroidism is currently unclear, but it represents an important advancement in the treatment of parathyroid deficiency, especially for children.

Another area of research in treatment of hypoparathyroidism is cellular replacement therapy (i.e. stem cells). Woods Ignatoski and colleagues used BG01 human stem cells and forced differentiation into parathyroid cells that expressed mRNA for calcium-sensing receptor on the parathyroid gland, CXCR4 (an epithelial marker), GCM2 (a parathyroid specific marker) and PTH [36]. These cells have been isolated and cultured in the long term and may represent the first step toward altering adult pluripotent stem cells to create parathyroid cells for therapeutic purposes.

Conclusion

Hypoparathyoidism is a very rare permanent sequela of thyroidectomy that can significantly affect the patient's quality of life. The risk of this occurring can be minimized by diligently looking for parathyroid glands during dissection, handling them with utmost care and preserving them with their blood supply.

References

1 Modarai B, Sawyer A, Ellis H. The glands of Owen, J R Soc Med 2004: 97: 494–5.

2 Pederson LC, Shapiro SE, Fritsche HA Jr, et al. Potential role for intraoperative gamma probe identification of normal parathyroid glands. Am J Surg 2003; 186: 711–17.

3 Grubbs EG, Mittendorf EA, Perrier ND, Lee JE. Gamma probe identification of normal parathyroid glands during central neck surgery can facilitate parathyroid preservation. Am J Surg 2008; 196(6): 931–5.

4 Chea WK, Arici C, Ituarte PHG, Siperstein AE, Duh QY, Clark OH. Complications of neck dissection for thyroid cancer. World J Surg 2002; 26: 1013–16.

5 Roh JL, Park JY, Park CI. Total thyroidectomy plus neck dissection in differentiated papillary thyroid carcinoma patients: pattern of nodal metastasis, morbidity, recurrence, and postoperative levels of serum parathyroid hormone. Ann Surg 2007; 245: 604–10.

6 Cavicchi O, Piccin O, Caliceti U, de Cataldis A, Pasquali R, Ceroni AR. Transient hypoparathyroidism following thyroidectomy: a prospective study and multivariate analysis of 604 consecutive patients. Otolaryngol Head Neck Surg 2007; 137: 654–8.

7 White ML, Gauger PG, Doherty GM. Central lymph node dissection in differentiated thyroid cancer. World J Surg 2007; 31: 895–904.

8 Pereira JA, Jimeno J, Miquel J, et al. Nodal yield, morbidity, and recurrence after central neck dissection for papillary thyroid carcinoma. Surgery 2005; 138: 1095–100.

9 Son YI, Jeong HS, Baek CH, et al. Extent of prophylactic lymph node dissection in the central neck area of the patients with papillary thyroid carcinoma: comparison of limited versus comprehensive lymph node dissection in a 2–year safety study. Ann Surg Oncol 2008; 15(7): 2020–6.

10 Lee YS, Kim SW, Kim SW, et al. Extent of routine central lymph node dissection with small papillary thyroid carcinoma. World J Surg 2007; 31: 1954–9.

11 Sywak M, Cornford L, Roach P, Stalberg P, Sidhu S, Delbridge L. Routine ipsilateral level VI lymphadenectomy reduces postoperative thyroglobulin levels in papillary thyroid cancer. Surgery 2006; 140: 1000–7.

12 Shindo M. Stern A. Total thyroidectomy with and without selective central compartment dissection: a comparison of complication rates. Arch Otolaryngol Head Neck Surg 2010; 136(6): 584–7.

13 Prim MP, de Diego JI, Hardisson D, Madero R, Gavilan J. Factors related to nerve injury and hypocalcemia in thyroid gland surgery. Otolaryngol Head Neck Surg 2001; 124: 111–14.

14 Pesce CE, Shiue Z, Tsai HL, *et al.* Postoperative hypocalcemia after thyroidectomy for Graves' disease. Thyroid 2010; 20(11): 1279–83.

15 Page C, Strunski V. Parathyroid risk in total thyroidectomy for bilateral, benign, multinodular goiter: report of 351 surgical cases. J Laryngol Otol 2007; 121: 237–41.

16 Thomusch O, Machens A, Sekulla C, Ukkat J, Brauckhoff M, Dralle H. The impact of surgical technique on postoperative hypoparathyroidism in bilateral thyroid surgery: a multivariate analysis of 5846 consecutive patients. Surgery 2003; 133: 180–5.

17 Urbano FL. Signs of hypocalcemia. Chvostek's and Trousseau's sign. Hosp Phys 2005; 36: 43–5.

18 Sam AH, Dhillo WS, Donaldson M, *et al.* Serum phosphate predicts temporary hypocalcaemia following thyroidectomy. Clin Endocrinol 2011; 74(3): 388–93.

19 Roh JL, Park JY, Park CI. Prevention of postoperative hypocalcemia with routine oral calcium and vitamin D supplements in patients with differentiated papillary thyroid carcinoma undergoing total thyroidectomy plus central neck dissection. Cancer 2009; 115(2): 251–8.

20 Bellantone R, Lombardi CP, Raffaelli M, *et al.* Is routine supplementation therapy (calcium and vitamin D) useful after total thyroidectomy? Surgery 2002; 132: 1109–12.

21 Noordzij JP, Lee SL, Bernet VJ, *et al.* Early prediction of hypocalcemia after thyroidectomy using parathyroid hormone: an analysis of pooled individual patient data from nine observational studies. J Am Coll Surg 2007; 205(6): 748–54.

22 Sands N, Young J, MacNamara E, *et al.* Preoperative parathyroid hormone levels as a predictor of postthyroidectomy hypocalcemia. Otolaryngol Head Neck Surg 2011; 144(4): 518–21.

23 Kara M, Tellioglu G, Krand O, *et al.* Predictors of hypocalcemia occurring after a total/near total thyroidectomy. Surg Today 2009; 39(9): 752–7.

24 Graff AT, Miller FR, Roehm CE, Prihoda TJ. Predicting hypocalcemia after total thyroidectomy: parathyroid hormone level vs. serial calcium levels. Ear Nose Throat J 2010; 89(9): 462–5.

25 Lombardi CP, Raffaelli M, Princi P. Early prediction of postthyroidectomy hypocalcemia by one single iPTH measurement. Surgery 2004; 136: 1236–41.

26 Payne R, Hier M, Tamilia M, Namara E, Young J, Black M. Same-day discharge after total thyroidectomy: the value of 6-hour serum parathyroid hormone and calcium levels. Head Neck 2005; 27: 1–7.

27 Jumaily JS, Noordzij JP, Dukas AG, *et al.* Prediction of hypocalcemia after using 1- to 6-hour postoperative parathyroid hormone and calcium levels: an analysis of pooled individual patient data from 3 observational studies. Head Neck 2010; 32(4): 427–34.

28 Lim JP, Irvine R, Bugis S, Holmes D, Wiseman SM. Intact parathyroid hormone measurement 1 hour after thyroid surgery identifies individuals at high risk for the development of symptomatic hypocalcemia. Am J Surg 2009; 197(5): 648–53; discussion 653–4.

29 Lam A, Kerr PD. Parathyroid hormone: an early predictor of postthyroidectomy hypocalcemia. Laryngoscope 2003; 113: 2196–200.

30 Fahad Al-Dhahri S, Al-Ghonaim YA, Sulieman Terkawi A. Accuracy of postthyroidectomy parathyroid hormone and corrected calcium levels as early predictors of clinical hypocalcemia. J Otolaryngol Head Neck Surg 2010; 39(4): 342–8.

31 Youngwirth L, Benavidez J, Sippel R, Chen H. Postoperative parathyroid hormone testing decreases symptomatic hypocalcemia and associated emergency room visits after total thyroidectomy. Surgery 2010; 148(4): 841–4.

32 Sabour S, Manders E, Steward DL. The role of rapid PACU parathyroid hormone in reducing post-thyroidectomy hypocalcemia. Otolaryngol Head Neck Surg 2009; 141(6): 727–9.

33 Wiseman JE, Mossanen M, Ituarte PH, Bath JM, Yeh MW. An algorithm informed by the parathyroid hormone level reduces hypocalcemic complications of thyroidectomy. World J Surg 2010; 34(3): 532–7.

34 Winer KK, Sinaii N, Reynolds J, *et al.* Long-term treatment of 12 children with chronic hypoparathyroidism: a randomized trial comparing synthetic human parathyroid hormone 1-34 versus calcitriol and calcium. J Clin Endocrinol Metab 2010; 95(6): 2680–8.

35 Newfield RS. Recombinant PTH for initial management of neonatal hypocalcemia. N Engl J Med 2007; 356(16): 1687–8.

36 Woods Ignatoski KM, Bingham EL, Frome LK, Doherty GM. Differentiation of precursors into parathyroid-like cells for treatment of hypoparathyroidism. Surgery 2010; 148(6): 1186–9.

CHAPTER 16

Cosmetic Complications

Melanie W. Seybt and David J. Terris

Department of Otolaryngology – Head and Neck Surgery, Georgia Health Sciences University, Augusta, GA, USA

Introduction

Cosmetic outcomes in thyroid surgery have been addressed in the literature since the 1970s [1]. Acknowledging that the majority of thyroid disease occurs in females and the ever-increasing societal focus on appearance, cosmesis in thyroid surgery is becoming an important factor in providing optimal patient care. Furthermore, excellent aesthetic results can be accomplished without compromising patient safety or surgical completeness [2].

A number of important principles have emerged that substantially affect cosmetic outcomes [3]. These are addressed in detail below.

Incision location

Planning the operative incision with the patient anaesthetized and in a supine position may result in a location lower than desired. Additionally, distortion by goitre or large nodule can make incision placement difficult. It is important that when planning the surgical incision, the patient be marked while sitting in an upright position. This is most easily performed in the holding area (Figure 16.1) and usually reveals a natural skin crease that may not be readily visualized after the patient is supine on the operating table. The incision should ideally be placed above the sternum in the depression created by the medial heads of the sternocleidomastoid muscle (Figure 16.2) and be parallel to relaxed skin tension lines [4]. The incision length should be customized to accommodate the size of the patient and disease [5], with an incision as small as possible to safely remove the thyroid gland. The incision length will vary depending on the patient's neck circumference and gland volume. However, it should be noted that the incision can almost always be smaller than the gland or nodule, as these structures can usually be manipulated through a small aperture (Figure 16.3). Furthermore, the surgeon should strive to place an incision so that a symmetrical scar results as this is typically most aesthetically pleasing.

Over the last decade, minimally invasive and endoscopic approaches have become increasingly embraced due to their ease of performance, decreased pain, faster recovery and superior cosmetic outcomes [6], in addition to the excellent functional outcomes [7]. More recently, surgeons have begun using remote-access incisions to approach the thyroid compartment, completely camouflaging incisions in the axilla [8], postauricular hairline [9,10] and areola [11]. These techniques were developed mainly in Asian countries where there is a cultural aversion to neck scars and a higher incidence of hypertrophic scarring.

Each of these approaches has potential cosmetic benefits but due to the extensive dissection necessary, there is often associated morbidity. In the transaxillary approach, frequent chest wall numbness and multiple brachial plexus injuries have been reported. In the breast approach, postoperative seroma formation requiring frequent aspiration has been reported. Shan *et al.* reported on a large, anterior chest wall seroma that ultimately formed a pseudo-bursa, creating a tumour-like effect on the anterior chest wall, severely compromising the cosmetic outcome [12].

Thyroid Surgery: Preventing and Managing Complications, First Edition. Edited by Paolo Miccoli, David J. Terris, Michele N. Minuto and Melanie W. Seybt.

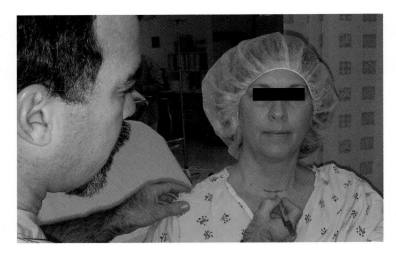

Figure 16.1 Optimal incision placement may be determined in the preoperative holding area with the patient sitting in an upright position. Reproduced from Terris *et al.* [3] with permission from Lippincott Williams and Wilkins.

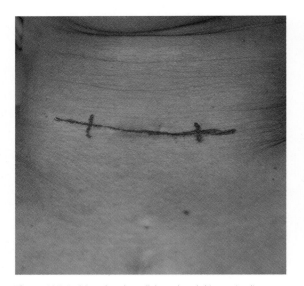

Figure 16.2 Incision placed parallel to relaxed skin tension lines between medial heads of sternocleidomastoid muscle.

Hypertrophic or hyperpigmented scarring

The thyroidectomy wound edges may be traumatized from stretching of the wound during gland delivery or tension from the retractors or inadvertent instrument trauma (electrocautery and ultrasonic energy burns), especially when a minimally invasive or endoscopic approach is used (Figure 16.4) and may result in a

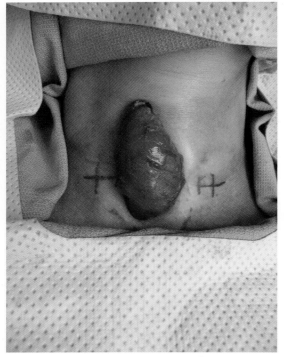

Figure 16.3 A hemithyroidectomy is accomplished in which the specimen is delivered through a incision which is smaller than the gland.

hypertrophic scar (Figure 16.5). Some surgeons prefer to cover the skin edges with an adhesive bandage or sterile towel, with varying levels of success. In order to provide a border of healthy tissue for wound closure, it is

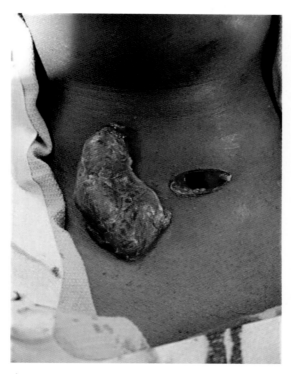

Figure 16.4 Traumatized thyroidectomy wound edges. Reproduced from Terris *et al.* [3] with permission from Lippincott Williams and Wilkins.

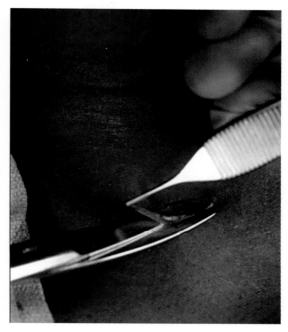

Figure 16.6 Excision of a small sliver of skin at the traumatized wound edge. Reproduced from Terris *et al.* [3] with permission from Lippincott Williams and Wilkins.

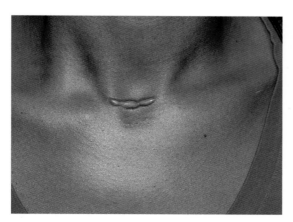

Figure 16.5 Hypertrophic scar resulting from traumatized wound edge in an endoscopic thyroidectomy.

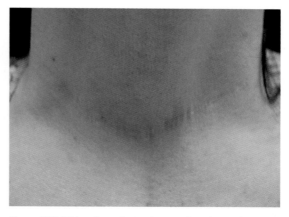

Figure 16.7 Widened scar due to downward traction on the incision in a patient with pendulous breasts.

advantageous to excise a small sliver of the traumatized or ischaemic wound edge (Figure 16.6). This freshened edge helps to ensure proper wound healing. During closure of the wound, the edges should be everted in order to minimize skin tension. These everted edges will flatten to form a thin scar as wound remodelling occurs. Patients with large breasts should wear a supportive garment during the early postoperative period in order to minimize downward traction on the lower skin edge (Figure 16.7). Patients should be encouraged to avoid sun exposure for 6–12 months in order to decrease the potential for hyperpigmentation. In patients with a propensity to form keloids, we have found it useful to inject the incision site with steroids prior to making the incision.

Skin closure

Monofilament sutures or staples can result in excellent wound healing but there is the potential of 'railroad tracking' when these techniques are employed, particularly in younger individuals (Figure 16.8). While subcuticular sutures avoid this possibility, it is difficult to achieve perfect apposition of the wound edges even in experienced hands. We have found the use of cyanoacrylate skin adhesives (Dermabond™, DermaFlex®, LiquiBand®) to be beneficial for reapproximating the skin edges after placement of one or two subcutaneous absorbable sutures to alleviate tension from the wound edge. An additional benefit of this technique is that the patient does not need to return to the surgeon at a specific interval for suture removal, making this convenient for both the patient and the surgeon. In fact, Amin *et al.* noted improved patient satisfaction with tissue adhesive as patients required no rigid follow-up for wound care and were allowed to shower on the day of surgery due to the occlusive nature of the adhesive [13].

Additionally, one should ensure that there is no potential for the skin to become tethered to the underlying subcutaneous tissues or adherent to the trachea, as this is not only cosmetically unappealing but can create a functional impairment as well. In order to circumvent this possibility, the strap muscles should be reapproximated in the midline prior to skin closure. This can easily be accomplished with a single figure-of-eight between the opposing strap muscles.

Drain placement

The use of drains in thyroid and parathyroid surgery remains widespread, despite many surgeons who advocate their limited utility. Tabaqchali *et al.* noted no difference in the incidence of bleeding or airway obstruction between patients who had drains and those who did not, and actually noted that patients who received post-thyroidectomy drains were more likely to develop wound infections [14]. Based on the literature and our own experience, we no longer use drains in thyroid and parathyroid surgery except in patients who require immediate postoperative anticoagulation due to the need for dialysis. When a drain is utilized, optimal cosmesis will occur when an active drain is placed by a sharp trocar immediately lateral to the cervical incision in the previously identified skin crease. In this location, a drain hole will often heal without a visible scar. A drain should never be placed along the manubrium or sternum, as this area is especially prone to hypertrophic scarring. Similarly, a passive drain placed through the middle of the incision may also create a widened scar at the exit point of the drain (Figure 16.9).

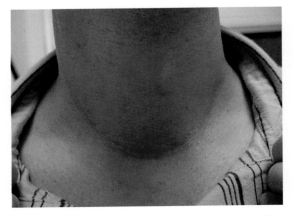

Figure 16.8 'Railroad tracking' resulting from wound closure with monofilament suture.

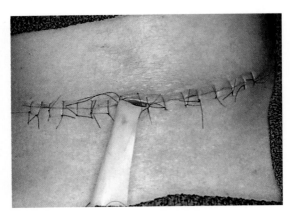

Figure 16.9 Drain location is poorly placed in the middle of the incision.

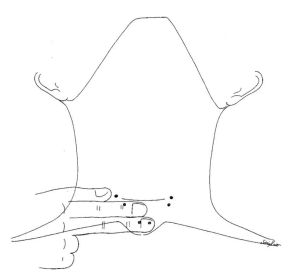

Figure 16.10 Correct positions of the incision and the drains.

In Figure 16.10, the correct positions of both the incision and the drains are shown.

Conclusion

Excellent cosmetic results can be obtained in thyroid and parathyroid surgery, especially when guided by principles of plastic surgery. Optimal incision placement along relaxed skin tension lines is critical and caution should be exercised with wound edges. When wound edges become macerated due to overzealous retraction or electrocautery burns, trimming a sliver of skin is useful and decreases the likelihood of hypertrophic and hyperpigmented scarring. Drains should be avoided when possible but if necessary, the exit point of the drain should be carefully chosen so as not to adversely affect the cosmetic outcome. Minimally invasive, endoscopic and remote-access thyroidectomy techniques are becoming more widely practised worldwide and may provide a significant cosmetic advantage in appropriately selected patients.

References

1 Chavatzas D. Cosmetic result in thyroid surgery. Ann R Coll Surg Engl 1975; 56: 270–3.
2 Miccoli P, Elisei R, Materazzi G, *et al.* Minimally invasive video-assisted thyroidectomy for papillary carcinoma: a prospective study of its completeness. Surgery 2002; 132: 1070–3.
3 Terris DJ, Seybt MW, Elchoufi M, Chin E. Cosmetic thyroid surgery: defining the essential principles. Laryngoscope 2007; 117(7): 1168–72.
4 McCarthy JG (ed). Plastic Surgery. Philadelphia: WB Saunders, 1990.
5 Terris DJ, Seybt MS. Classification system for minimally invasive thyroid surgery. ORL 2008; 70(5): 287–91.
6 Miccoli P, Berti P, Raffaelli M, *et al.* Comparison between minimally invasive video-assisted thyroidectomy and conventional thyroidectomy: a prospective randomized study. Surgery 2001; 130: 1039–43.
7 Lombardi CP, Raffaelli M, d'Alatri L, *et al.* Video-assisted thyroidectomy significantly reduces the risk of early postthyroidectomy voice and swallowing symptoms. World J Surg 2008; 32(5): 693–700.
8 Kang SW, Lee SC, Lee SH, *et al.* Robotic thyroid surgery using a gasless, transaxillary approach and the da Vinci S system: the operative outcomes of 338 consecutive patients. Surgery 2009; 146(6): 1048–55.
9 Terris DJ, Singer MC, Seybt MW. Robotic facelift thyroidectomy: I. pre-clinical simulation and morphometric assessment. Laryngoscope 2011 (In press).
10 Terris DJ, Singer MC, Seybt MW. Robotic Facelift Thyroidectomy: II. Clinical Feasibility and Safety. Laryngoscope 2011; 121(8): 1631–5.
11 Choe JH, Dim SW, Chung, KW, *et al.* Endoscopic thyroidectomy using a new bilateral axillo-breast approach. World J Surg 2007; 31(3): 601–6.
12 Shan CX, Zhang W, Jiang DZ, *et al.* Prevalence, risk factors, and management of seroma formation after breast approach endoscopic thyroidectomy. World J Surg 2010; 34(8): 1817–22.
13 Amin M, Glynn F, Timon C. Randomized trial of tissue adhesive vs staples in thyroidectomy integrating patient satisfaction and Manchester score. Otolaryngol Head Neck Surg 2009; 140(5): 703–8.
14 Tabaqchali MA, Hanson JM, Proud G. Drains for thyroidectomy/parathyroidectomy: fact or fiction? Ann R Coll Surg Engl 1999; 81: 302–5.

PART IV

Intraoperative Complications: The Rare Ones

CHAPTER 17

Management and Prevention of Laryngotracheal and Oesophageal Injuries in Thyroid Surgery

Eran E. Alon[1] and Mark L. Urken[2]

[1] Department of Otolaryngology – Head and Neck Surgery, Chaim Sheba Medical Center, Tel, Hoshomer, Israel

[2] Department of Otorhinolaryngology – Head and Neck Surgery, Albert Einstein College of Medicine; Director of Head and Neck Surgery, Continuum Cancer Centers of New York; Department of Otolaryngology – Head and Neck Surgery, Beth Israel Medical Center, New York, NY, USA

Introduction

The incidence of invasive well-differentiated thyroid cancer ranges between 1% and 23%, in various series. As the incidence of early-stage thyroid cancer has continued to increase, the result is that the percentage of patients with invasive disease has decreased. The important effect of this change is that surgeons who are not accustomed to dealing with invasive thyroid cancer are more likely to be *taken off guard* and may be ill prepared to manage it at the time of the initial surgery.

However, in those series that have evaluated the patients who developed invasive thyroid cancer, it is instructive to identify which structures are most commonly involved. In the Mayo Clinic series which reviewed 859 patients with papillary thyroid carcinoma, 138 (16%) had invasion of upper aerodigestive tract structures [1]. More than half of associated deaths from thyroid cancer are due to airway obstruction or bleeding [2]. In patients with invasive disease, involvement of the recurrent laryngeal nerve (RLN) was seen in 47%, the trachea in 60%, the larynx in 34%, the oesophagus in 17% and the strap muscles or platysma in 43% [1]. In other series of invasive thyroid disease, RLN involvement ranges from 33% to 61%, tracheal involvement ranges from 33% to 61%, and oesophageal involvement was found in 9–31%. Thus, encroachment on the trachea, larynx and oesophagus represent a significant percentage of the structures that are involved in patients with invasive disease and often more than one structure may be invaded in the central neck compartment. Many studies have now shown that aerodigestive tract invasion is a negative prognostic factor lowering long-term survival [3–5].

Various mechanisms of invasion have been proposed. In general, locally invasive thyroid disease in the central neck can be explained by one of two mechanisms. The first is extrathyroidal extension (ETE), in which disease can extend directly through the thyroid capsule [6,7]. Involvement of the central compartment visceral and neural structures includes the anterior and lateral walls of the trachea, recurrent and superior laryngeal nerves, anterior and lateral aspects of the cricoid and thyroid cartilages, the oesophagus and, of course, the adjacent musculature. Extracapsular extension of metastatic nodal disease may involve the pretracheal or prelaryngeal lymph nodes, which may in turn extend to the viscera of the central neck [8].

Thyroid Surgery: Preventing and Managing Complications, First Edition. Edited by Paolo Miccoli, David J. Terris, Michele N. Minuto and Melanie W. Seybt.

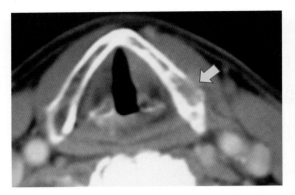

Figure 17.1 CT image that demonstrates a metastatic focus of papillary thyroid cancer in a patient who underwent a total thyroidectomy 11 years before (*arrow*). In addition, the patient has evidence of other systemic disease.

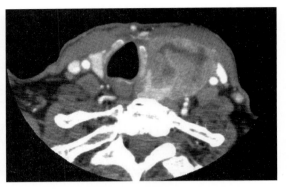

Figure 17.2 Cross-sectional imaging demonstrates a large papillary thyroid cancer involving the thyroid lobe and encroaching on the lateral wall of the trachea. Although there is no evidence of intraluminal involvement, the surgeon should be aware of the potential for cartilage involvement.

Alternatively, invasive disease that spreads to the paratracheal lymph nodes may extend to involve the oesophagus or the lateral aspect of the trachea. Rarely, there can be a metastasis directly to the cartilage (Figure 17.1).

Patients at risk for disease invading the upper aerodigestive tract include those with ETE, and central lymph node metastases. Recurrent differentiated thyroid cancer (DTC), extensive nodal disease, older patients and distant metastases are all associated with locally advanced disease. Even though DTC is more common in women, locally advanced disease is more commonly found in men [9–11]. DTC invading the trachea and oesophagus is associated with a grim prognosis. Tsumori and associates have demonstrated that poorly differentiated tumours are seen in 50% of papillary and follicular tumours invading the airway compared to 11.4% when they are restricted to the gland. They hypothesized that airway invasion and loss of differentiation are related phenomena [12]. These findings were also confirmed by McCaffrey *et al.* and Ito *et al.* Shin *et al.* further demonstrated that the depth of tracheal involvement also predicts outcome, with shorter survival in patients with transmural invasion and macroscopic disease involvement of the lumen [6]. This information is extremely important with respect to the surgeon's mindset when managing such patients. An awareness that less well-differentiated thyroid cancer is unlikely to be treated effectively with radioactive iodine helps the surgeon to make the correct decisions with respect to the completeness of the ablative procedure.

As many patients with invasive thyroid cancer do not present with symptoms, the surgeon should be aware of the signs and symptoms that may point to invasive disease but a high index of suspicion in virtually every thyroid operation will serve the surgeon well. Obvious hoarseness, dyspnoea, dysphagia, stridor and haemoptysis suggest invasive disease [13]. However, up to two-thirds of patients with vocal cord paralysis will not report a change in their voice [14]. Physical examination revealing a fixed mass or skin involvement also suggests invasion of central neck structures. Patients with suspected invasive disease require further cross-sectional assessment with either a computed tomography (CT) or magnetic resonance imaging (MRI) scan, apart from a comprehensive ultrasound exam of the neck (Figure 17.2). An MRI has the advantage of a detailed anatomical evaluation without the need for iodine contrast (which may delay postoperative radioactive iodine treatment). In addition, if invasive disease is suspected, all patients should undergo office-based or intraoperative bronchoscopy and oesophagoscopy [15]. Identification of mucosal erythema or gross tracheal invasion will raise awareness of the possibility of invasive disease. Careful preoperative evaluation will allow for optimal assessment and determination of the extent of surgery required, as well as allowing for a more informed preoperative discussion with the patient.

There have been two schools of thought as to the extent of surgical resection required in invasive thyroid cancer. There have been compelling data at both ends of the spectrum, showing on the one hand that conservative surgery with only resection of gross disease and the addition of adjuvant therapy can achieve long-term survival similar to complete resection of the disease, through more extensive local surgery [16–18]. On the other hand, other studies have shown a significant benefit to a more aggressive surgical approach [19–21]. Suffice it to say that complete surgical resection with negative or at least microscopically positive margins has been shown to affect prognosis. Incomplete resection in patients with extrathyroidal extension above the age of 45 years has been shown to have a negative predictive value [15,16]. In contrast with squamous cell carcinomas of the head and neck, the resection of well-differentiated thyroid cancer does not usually require a 1 cm margin. However, the oncological surgeon should not rely upon radioactive iodine to ablate gross residual disease [16]. In addition, frozen section pathology plays a key role in identifying the appropriate margins prior to performing major reconstructive procedures.

Injury to the trachea, oesophagus or larynx can occur via two mechanisms. The first is related to the underlying biology of the disease with local invasion and destruction resulting from the primary disease, residual disease left behind after incomplete resection or the development of recurrence. The second mechanism is due to iatrogenic injury at the time of surgery for non-invasive disease.

As most thyroid surgeries require only a total thyroidectomy, the head and neck surgeon who is unaccustomed to managing invasive disease may not be prepared to address unexpected invasive disease, either leaving gross disease behind or achieving suboptimal reconstruction. Regardless of the mechanism of injury, head and neck surgeons must be prepared for the unexpected, closely adhering to sound oncological surgical principles while offering their patients suitable reconstruction.

To date, there is no classification when dealing with the extent of laryngotracheal invasion by thyroid cancer when considering reconstruction options. The only staging system available was devised by Shin and associates, in which they found a relationship between depth of invasion of the trachea and prognosis. In this chapter, we will discuss techniques to repair tracheal, oesophageal and laryngeal injuries. The management of injuries to the recurrent laryngeal nerve is discussed in Chapter 13.

Injuries to the laryngotracheal complex

The use of sound surgical technique will help thyroid surgeons to avoid inadvertent injury to the laryngotracheal

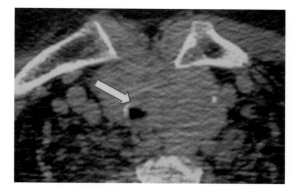

Figure 17.3 Irregularity in the lumen of the trachea provides clear evidence of transmural involvement by the thyroid malignancy (*arrow*).

complex in patients without invasive disease. It is often helpful for the surgeon to be well versed in multiple approaches to identification of the recurrent laryngeal nerve as well as various options for implementing the resection of a portion or all of the thyroid gland. This is especially true in surgical intervention for thyroid disease that is recurrent or has been previously operated upon. Often it is helpful to establish the plane of the trachea or the laryngeal cartilages from an area that is uninvolved in order to more safely approach the area of greatest scarring or invasion.

Appropriate cross-sectional imaging of the laryngotracheal complex should be obtained in patients with recurrent disease; patients with local symptoms related to voice, swallowing or an abnormal airway; patients with an abnormal physical exam, in particular the identification of a paralysed or paretic vocal cord or visualization of a mass encroaching on the lumen of the laryngopharynx, subglottis or trachea (Figure 17.3). In addition, patients who present with documented distant metastases should undergo more detailed imaging studies due to the association of distant metastases with locally invasive cancer.

With detailed cross-sectional imaging, the surgeon can better plan ablative surgery as well as potential reconstructive surgery. Involvement of the tracheal wall varies with respect to the depth of invasion. Superficial invasion may be effectively managed with a shave excision. Unfortunately, it is often difficult to determine the exact extent of the tracheal wall involvement, especially when the cartilaginous involvement is unexpectedly encountered by the unsuspecting surgeon. In patients who undergo appropriate preoperative imaging, transmural involvement with gross disease in the lumen undoubtedly mandates that a segmental resection or a window resection of the trachea be performed.

Shave resection is usually performed tangentially with a knife, leaving a layer of cartilage. There is growing evidence that shave resection does not remov all tumour cells, with an expected high rate of local failure [13,21–24]. In fact, local recurrence after shave procedures may be higher by a factor of 8 compared to segmental resection. This may be due to the fact that the peritracheal fascia is continuous with the dense fibrous tissue between the tracheal rings. In addition, the perithyroidal adventitia and lymphatics of the tracheal mucosa communicate via the intercartilagnous spaces [6]. Arguably, the fact that overall survival rates do not decline in younger patients with invasive disease does not change the fact that residual disease may grow over time, lead to invasion of other structures, metastasize and even dedifferentiate. One must measure success not only by overall survival but, more importantly, by disease-free survival. Shave resection should be limited to those cases where the tumour only abuts the tracheal rings in order to achieve a clear margin [24,25].

Despite visualization of the tracheal lumen by bronchoscopy, the surgeon is often at a loss as to the full extent of tumour involvement of the tracheal wall based on observation of the disease on the external portion of the wall of the trachea. Ozaki identified that the extent of the tumour on the outside wall of the trachea most often accurately predicts the longitudinal extent of the tumour within the wall or on the inside of the tracheal lumen [21]. However, the extent of the circumferential involvement is often underestimated. Hence, the performance of a segmental resection of the tracheal wall is often more advisable than a window resection. Frozen section is mandatory in whichever procedure is undertaken.

When a partial resection of the trachea is performed, there are a number of options for reconstructing the anterior or lateral wall. When a limited window of the trachea is resected, a sliding tracheoplasty can be performed. If the resection involves less than one-third of the circumference of a few tracheal rings, a tracheotomy tube may be placed in the defect and removed 3–4 days later, as with any tracheostomy. However, when closer to 50% of the tracheal circumference is removed, more elaborate techniques for reconstruction are usually required. A

number of approaches have been described, including the use of various rotation flaps such as the sternocleidomastoid myoperiosteal flap or pectoralis flap.

The ideal tissue to replace a portion of the wall of the trachea is undoubtedly the trachea itself. Alternatively, that tissue should include well-vascularized epithelium and a firm structure to replace the native cartilage. The importance of introducing well-vascularized skin or mucosa is that it will heal primarily and prevent the formation of granulation. The development of granulation tissue encroaches on the lumen and leads to tracheal stenosis. Alternative options have been developed in order to achieve more rigid structural support so as to avoid dynamic movement of the tracheal wall when negative pressure is generated with inspiration. This can be readily achieved with the principle of creating a *prefabricated flap* composed of epithelium for lining and a rigid implant to provide support. This can be accomplished with a delayed reconstruction in a three-step approach. At first, a formal epithelium-lined stoma is created by suturing the cervical skin to the mucosal edges through the defect in the cartilaginous wall of the trachea. Approximately 3 weeks later, when the stoma has healed, either cartilage or titanium mesh is placed in a subcutaneous pocket at the stomal edge. Access for placement of either the cartilage or titanium is achieved through a circumferential incision that will be used to turn in skin with the underlying structural support as a composite flap. Finally, the third stage requires folding over of the skin flap with the buried cartilage or mesh to recreate the tracheal wall (Figure 17.4). The defect in the overlying skin can then be closed primarily or with the use of a deltopectoral flap [26].

The removal of a circumferential section of the trachea, otherwise known as a segmental resection of the trachea, is a safe procedure in experienced hands. The reported mortality excluding high-risk patients (previously radiated, cervical exenteration) is 1.4% [20,24]. Common complications include need for long-term tracheostomy due to bilateral recurrent laryngeal nerve injury, and airway stenosis. Repair of the trachea following segmental resection is best accomplished by end-to-end anastomosis, the technique for which is well delineated in standard texts and articles. The essentials of that technique are that the repair must be accomplished without tension and the sutures must be placed in a precise, interrupted fashion around the circumference of the repair (Figure 17.5). Most often, the

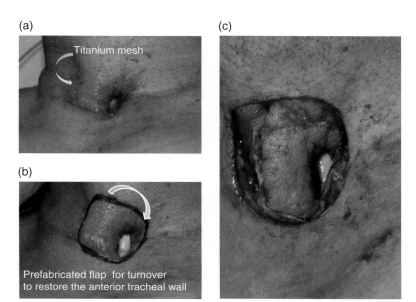

Figure 17.4 Third stage closure of a window resection of the tracheal wall. (a) During stage 2 a piece of titanium mesh is placed deep to the skin on the right side of the formal stoma. (b) At the third stage the prefabricated flap is incised and the skin and structural support are turned over to suture to the circumferential suture line as shown (*arrow*). (c) The plane of dissection is along the muscle plane in order to raise the flap with the mesh, but without exposing the mesh. The secondary defect in the cervical skin is closed with either advancement of the surrounding skin or transposition of a deltopectoral flap, often with an island design.

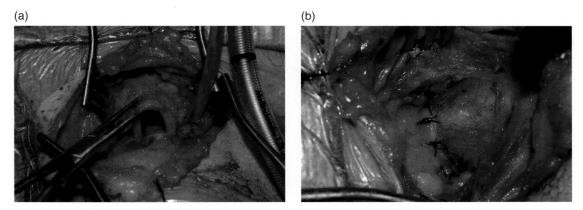

Figure 17.5 A segmental resection of the trachea has been performed for an invasive thyroid cancer. (a) The distal end of the trachea is shown. (b) Interrupted sutures are placed around the circumference of the repair, with the knots positioned on the outside of the lumen.

resected segment is not more than a few tracheal rings long. Mobilization of the remaining trachea is usually adequate to achieve a tension-free closure. However, obtaining an anastomosis free of tension when longer segments are resected will require further mobilization of the laryngotracheal complex, including a suprahyoid release in which the strap muscles attached to the hyoid are transected. This technique allows the larynx to be released from the suspension to the hyomandibular muscle complex, permitting a larger segment of trachea to be removed and primarily repaired. Transection of the suspensory muscles of the larynx may produce temporary dysphagia. It is only under unusual circumstances that a hilar release is required to complete the tension-free repair.

When primary anastomosis is performed, care must be taken when freeing the trachea not to injure the recurrent laryngeal nerves and to ensure that the blood supply to the trachea is maintained. Overnight intubation facilitates wound healing and prevents the development of immediate subcutaneous emphysema due to increased tracheal pressure secondary to cough and Valsalva manoeuvres. When there is concern about tension on the anastomosis, a suture may be placed from the mentum to the chest, also known as the 'Grillo stitch', which will restrict the patient's ability to extend their neck and place early undue tension on the repair. In such instances, the stitch should be kept in place for approximately 1 week. The use of precise surgical technique cannot be emphasized enough when approximating the tracheal ends in order to restore the lumen of the trachea. A significant air leak can place the patient at risk for a neck infection, abscess formation, significant mediastinitis as well major vascular erosion and life-threatening bleeding. Any signs or symptoms of a leak require immediate attention.

The laryngeal complex may be involved by invasive cancer through anterior penetration at the cricothyroid space or more commonly around the posterior aspect of the thyroid ala. One thyroid ala can be resected, without incident, when the lateral aspect of the cartilage is involved without transcartilaginous extension to involve the pyriform sinus mucosa. A variety of partial laryngectomy procedures have been described over the years, primarily for use in resection of mucosa-based neoplasms. However, the same basic principles can be utilized in the resections and reconstructions for patients with invasive thyroid cancer. The most commonly utilized approach is the vertical hemilaryngectomy, but this can be extended to include the hemicricoid cartilage as well [27]. In these instances, the patient requires a temporary tracheotomy. More sophisticated reconstructive procedures are required to bring vascularized lining and support when larger portions of the larynx are removed.

McCaffrey and Lipton advocated total laryngectomy when more than one-third of the cricoid cartilage is involved [8] but others have advocated total laryngectomy when over 50% of the laryngeal framework is involved [28]. The fundamental ingredient for restoring function is to have an intact and mobile cricoarytenoid unit. However, the desire to restore the larynx in this

setting, although technically feasible with the use of contemporary reconstructive techniques, must be tempered by awareness of the biological aggressiveness of the tumour and the likely necessity of adding adjuvant external beam radiation therapy. The performance of a total laryngectomy with a tracheo-oesophageal puncture for placement of a speaking valve is a very effective means of eradicating disease and restoring speech and swallowing function, albeit with a permanent tracheal stoma.

Injuries to the cervical oesophagus

The cervical oesophagus is often superficially involved by invasive thyroid cancer and transmural involvement is not very common. Invasive disease identified prior to surgery with cross-sectional imaging can identify those patients in whom the oesophagus is most likely to be at risk. However, there are also patients with benign disease that is both very large and with posterior extension that may place the oesophagus at risk (Figure 17.6). The best way to prevent transmural oesophageal wall resection is by placing a bougie into the cervical oesophagus in order to provide a stent to facilitate surgical resection. With the bougie in place, the surgeon can safely remove the attached oesophageal musculature and dissect in the submucosal plane (Figure 17.7).

If a defect is created in the wall of the oesophagus, then primary repair can be performed provided that the calibre of the lumen around the bougie is maintained (prefer-

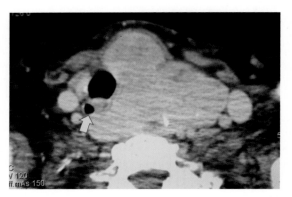

Figure 17.6 Benign thyroid enlargement with posterior extension has caused displacement of the oesophagus and intimate association of the tumour to the muscular layer of the oesophagus (*arrow*).

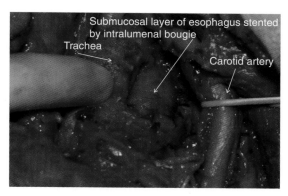

Figure 17.7 Invasive thyroid cancer has involved the muscular layer of the oesophagus. The placement of a bougie into the lumen of the oesophagus facilitates dissection in the submucosal plane to help prevent a transmural resection and the need to perform either a direct repair or reconstruction with a flap.

ably a size 38 Fr or larger will be utilized). Alternatively, if the defect in the wall does not permit safe primary repair, then reconstruction will require importation of new, healthy tissue from another part of the body. The authors most commonly do this by transfer of thin, pliable tissue from such donor sites as the radial forearm, anterolateral thigh or lateral arm, using microvascular techniques. Partial or circumferential defects can be repaired in this manner.

Conclusion

Thyroid cancer invading the airway has been clearly shown to have a negative prognostic impact on local control. As thyroid cancer may be seen in otherwise young healthy patients with a life expectancy which exceeds 20 years, our aim is not only to achieve long-term overall survival but also long-term disease-free survival. Thus, the surgeon should try to perform an appropriate surgical resection as outlined above. Patients with airway invasion should be identified preoperatively as operative surprises often translate into inappropriate surgeries. Transmural involvement of the oesophagus is rare and most cases of thyroid cancer can be managed with removal of the muscular layer only. Finally, the thyroid surgeon who is not accustomed to managing patients with invasive disease should refer those patients to centres that have experience in managing both the ablative and reconstructive

aspects of this disease. In addition, the surgeon should maintain a high index of suspicion in the population of patients who are most likely to have invasive disease: the older population, patients with preoperative suspicious signs and symptoms, patients with recurrent central compartment disease, and patients with documented metastatic disease.

References

1 McConahey WM, Hay I, Woolner L, *et al*. Papillary thyroid cancer treated at the Mayo Clinic, 1946 through 1970: initial manifestations, pathologic findings, therapy, and outcome. Mayo Clin Proc 1986; 61(12): 978–96.

2 Ishihara T, Yamazaki S, Kobayashi K, *et al*. Resection of the trachea infiltrated by thyroid carcinoma. Ann Surg 1982; 195(4): 496–500.

3 Czaja JM, McCaffrey TV. The surgical management of laryngotracheal invasion by well-differentiated papillary thyroid carcinoma. Arch Otolaryngol Head Neck Surg 1997; 123(5): 484–90.

4 McCaffrey JC. Aerodigestive tract invasion by well-differentiated thyroid carcinoma: diagnosis, management, prognosis, and biology. Laryngoscope 2006; 116(1): 1–11.

5 Ito Y, Tomoda C, Uruno T, *et al*. Prognostic significance of extrathyroid extension of papillary thyroid carcinoma: massive but not minimal extension affects the relapse-free survival. World J Surg 2006; 30(5): 780–6.

6 Shin DH, Mark E, Suen H, Grillo H. Pathologic staging of papillary carcinoma of the thyroid with airway invasion based on the anatomic manner of extension to the trachea: a clinicopathologic study based on 22 patients who underwent thyroidectomy and airway resection. Hum Pathol 1993; 24(8): 866–70.

7 Machens A, Hinze R, Lautenschlager C, Thomusch O, Dralle H. Thyroid carcinoma invading the cervicovisceral axis: routes of invasion and clinical implications. Surgery 2001; 129(1): 23–8.

8 McCaffrey TV, Lipton RJ. Thyroid carcinoma invading the upper aerodigestive system. Laryngoscope 1990; 100(8): 824–30.

9 Ortiz S, Rodriguez J, Soria T, *et al*. Extrathyroid spread in papillary carcinoma of the thyroid: clinicopathological and prognostic study. Otolaryngol Head Neck Surg 2001; 124(3): 261–5.

10 Segal K, Shpitzer T, Hazan A, *et al*. Invasive well-differentiated thyroid carcinoma: effect of treatment modalities on outcome. Otolaryngol Head Neck Surg 2006; 134(5): 819–22.

11 Borson-Chazot F, Causeret S, Lifante J, *et al*. Predictive factors for recurrence from a series of 74 children and adolescents with differentiated thyroid cancer. World J Surg 2004; 28(11): 1088–92.

12 Tsumori T, Nakao K, Miyata M, *et al*. Clinicopathologic study of thyroid carcinoma infiltrating the trachea. Cancer 1985; 56(12): 2843–8.

13 McCarty TM, Kuhn J, Williams W Jr, *et al*. Surgical management of thyroid cancer invading the airway. Ann Surg Oncol 1997; 4(5): 403–8.

14 Randolph GW, Kamani D. The importance of preoperative laryngoscopy in patients undergoing thyroidectomy: voice, vocal cord function, and the preoperative detection of invasive thyroid malignancy. Surgery 2006; 139(3): 357–62.

15 Gillenwater AM, Goepfert H. Surgical management of laryngotracheal and esophageal involvement by locally advanced thyroid cancer. Semin Surg Oncol 1999; 16(1): 19–29.

16 McCaffrey TV, Bergstralh EJ, Hay ID. Locally invasive papillary thyroid carcinoma: 1940–1990. Head Neck 1994; 16(2): 165–72.

17 Lipton RJ, McCaffrey TV, van Heerden JA. Surgical treatment of invasion of the upper aerodigestive tract by well-differentiated thyroid carcinoma. Am J Surg 1987; 154(4): 363–7.

18 Breaux GP Jr, Guillamondegui OM. Treatment of locally invasive carcinoma of the thyroid: how radical? Am J Surg 1980; 140(4): 514–17.

19 Park CS, Suh KW, Min JS. Cartilage-shaving procedure for the control of tracheal cartilage invasion by thyroid carcinoma. Head Neck 1993 15(4): 289–91.

20 Gaissert HA, Honings J, Grillo H, *et al*. Segmental laryngotracheal and tracheal resection for invasive thyroid carcinoma. Ann Thorac Surg 2007; 83(6): 1952–9.

21 Ozaki O, Sugino K, Mimura T, Ito K. Surgery for patients with thyroid carcinoma invading the trachea: circumferential sleeve resection followed by end-to-end anastomosis. Surgery 1995; 117(3): 268–71.

22 Djalilian M, Beahrs O, Devine K, *et al*. Intraluminal involvement of the larynx and trachea by thyroid cancer. Am J Surg 1974; 128(4): 500–4.

23 Frazell EL, Foote FW Jr. Papillary cancer of the thyroid; a review of 25 years of experience. Cancer 1958; 11(5): 895–922.

24 Honings J, Stephen A, Marres H, Gaissert H. The management of thyroid carcinoma invading the larynx or trachea. Laryngoscope 2010; 120(4): 682–9.

25 Nishida T, Nakao K, Hamaji M. Differentiated thyroid carcinoma with airway invasion: indication for tracheal resection based on the extent of cancer invasion. J Thorac Cardiovasc Surg 1997; 114(1): 84–92.

26 Sugenoya A, Matsuo K, Asanuma K, *et al*. Management of tracheal wall resection for thyroid carcinoma by tracheocutaneous fenestration and delayed closure using auricular cartilage. Head Neck 1995; 17(4): 339–42.

27 Urken ML, Blackwell K, Biller HF. Reconstruction of the laryngopharynx after hemicricoid /hemithyroid cartilage resection: preliminary functional results. Arch Otolaryngol Head Neck Surg 1997; 123(11): 1213–22.

28 Friedman M. Surgical management of thyroid carcinoma with laryngotracheal invasion. Otolaryngol Clin North Am 1990; 23(3): 495–507.

CHAPTER 18
Injury of the Major Vessels

Lourdes Quintanilla-Dieck and Neil D. Gross
Department of Otolaryngology – Head and Neck Surgery,
Oregon Health and Science University, Portland, OR, USA

Anatomy of the great vessels of the neck

Injury to the great vessels is a feared complication of any surgery involving the neck. This is particularly true for surgeries that involve the central low neck, most notably thyroid surgery. Injury to the great vessels can lead to devastating consequences, including massive haemorrhage, stroke, air embolism and/or even death. It is therefore incumbent upon the head and neck endocrine surgeon to have a thorough understanding of the anatomy of the great vessels of the neck (Figure 18.1). It is especially important for the surgeon to be aware of possible anomalies of the great vessels that can be encountered during head and neck endocrine surgery.

Understanding the anatomy of the great vessels is important even though the risk of injury is low. The great vessels of the neck serve as landmarks for finding other important structures. For example, preservation of the recurrent laryngeal nerve (RLN) is one of the important goals of any thyroid surgery. The surgeon must be aware of the relationship between the nerve and the common carotid and subclavian arteries. Importantly, the surgeon must be aware of the anatomical differences between the courses of the right and the left RLNs. The right RLN branches off the right vagus nerve which passes superficial to the right subclavian artery. The right RLN then curves deep to the subclavian artery, and angles superomedially deep to the thyroid gland. The left RLN, on the other hand, branches off the left vagus nerve as it passes superficial to the aortic arch. The left RLN then passes deep to the aorta at the level of the ligamentum arteriosum. It ascends cephalad and medially towards the thyroid gland, staying in the tracheo-oesophageal groove for the majority of its upward course. Because of this relationship with the aortic arch, the left RLN is longer and in a deeper and more vertical position than the right RLN.

It is equally important for the endocrine head and neck surgeon to be aware of the common anatomical variants of the great vessels of the neck (Table 18.1). Aberrant vascular anatomy is a major risk factor for life-threatening bleeding from inadvertent injury during surgery. The most common vascular aberrations are tortuous versions of normally positioned vessels. Advanced age and atherosclerosis can lead to dramatic tortuousness of major arteries of the central low neck. Specifically, the innominate artery, the right and left common carotid arteries and the right subclavian artery are prone to being displaced in elderly patients.

An aberrant right subclavian artery is one of the most common vascular anomalies of the great vessels of the neck. An aberrant right subclavian artery most commonly courses behind the oesophagus (Figure 18.2). Interestingly, a retro-oesophageal subclavian artery can be found between the oesophagus and the trachea in up to 15% of cases [1]. The clinical relevance of recognizing a retro-oesophageal subclavian artery cannot be overstated as this anomaly is coincident with the presence of a non-recurrent RLN on the right (Figure 18.3). This phenomenon can occur on either side. Therefore, preoperative knowledge of an aberrant right subclavian artery can be immensely beneficial. A left common carotid artery

Thyroid Surgery: Preventing and Managing Complications, First Edition. Edited by Paolo Miccoli, David J. Terris, Michele N. Minuto and Melanie W. Seybt.
© 2013 John Wiley & Sons, Ltd. Published 2013 by John Wiley & Sons, Ltd.

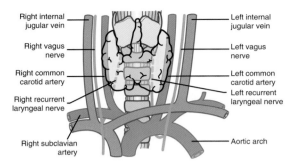

Figure 18.1 Major vessels of the anterior neck and their relationship to the recurrent laryngeal nerves.

arising from the innominate can be found in 7–27% of patients [2]. However, there is little clinical consequence of this anomaly since the artery essentially remains in a normal anatomical position.

An aberrant innominate artery (also known as the brachiocephalic trunk) is also commonly observed during surgery of the central low neck. The innominate artery normally arises as the first and largest branch of the aortic arch. It originates at the level of the superior border of the second right costochondral junction and crosses the anterior trachea most commonly at the level of the ninth tracheal ring. The point where the innominate artery crosses the trachea can vary between the sixth and 13th tracheal rings [3]. It then courses posterosuperiorly to the right, where it divides into the right common carotid and right subclavian arteries. This division occurs posterior to the right sternoclavicular joint in the root of the neck. However, there can be considerable anatomical variability. Congenital anomalies of the innominate artery, such as a left innominate artery or a retro-oesophageal innominate artery, have been associated with a right aortic arch [4]. A high-riding innominate artery, reaching up to the level of the upper tracheal rings or the cricoid cartilage, has also been occasionally identified [3] (Figure 18.4). Damage to the innominate artery resulting in bleeding during surgery can be catastrophic. Even normal anatomy can be distorted by maximal neck extension, which tends to elevate the artery to just below the sternal notch. Therefore, it is good practice to routinely palpate below the sternal notch prior to dividing the midline fascia deep to the anterior strap muscles to ensure that the innominate artery is avoided.

The location of the thyroid gland itself can be the cause for a vascular variant. An ectopic thyroid gland can have an anomalous vascular supply. Although very rare, an ectopic thyroid can be isolated to the mediastinum and have the entire blood supply from thoracic vessels. The inferior thyroid artery is absent on the left side in 5% of patients and absent on the right in 2%. In these cases, the thyroid and parathyroid glands are supplied directly by branches of the left subclavian artery. The thyroidea ima artery is present in a small portion of the population. The thyroidea ima artery can arise deep to the manubrium and if injury occurs, bleeding is difficult to control [5].

Management of intraoperative haemorrhage: general principles

Significant intraoperative haemorrhage occurs rarely in thyroid and parathyroid surgery [6]. The risk of bleeding

Table 18.1 Aberrant pathways of the great vessels of the neck.

Vessel	Expected pathway	Aberrant pathway	Clinical findings
Right subclavian artery (arteria lusoria)	Anterior to oesophagus and trachea	**a** Retro-oesophageal **b** Between oesophagus and trachea	Absent innominate Strong pulsation anterior or posterior to oesophagus
Innominate artery	First branch of the aortic arch; crosses the anterior trachea at the level of the 9th tracheal ring and courses superiorly to the right	**a** High-riding, crossing the anterior trachea as high as the cricoid cartilage **b** Coursing horizontally anterior to the trachea	Pulsatile horizontal mass at the suprasternal notch upon neck extension
Left common carotid artery	Arising from the aortic arch	Arising from the innominate artery	

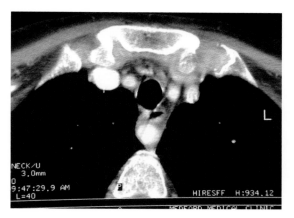

Figure 18.2 Aberrant retro-oesophageal right subclavian artery.

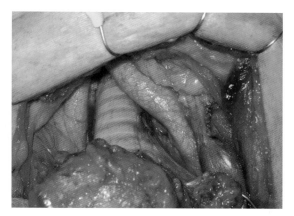

Figure 18.4 High-riding innominate artery.

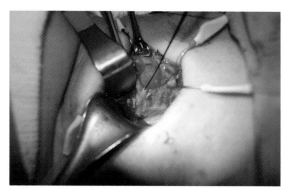

Figure 18.3 Non-recurrent right recurrent laryngeal nerve (identified by nerve monitoring probe).

is probably greatest during a neck dissection which often accompanies thyroid cancer surgery. If injury occurs to a great vessel during thyroidectomy, management of bleeding depends significantly on which vessel is injured. The most important initial step is for the surgeon to maintain composure. Bleeding from most vascular injuries can be controlled with direct pressure from a single, well-positioned finger. Once the bleeding has stopped, or at least slowed down significantly, then attention can be paid to general precautions, including important communications with anaesthesia and operating room staff. For example, during a bleeding episode it is often helpful to request a paediatric vascular tray since vascular clamps are often not part of a standard thyroidectomy tray. Large-bore intravenous access should be established and blood products may be ordered. Intraoperative

consultation from vascular and/or thoracic surgery may even be considered, depending on the specific injury.

It is usually possible to determine if the bleeding is venous or arterial. Of course, arterial bleeding is pulsatile and tends to project out of the surgical wound, compared to venous bleeding which more often 'fills' the wound. Brisk venous bleeding can be as alarming and dangerous as arterial bleeding. It is often also more difficult to control. Thin-walled veins are fragile and can tear during attempts to control bleeding. A linear tear in a large vein can be difficult to control, particularly if the injury is deep to the clavicle or sternum. Therefore, a calm and measured approach to bleeding from a great vessel is always advised to minimize the risk of exacerbating the initial injury.

The first critical decision to make once bleeding from a great vessel is identified is whether or not the exposure is adequate for evaluation and repair of the injury. This is particularly true for injuries involving the innominate artery or vein. The innominate artery can be exposed by division of the cervical thymus with superior retraction of the innominate vein [7]. A sternotomy or partial sternotomy may be required to repair a 'low' innominate injury caudal to the upper sternum and/or clavicle. Methods for improved exposure could be as simple as enlarging the incision or dividing the strap muscles. On rare occasions, a specialized sternal retractor may be useful to improve exposure (e.g. Rultract™ retractor [8]). However, the time required to obtain and deploy such a retractor may be unacceptable to the surgical team. Of course, adequate suction and lighting are requisite to successful control of haemorrhage from any great vessel in the neck.

The next crucial step in managing intraoperative haemorrhage from a great vessel during neck surgery is to obtain proximal and distal control of the vessel if possible. This can be achieved by dissecting circumferentially around the injured vessel cephalad and caudad to the bleeding site. Typically, vessels loops or vascular clamps are used. This manoeuvre is easily performed in common carotid artery injuries but may be more challenging, or unsafe to attempt, in injuries involving the innominate artery or vein. Innominate vein injuries can usually be isolated using a curved vascular clamp around the site of the injury while maintaining partial flow through the vessel. Then, the site of injury can be oversewn using a vascular suture (e.g. 5-0 Prolene). Proximal control of an innominate artery injury is sometimes impossible without a sternotomy. Therefore, if transcervical access is adequate then attempted suture repair of an innominate artery is reasonable without proximal control.

Management of postoperative haemorrhage: general principles

Significant postoperative haemorrhage after thyroid or parathyroid surgery can be life-threatening even if the great vessels of the neck are not involved. For example, a simple haematoma can cause airway obstruction. Therefore, postoperative haemorrhage from a great vessel in the neck is always a dire scenario. Postoperative haemorrhage can be chaotic compared to intraoperative haemorrhage where the airway is controlled, equipment is available and exposure is immediately possible. Therefore, it is important to be prepared for postoperative bleeding after any thyroid surgery and have an established management algorithm. Similar to a 'code' situation, the ABCs of cardiopulmonary resuscitation are paramount. The airway should be maintained and secured. The patient should either be transorally intubated or, if they have a tracheostomy site or postlaryngectomy stoma, a tracheostomy or endotracheal tube should be inserted and secured, with the cuff inflated. Overinflation of the cuff can help serve as a mechanism for bleeding control in the case of a tracheo-innominate fistula.

Once the airway is secured and breathing achieved, then attention can be directed to circulation. It is imperative that the patient have adequate intravenous access ideally via two different routes, suitable for large-volume resuscitation. Packed red blood cells should be typed and crossed immediately.

Acute postoperative haemorrhage from a major vessel such as the carotid artery is a rare but feared complication after any deep neck surgery. Large, life-threatening bleeds are often preceded by a smaller sentinel bleed. It is important to recognize a possible sentinel bleed promptly and have a high suspicion for the potential for further massive bleeding, especially in patients with risk factors such as history of radiation to the neck, mucocutaneous fistula or wound infection [9].

In patients with either a sentinel bleed or active bleeding, the choice of definitive treatment should be made promptly. This would include either a return to the operating room, for identification and control of haemorrhage, or transfer to the angiography suite. The latter is increasingly preferred, given the ease and effectiveness of intravascular techniques. This is particularly true in patients who have had a sentinel bleed without an obvious source identified on clinical examination. Angiography can be helpful for the diagnosis of the site of injury. Further, contemporary endovascular techniques allow for the deployment of arterial stents and/or coils and for possible balloon occlusion testing. Arterial stents have become progressively popular since they allow maintenance of blood flow and may decrease the incidence of stroke [9]. If the patient is taken to the operating room, then a critical intraoperative decision is whether the repair should be made with permanent interruption of blood flow or maintenance of blood flow. Some of the definitive methods that involve interruption of flow include vessel resection, ligation, clipping, division and primary suture.

Management of tracheo-innominate fistula

One of the most feared complications of a thyroidectomy is a tracheo-innominate fistula (TIF). The close juxtaposition of the proximal trachea and the innominate artery can predispose to the formation of a fistula after thyroid or parathyroid surgery [7]. Common mechanisms for development of TIF include mechanical irritation (e.g. ill-fitting tracheostomy), infectious exposure and/or malignancy. Other risk factors include frequent or prolonged episodes of hypotension, use of vasopressive agents, radiation treatment, steroid treatment and malnutrition [7]. The common final pathway in the development of TIF is most frequently chronic air and/or saliva exposure to the outer vessel wall. While a long-standing suction drain could theoretically result in TIF, it is highly unlikely to be the primary cause. Chronic saliva exposure occurs as the result of a pharyngeal wound dehiscence (e.g. fistula formation after laryngectomy). Chronic air exposure is most frequently facilitated by either tracheostomy or subcutaneous emphysema from a tracheal injury (Figure 18.5).

There are few options to control postoperative bleeding from a TIF. As mentioned previously, immediate intubation through a laryngectomy stoma or tracheostomy site can allow overinflation of an endotracheal tube to temporarily tamponade the innominate artery or vein. If bleeding persists in this case, the tube can be slowly withdrawn with pressure directed towards the anterior tracheal wall. Similarly, direct finger pressure can be applied aggressively under the sternal notch and along the anterior surface of the trachea in order to occlude the innominate vessels against the upper sternum. It is even possible to apply pressure with a finger in the lumen of the trachea if the airway is secured distally. Finally, bedside wound exploration and extensive packing have been described [10].

Regardless of the technique used for immediate management, few patients with significant postoperative bleeding from TIF survive. That is because even temporary control of bleeding, with airway management and fluid resuscitation, is rarely achieved. Patients with TIF who are stabilized will require definitive management in the operating room. The application of an endovascular stent is possible as a temporizing measure but is no substitute for surgically correcting the underlying cause of TIF. A median sternotomy is invariably necessary followed by ligation or graft repair of the damaged vessel. The authors of one of the largest series reported in the literature advocate routine ligation of the innominate artery after TIF despite the small risk of stroke [10]. A soft tissue interposition graft is also advisable in any patient with TIF. For example, a sternocleidomastoid flap can be interposed between the trachea and innominate artery in the case of an ill-fitting tracheostomy with erosion of the anterior tracheal wall as the cause of bleeding.

Management of carotid artery rupture

Carotid artery injury is a risk associated with any deep neck surgery including thyroid and parathyroid surgery.

Carotid artery injury during surgery is rare even among inexperienced surgeons. Prior surgeries and/or radiation can predispose to injury as the normal dissection planes can be disrupted. Even so, it is the responsibility of the head and neck endocrine surgeon to avoid injury by being properly prepared (including a careful review of any imaging), maintaining a thorough knowledge of the anatomy and using meticulous surgical technique. The general management principles outlined above should be used in the event of a carotid injury or rupture encountered during surgery. Finger occlusion of the bleeding should be followed by proximal and distal control of the vessel, which can be easily achieved with vessel loops. The risk of stroke is low with temporary occlusion of the proximal carotid artery but repair should be performed expeditiously. To this end, intraoperative vascular surgery consultation can be very helpful. The site of injury can be oversewn using a vascular suture (e.g. 5-0 Prolene). An interposition vein graft is rarely needed except possibly in the event of a complete transaction. In that case, the internal or external jugular vein can be readily sacrificed and used for the repair.

While carotid rupture can be managed quickly and effectively, postoperative bleeding from the carotid artery is often catastrophic. Factors also associated with carotid rupture after surgery include wound infection, dehiscence and/or pharyngocutaneous fistula. Immediate recognition and decisive intervention are needed in the event of carotid artery rupture if the patient is to survive. Finger occlusion of the bleeding site followed by aggressive airway management and fluid resuscitation should be undertaken. Bedside wound exploration is ill advised. Rather, exploration in the operating room or endovascular stent placement by interventional radiology should be performed [11]. Definitive soft tissue coverage is required regardless of the technique used for short-term control of bleeding.

Management of internal jugular bleeding

The internal jugular vein is at great risk of injury during thyroid and parathyroid surgery. This is particularly true for thyroid cancer cases that include bulky level IV metastatic adenopathy. Enlarged lymph nodes can displace the vein. In some cases, the vein may be adherent to a lymph node or directly invaded by metastatic tumour.

Control of internal jugular bleeding is usually easily achieved following the general principles outlined above. Generally, an injury to the vein can be suture-repaired while maintaining the integrity of the vessel. However, there are occasions when the internal jugular vein is sacrificed as the most reliable means of extirpating disease and maintaining haemostasis. The most difficult internal jugular vein injuries to control are those located low in the neck as the vein branches from the innominate vein. In these cases, deliberate sacrifice of the internal jugular vein is often the most prudent course rather than attempted suture repair.

Transaxillary endoscopic and robotic-assisted procedures place the internal jugular vein at increased risk of injury. In these cases, the lateral surgical approach closely approximates the internal jugular vein. The dissection ideally occurs from lateral to medial between the sternal and clavicular heads of the sternocleidomastoid muscle. Dissection too posterior into the muscle can place the internal jugular vein in the centre of the working space where instrumentation can cause injury. Internal jugular vein bleeding in these cases can be alarming since direct pressure is not an option for control of haemorrhage. It is, however, possible to tamponade the vein using suction and/or long Debakey forceps. In these cases, endoscopic surgical clip appliers are essential for controlling the bleeding. Conversion to an open approach may also be required to ensure adequate haemostasis.

Management of a sentinel bleeding event

Most patients who experience significant postoperative bleeding associated with TIF or carotid artery rupture will have a history of a sentinel bleeding event. The typical story will include a description of a sudden but brief rush of brisk bleeding from the neck wound. Quantification of the volume of bleeding can be difficult for patients to communicate and easy for caregivers to minimize. Therefore, any bleeding from the neck should be taken seriously after neck surgery. A history suspicious for sentinel bleeding, usually at least a shotglass-full volume of blood, should be evaluated aggressively. Any such patient should be admitted for observation. Anatomical imaging, most commonly computed tomography (CT), is important to rule out pathology such as an occult aneu-

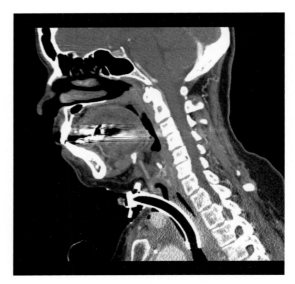

Figure 18.5 CT scan showing air around the innominate artery in a patient with a tracheostomy.

rysm, abscess or fistula. A finding of air immediately adjacent to the great vessels can be a harbinger of impending bleeding (see Figure 18.5). Management should be tailored to correct any identified abnormality, ranging from intravenous antibiotics to prophylactic reconstructive surgery.

Prevention

Of course, prevention of injury to the great vessels is a top priority of any neck surgery. Preoperative planning is the cornerstone of prevention of injury during and after surgery. A detailed physical examination and review of imaging can be helpful in identifying and ruling out vascular anomalies prior to surgery. Pulsation in the neck is a sign that should be sought on physical exam. Pulsation in the low, central anterior neck is rare and should be considered a vascular anomaly (e.g. high-riding innominate artery) until proven otherwise. Preoperative imaging can also assist in ruling out a vascular anomaly (e.g. retro-oesophageal right subclavian artery). Unusual vascular findings identified on examination or imaging can be further worked up using Doppler ultrasound, magnetic resonance angiography (MRA) or conventional angiography as needed.

A detailed surgical plan is also critical for preventing injury to the great vessels during neck surgery. For example, surgery to remove a locally aggressive thyroid cancer with possible tracheal involvement should include a plan for possible immediate airway reconstruction. The extent of surgery and potential risks of dissection should be fully anticipated before entering the operating room, particularly in reoperative cases. Likewise, proper skin flap design can help prevent wound complications that can compromise the great vessels. For instance, incisions overlying the carotid artery should be minimized, particularly if a level V neck dissection or sacrifice of the sternocleidomastoid muscle is expected. During surgery, adequate exposure is essential for prevention of injury to the great vessels. Exposure is also critical should severe haemorrhage be encountered. Prevention of bleeding also includes careful attention to the inferior thyroid vessels, possibly including the thyroidea ima artery. Retraction of inferior thyroid vessels into the mediastinum can result in bleeding that is difficult to control.

Excellent exposure is also essential whenever ectopic thyroid is encountered, given the increased chance of simultaneous vascular anomalies. It is important to note that exposure is not synonymous with extent of incision. Poor visualization of anatomy through a small incision can be extremely hazardous with an increased risk of injury to the great vessels. In experienced hands, excellent exposure can be achieved with both conventional and minimally invasive techniques.

Soft tissue coverage may be necessary to prevent postoperative injury to the great vessels. Patients with a history of radiation to the neck and/or prior neck surgeries are most likely to benefit from soft tissue coverage. In addition, special consideration should be given to any patients with a tracheal disruption adjacent to the innominate artery [7] or a tracheostomy tube that lies adjacent to a high-riding innominate artery. In these cases, strap muscle, thymus or sternocleidomastoid muscle can be used to protect the artery of concern. Rarely, in larger neck procedures, a pedicled pectoralis muscle flap or microvascular free tissue transfer reconstruction can be considered for a more robust soft tissue coverage. For example, aggressive soft tissue coverage may be beneficial for the rare patient who requires external beam radiation after surgery for thyroid cancer.

Conclusion

Haemorrhage from a great vessel during surgery of the neck is a feared complication, whether it be intraoperative or postoperative. A thorough knowledge of normal and aberrant neck anatomy, patient-specific preoperative planning and a step-wise approach to management of both minor and major bleeding events aid in prevention of long-term injury to the patient.

References

1 Henry JF, Audiffret J, Denizot A. The nonrecurrent inferior laryngeal nerve: review of 33 cases, including two on the left side. Surgery 1988; 104: 977.

2 Upadhyaya PK, Bertellotti R, Laeeq A, *et al*. Beware of the aberrant innominate artery. Ann Thorac Surg 2008; 85: 653–4.

3 Netzer A, Ostrovsky D, Bar R, Westerman ST, Golz A. Protection of high-riding aberrant innominate artery during open tracheotomy. J Laryngol Otol 2010; 124: 892–5.

4 Ozlugedik S, Ozcan M, Unal A, *et al*. Surgical importance of highly located innominate artery in neck surgery. Am J Otolaryngol 2005; 26: 330–2.

5 Caldarelli DD, Holinger LD. Complications and sequelae of thyroid surgery. Otolaryngol Clin North Am 1980; 13: 85.

6 Matthews TW, Briant TD. The use of fibrin tissue glue in thyroid surgery: resource utilization implications. J Otolaryngol 1991; 20: 276.

7 Allan JS, Wright CD. Tracheoinnominate fistula: diagnosis and management. Chest Surg Clin North Am 2003; 13: 331–41.

8 Komanapalli CB, Person TD, Schipper P, *et al*. An alternative retractor for transcervical thymectomy. J Thorac Cardiovasc Surg 2005; 130(1): 221–2.

9 Powitzky R, Vasan N, Krempl G, *et al*. Carotid blowout in patients with head and neck cancer. Ann Otol Rhinol Laryngol 2010; 119: 476–84.

10 Jones JW, Reynolds M, Hewitt RL, *et al*. Tracheo-innominate artery erosion: successful surgical management of a devastating complication. Ann Surg 1976; 184(2): 194–204.

11 Warren FM, Cohen JI, Nesbit GM, *et al*. Management of carotid 'blowout' with endovascular stent grafts. Laryngoscope 2002; 112: 428–33.

CHAPTER 19

Lesions Following Lateral Neck Dissection: Phrenic, Vagus and Accessory Nerve Injury, and Chyle Leak

Clive S. Grant

Department of Surgery, College of Medicine, Mayo Clinic, Rochester, MN, USA

Introduction

In order to provide sound advice to patients with lateral neck lymph node metastases (LNM) from papillary thyroid carcinoma (PTC), an in-depth understanding of practical and biological implications is necessary. Only then can an optimal operation be undertaken, balancing the attendant risks of complications against the potential benefits. The principles of neck dissection for medullary thyroid carcinoma (MTC) are quite similar to PTC, with the exception that MTC nodes tend to have more adherence or invasiveness than do PTC nodes. In addition, the extent of dissection more commonly involves compartments II–Vb for MTC where it is often more limited in LNM from PTC. Because PTC is overwhelmingly more common than MTC, the concepts and management described are focused on PTC.

Lymph node metastases are extremely common in PTC. The frequency and distribution of PTC LNM are highly dependent on the diligence of and methods used for detection. With routine lateral neck dissection of the internal jugular lymph nodes, as many as 90% [1,2] of patients will harbour at least microscopic LNM, and more than 50% of lymph nodes interpreted as free of metastases by standard haematoxylin and eosin (H&E)

light microscopy can be found to contain LNMs by immunohistochemistry stained for cytokeratin [3]. There are data supporting a sequential, reasonably predictable pattern of spread of PTC to lymph nodes. Initially, and quite early in the presence of PTC, compartment VI lymph nodes will be involved. From a clinical perspective (macroscopic lymph nodes identified by palpation or high-resolution ultrasound), compartments IV and III subsequently become involved, and still later compartments II and V. Compartment IIb rarely has LNM without IIa being 'positive', and compartments I and Va rarely contain LNM from PTC. Additionally, the submental, parotid and retro-auricular nodes are virtually never dissected in PTC.

Quite different from the biological implications of lymph node metastases in such malignancies as breast and colon cancer, LNM in PTC are frequently not associated with lethal disease. These LNM are found frequently in children and young adults, yet these patients rarely suffer a lethal outcome. Other prognostic factors, such as extrathyroidal tumour invasion and elderly age, pose far greater mortality risk. Nevertheless, technological advances in high-resolution ultrasonography now commonly used by endocrinologists, and the ability to detect nanogram levels of the PTC tumour marker thyroglobulin as part of

Thyroid Surgery: Preventing and Managing Complications, First Edition. Edited by Paolo Miccoli, David J. Terris,
Michele N. Minuto and Melanie W. Seybt.

intensive postoperative disease surveillance, have facilitated detection of miniscule disease recurrence. This usually takes the form of residual lymph node disease, and despite the usually very low risk of life-threatening implications, attempting to reassure a patient with the 'cancer' recurrence, unless excised, is rarely possible.

While in previous years, a 'node-picking' approach to lateral neck dissection was favoured by some surgeons, general consensus now strongly favors an '*en bloc*' dissection of LNM in a compartment-oriented manner (Table 19.1, Figure 19.1). Recurrent LNMs were significantly more frequent with the node-picking approach [4]. The indications for lateral neck dissection usually include the presence of LNM, detected either by palpation or preoperatively performed imaging studies. There seems no controversy among internationally recognized authorities in thyroid cancer and specialty societies that surgical lymphadenectomy is the preferred approach to cervical LNM [5–7].

The most recent American Thyroid Association guidelines for the management of PTC [8] include the following: '(R21) Preoperative neck ultrasound for the contralateral lobe and cervical (central and especially lateral compartments) lymph nodes is recommended for all patients undergoing thyroidectomy for malignant cytologic findings on biopsy'. Specifically with reference to lateral neck compartment lymph nodes, the guidelines state: '(R27) for those patients in whom nodal disease is evident clinically, on preoperative ultrasound, or at the time of surgery, surgical resection may reduce the risk of recurrence and possibly mortality. (R28) Lateral neck compartmental lymph node dissection should be performed for patients with biopsy-proven metastatic lateral cervical lymphadenopathy'. Both the American Association of Clinical Endocrinologists and the American Association of Endocrine Surgeons have endorsed similar recommendations [9]. Moreover, a recent report favoured an even more aggressive approach including routine dissection of levels III and IV at the time of thyroidectomy, even if preoperative ultrasound did not identify LNM [10].

The classic, compartment I through V radical neck dissection dates back to Crile in 1906 [11]. His description not only incorporated the lymph nodes but also sacrificed the sternocleidomastoid muscle (SCM), internal jugular vein (IJV) and the spinal accessory nerve (cranial nerve XI, C-XI). Based on extensive anatomical studies, Suarez [12] and Bocca [13–15] determined that the lymphatic system of the neck is contained within a complex system of aponeurotic partitions that could be dissected safely and completely, while preserving important functional structures. Specifically, the spinal accessory nerve, although crossing intra-aponeurotic spaces, could be dissected free. The term *modified radical neck dissection* was recommended by Bocca and Pignataro [13] for the more conservative approach in which the SCM, IJV and C-XI were preserved. More favoured terms such as selective neck dissection and functional neck dissection are also used to describe variations of compartment-oriented neck dissections.

Lymph node dissection in papillary thyroid carcinoma

Prevalent throughout the extensive published literature regarding lateral neck dissection for PTC is the admonishment that for complications, *prevention* is the key. Without further details, this is merely an empty

Table 19.1 Compartments/levels of cervical lymph nodes.

Level (compartment)	Location
I (Submandibular triangle)	Bounded by anterior and posterior bellies of digastric muscle and interior ramus of mandible
II (Upper jugular)	Extending from base of skull to bifurcation of carotid artery or the hyoid bone. Posterior border of the sternocleidomastoid, anterior border of the sternohyoid muscle. IIa superior to spinal accessory nerve; IIb inferior to spinal accessory nerve
III (Middle jugular)	Inferior border of level II to omohyoid muscle or cricoid cartilage; anterior borders same as II
IV (Lower jugular)	Inferior border of level III to clavicle; anterior and posterior borders same as II and III
V (Posterior triangle)	Around lower aspect of spinal accessory nerve and transverse cervical vessels, bounded by clavicle inferiorly, trapezius muscle posteriorly, sternocleidomastoid anteriorly. Va superior to level of cricoid cartilage; Vb inferior to level of cricoid cartilage

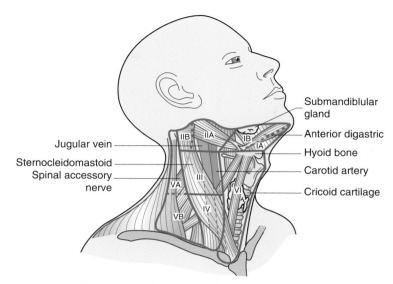

Figure 19.1 Compartments of the neck. Reproduced from Cooper *et al.* [8], with permission from American Thyroid Association.

statement. It follows, therefore, that a reasonably detailed explanation of a compartment-oriented lateral neck dissection, with emphasis on complication avoidance, should be presented. A few initial general comments seem appropriate.

• Reoperation is potentially far more difficult and dangerous than the initial dissection. Therefore, an *en bloc*, compartment-oriented thorough clearance of the lymph node packet is routine.

• Preoperative imaging (our strong preference for LNM in the lateral neck is ultrasound) is recommended, even if palpably worrisome lymph nodes are present.

• The key lateral compartments are IV, III and the anterior aspect of compartment V (posterior to the SCM, but not formally extending the dissection to the trapezius muscle). These compartments are routinely dissected whenever the lateral neck contains LNM.

• Compartment II is added to compartments III, IV and anterior V whenever LNM are found in or near that compartment.

• Long-acting muscle relaxant is not used to allow normal motor nerve conduction and muscle contraction throughout the neck dissection.

Incision

The extent of the incision is dependent on the extent of the lateral neck dissection and the patient's body habitus.

If compartment II is not dissected, the standard transverse collar incision used for the thyroidectomy can be further extended laterally and somewhat superiorly with extensive subplatysmal flaps developed. If compartment II is to be dissected, given the vulnerability and consequences of damage to the spinal accessory nerve, a more pronounced vertical extension of the incision along the anterior border of the SCM is usually employed.

Exposure of the internal jugular vein, carotid artery and vagus nerve

The plane between the strap muscles and the SCM is dissected with cautery, extending the dissection from the clavicle superiorly as far as indicated (Figure 19.2). The omohyoid muscle is uncovered by this dissection, and can be isolated superiorly and inferolaterally, and resected. Immediately underlying the omohyoid is the IJV within the carotid sheath. With the strap muscles retracted medially and the SCM laterally, the lateral border of the IJV is elevated with forceps and the areolar tissue is dissected away from it. This dissection is carried around posterior to the vein to the end of the areolar tissue that drops down and away from the vein. The dissection is started in a safe zone about 2 cm above the clavicle and is extended both superiorly and inferiorly, staying somewhat above the base of the neck to avoid injury to the thoracic duct (Figure 19.3). A vein retractor facilitates

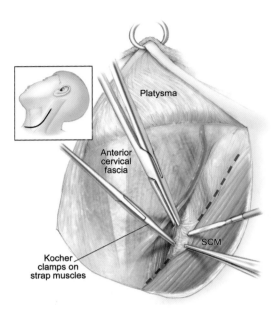

Figure 19.2 Incision and dissection between sternocleidomastoid muscle (SCM) and strap muscles in modified radical neck dissection. Reproduced with permission from Porterfield *et al.* [32].

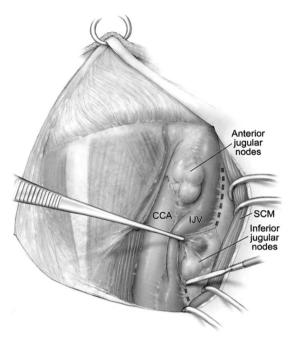

Figure 19.3 Initial dissection along lateral border of internal jugular vein (IJV). CCA, common carotid artery; SCM, sternocleidomastoid muscle. Reproduced with permission from Porterfield *et al.* [32].

elevation of the IJV during this step. Rarely, PTC LNM can invade the IJV, requiring resection of the vein. This is not a problem if unilateral. Care must be taken to avoid inadvertent tear of the vein with resultant bleeding or air embolism. The vagus nerve is located between and posterior to the carotid artery and IJV, within the carotid sheath. Damage to the vagus nerve should be an extreme rarity as it is bordering but not really within the area of dissection.

Exposure of the floor of the neck and phrenic nerve

As the areolar 'edge' is developed behind the IJV, this tissue is easily elevated off the 'floor of the neck' – the deep cervical fascia, which is overlying the anterior scalene muscle. Dissection should not be carried posterior to the carotid artery to avoid damage to the cervical sympathetic chain. Careful blunt dissection behind the areolar tissue exposes the transverse cervical artery (a branch of the thyrocervical trunk) coursing laterally across the anterior scalene muscle, and anterior to the vertically running phrenic nerve. The artery may be sacrificed if needed. The phrenic nerve is probably the most vulnera-

ble nerve throughout the dissection as it courses along the deep aspect of the dissection (Figure 19.4). Continued anterior traction on the lymphatic packet helps avoid injury to this structure.

Exposure and management of the thoracic duct

As the dissection is extended inferiorly along the lateral border of the IJV, care must be taken to uncover its confluence with the subclavian vein. LNMs from PTC are very common in this area, jeopardizing the thoracic duct as it loops up a short distance behind the IJV from medial to lateral, and descends to enter the confluence of the IJV and subclavian vein (Figure 19.5). The fluid within the duct is either clear or slightly blood-tinged, but rarely milky because the patient has fasted. Preferably, the adjacent tissue should be dissected from the duct, controlling all the lymphatic tributaries. If, however, the thoracic duct is injured or must be removed due to disease, the duct can be transected and ligated without harm in the

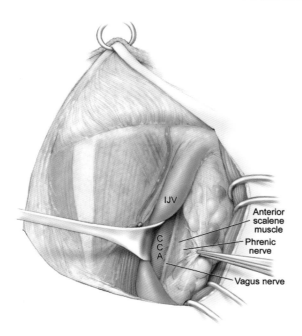

Figure 19.4 Exposure of anterior scalene muscle, vagus and phrenic nerves. IJV, internal jugular vein; CCA, common carotid artery. Metastatic PTC LNMs often have blue discoloration. Reproduced with permission from Porterfield *et al.* [32].

adult patient. If multiple tributaries are encountered in this area, *en masse* control with ligature is better than suture ligation. CAUTION: protect the underlying phrenic nerve! The lymphatic packet is then dissected laterally across at the level of or behind the clavicle, controlling small veins. The anterior scalene is fully exposed, and further lateral blunt dissection posteriorly onto the base of the neck exposes the brachial plexus, coursing between the anterior and middle scalene muscles. These nerves should be easily protected.

Dissection of the cervical plexus and spinal accessory nerves

The packet of tissue is then retracted anteriorly and medially, with retractors under the SCM, displacing it laterally. As the packet is dissected from its lateral attachments under the SCM, coursing superiorly, the individual sensory cervical plexus nerves are identified and preserved (Figure 19.6). As dissection proceeds superiorly, with cautery on very low power or with the aid of a nerve

stimulator, the spinal accessory nerve will be stimulated, causing obvious contraction of the SCM and trapezius muscle. With muscle contraction, instrument dissection should be used to uncover the nerve as it courses in an oblique vertical manner. The nodes need to be dissected away from the nerve without use of the cautery, with the dissection encompassing the posterior IIb nodes only as necessary. The superior border of the dissection is the posterior belly of the digastric muscle.

Dissection of nodes anterior to the internal jugular vein

Overlying the IJV on its anterior surface at about the level of the large anterior facial vein branch is a packet of lymph nodes that are commonly involved in patients with PTC. These nodes may be obscured from view by overlying fascia, but need to be dissected and removed. These may represent first-echelon draining lymph nodes from PTC located in the superior pole of the thyroid gland. Because the facial vein branch off the IJV is not transected nor the carotid artery displaced, the hypoglossal nerve should not really be threatened.

Complications

Phrenic nerve

Damage to the phrenic nerve anywhere along its course results in unilateral elevation of the diaphragm and possible compromise to respiratory function. In a report from The Netherlands, the frequency of phrenic nerve damage was 8% [16]. Although no patient suffered severe symptoms, there were a higher number of patients with atelectasis and pulmonary infiltrates complicating the procedures. Bilateral phrenic nerve paralysis has been reported [17] with consequent respiratory failure.

Vagus nerve

If the vagus nerve (cranial nerve X) is injured in the neck, unilateral vocal cord paralysis will result, as the recurrent laryngeal nerve is part of the vagus at this level. Unless co-morbid conditions exist regarding the heart, no significant cardiac complications should occur. Similarly, a unilateral vagus transection or damage should have little effect on the gastrointestinal tract.

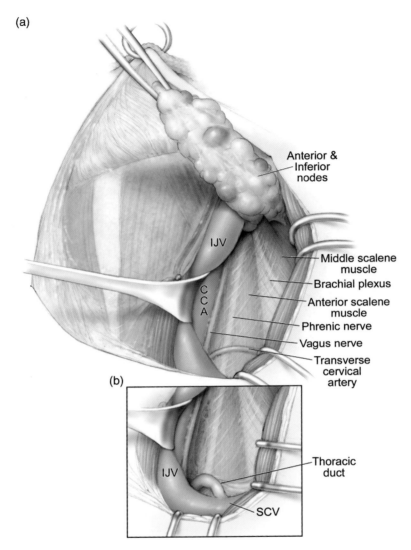

Figure 19.5 *En bloc* dissection of lymph nodes adjacent to internal jugular vein (IJV); exposure of anterior and middle scalene muscles with intervening brachial plexus nerves; phrenic nerve coursing on anterior scalene muscle. Thoracic duct coursing behind IJV, anterior to anterior scalene muscle to enter confluence of IJV and subclavian vein (SCV). CCA, common carotid artery. Reproduced with permission from Porterfield *et al.* [32]. © 2009 American Medical Association. All rights reserved.

Spinal accessory nerve

The most intensely studied complication of neck dissection is injury to the spinal accessory nerve, these reports frequently relating to malignancies of the head and neck separate from the thyroid gland. This nerve provides the motor supply to the SCM and trapezius muscles. Sacrifice of the spinal accessory nerve usually causes the 'shoulder syndrome' [18]. This is characterized by pain, weakness and atrophy of the shoulder girdle, with restriction of arm abduction and frontal flexion. The scapula is inadequately stabilized during shoulder movements (can result in 'winged scapula'), which can lead to a mechanical

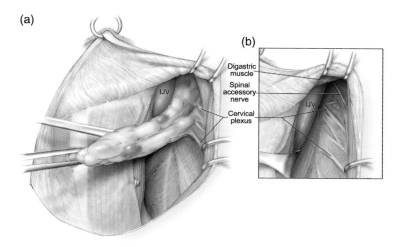

Figure 19.6 Cervical plexus and spinal accessory nerves coursing obliquely through lymph node packet with retraction laterally on sternocleidomastoid muscle. Posterior belly of digastric muscle as superior border of lymph node dissection. IJV, internal jugular vein. Reproduced with permission from Porterfield *et al*. [32]. © 2009 American Medical Association. All rights reserved.

overloading of different shoulder structures. Specifically, strain on the levator scapulae and the rhomboids may result in pain. Furthermore, secondary periarthritis may lead to a 'frozen shoulder' [19]. Interestingly, however, the trapezius muscle also has variable innervation by the second, third and fourth branches of the cervical plexus (C2–4), preserving some function in some patients when the spinal accessory nerve is sacrificed. Conversely, sacrifice of C2–4 rami of the cervical plexus causes worse dysfunction of the trapezius if combined with damage to or transection of the spinal accessory nerve [20,21].

The body of literature reviewing neck dissection has generally concluded that shoulder function is better following selective neck dissection than modified radical neck dissection [22]. This difference has been attributed to lack of dissection of level V in the area of the spinal accessory nerve in selective neck dissections. Even if the accessory nerve is preserved during dissection of the entire course of the nerve, temporary or even permanent dysfunction of the nerve may result [22]. One report, utilizing the Disability of Arm, Shoulder and Hand (DASH) questionnaire, found moderate to severe upper limb dysfunction in some patients, even when the spinal accessory nerve had been preserved [23]. In fact, over 75% of the patients had some long-term symptoms. Correlating with both motor and sensory nerve damage and consequent dysfunction and pain are corresponding negative

effects on patient quality of life [21]. Of particular interest relative to thyroid cancer is a report of outcome when only levels III and IV were dissected unilaterally [24]. In this patient group, mean scores for shoulder dysfunction were similar to patients who did not undergo neck dissection. However, patients with unilateral level V and bilateral level III and IV dissections reported much worse scores on average [25].

The unmistakable conclusion from all of these reports is that even careful, nerve-preserving dissection of the spinal accessory nerve, most notably in the posterior triangle, can and often does lead to significant shoulder disability. Because LNMs from PTC are very rarely found in this compartment, dissection of compartment V in this area should be avoided. Therefore, the lateral neck dissection technique often applied to head and neck cancers should be modified when dealing with PTC.

Most literature reports addressing repair of the injured spinal accessory nerve describe delayed exploration and repair, as the injury is seldom recognized at the time of operative damage. This delayed procedure is beyond the scope of this chapter, but if damage to the nerve is recognized intraoperatively, repair should be undertaken. If a sharp transection has occurred, then no loss of nerve length complicates the repair, and microsurgical reapproximation is appropriate. If a segment of the nerve has been resected or a portion damaged with electrocautery, the damaged segment should be resected and a judgement made about whether tension on the anastomosis would preclude a satisfactory direct repair. If a nerve graft is necessary to allow a tension-free anastomosis, either the greater auricular nerve or a sural nerve graft can be harvested. Using the operating microscope, the nerve ends should be anastomosed with fine (8-0 to 10-0) sutures, incorporating only the epineurium – not the substance of the nerve itself – to coapt the nerve ends. This usually requires 3–5 sutures.

Thoracic duct

Whereas chyle leaks following neck dissection are uncommon, in the range 1–2.5% [18], they can present significant treatment challenges. Between 2 and 4 L of chyle flow through the thoracic duct every day [26]. Chyle leak may lead to malnutrition, immune compromise, electrolyte abnormalities, hypoalbuminaemia and infection. A large proportion of total body protein is transported in chylous fluid, which, with a prolonged chylous leak, could result in serious protein loss. Moreover, if left uncontrolled, chyle leak can lead to necrosis of the overlying skin and eventual carotid artery damage [27]. Chyle leaks most often occur after neck dissection on the left side, but right-sided leaks from prominent lymphatics have been reported.

Diagnosis is usually not difficult or subtle; milky white effluent from a drain or on aspiration of a fluid collection is obvious. A more specific measure of fluid containing >100 mg/dL of triglycerides is considered indicative of chyle leak. Both medical and surgical options exist for resolution of the problem. Following neck dissection, drainage of 200–300 cc/day of milky fluid may resolve with continued catheter drainage. Restriction of oral intake completely or to 'fat-free' or only medium chain triglycerides may be attempted, with supplementation of intravenous nutrition. The use of octreotide injections has met with stunning successes at times. The theorized mechanism for this relates to reduced lymphatic and splanchnic blood flow. Chyle outputs in excess of 1.5 L/day for more than 5 days usually mandate intervention. Fibrin sealant [28], surgical muscle transpositions [29] and radiological intervention with occlusion of the thoracic duct are additional treatment options [30].

From a practical perspective, if a chyle leak in excess of 150–200 cc/day persists beyond 2–3 days, most surgeons would advocate re-exploration and ligation of the draining lymphatics or the actual thoracic duct if necessary. Drainage beyond 7–10 days would likely have generated a local inflammatory response, precluding any type of simple surgical approach. Rather, use of octreotide would be a reasonable next step. The most important emphasis should be on meticulous prevention of lymphatic leak at the initial operation.

Conclusion

Lymph node metastases from papillary thyroid carcinoma, involving compartments II–V, are detectable in 20–30% of patients by palpation or preoperative imaging. The internal jugular vein, carotid artery, vagus, cervical sympathetic, phrenic, cervical plexus, brachial plexus and C-XI nerves, and the thoracic duct are jeopardized by lateral neck dissection. These structures can almost always be preserved, as lymph node metastases from PTC have more characteristic 'pushing' rather than infiltrating borders. All of the important structures either border or are located deep to the lymph node 'packet', with the exceptions of C-XI and the cervical plexus nerves that course through it. Because compartment IV LNM are common in PTC, the thoracic duct is especially at risk for disruption, but can be ligated if necessary without harm. In contrast, even careful preservation of C-XI, if exposed and dissected throughout its entire course, can lead to significant shoulder symptoms. To avoid this complication, dissection should usually be limited to compartment II, without dissection of compartment Va.

Despite the number of important structures in the lateral neck, dissection can be accomplished with few complications by expert surgeons [31]. The precision and diligence necessary to carry out a safe thyroidectomy, preserving the parathyroid glands, recurrent laryngeal and external branch of the superior laryngeal nerves, should be extended to dissection of the lateral neck. Because prevention of complications should be the emphasis, the details of compartment-oriented dissection are described and illustrated, as well as the consequences of damage to the phrenic, vagus and accessory nerves and chyle leak.

References

1 Noguchi S, Murakami N. The value of lymph–node dissection in patients with differentiated thyroid cancer. Surg Clin North Am 1987; 67(2): 251–61.

2 Noguchi S, Noguchi A, Murakami N. Papillary carcinoma of the thyroid. Developing pattern of metastasis. Cancer 1970; 26: 1053–60.

3 Qubain S, Nakano S, Baba M, Takao S, Aikou T. Distribution of lymph node micrometastasis in .N0 well-differentiated thyroid carcinoma. Surgery 2002; 131: 249–56.

4 Hay I, Bergstralh E, Grant C, et al. Impact of primary surgery on outcome in 300 patients with pathologic tumor-node-metastasis stage III papillary thyroid carcinoma treated at one institution from 1940 through 1989. Surgery 1999; 126: 1173.

5 Schlumberger M. Papillary and follicular thyroid carcinoma. N Engl J Med 1998; 338(5): 297–306.

6 Mazzaferri E, Kloos R. Clinical review 128: current approaches to primary therapy for papillary and follicular thyroid cancer. J Clin Endocrinol Metab 2001; 86: 1447–63.

7 American Thyroid Association Guidelines Taskforce. Management guidelines for patients with thyroid nodules and differentiated thyroid cancer. Thyroid 2006; 16(2): 1–33.

8 Cooper D, Doherty G, Haugen B, et al. Revised American Thyroid Association management guidelines for pateints with thyroid nodules and differentiated thyroid cancer. Thyroid 2009; 19(11): 1167–214.

9 American Association of Clinical Endocrinologists. 2001 AACE/AAES medical/surgical guidelines for clinical practice: management of thyroid carcinoma. Endocr Pract 2001; 7: 202–20.

10 Bonnet S, Hartl D, Leboulleux S, et al. Prophylactic lymph node dissection for papillary thyroid cancer less than 2 cm: implications for radioiodine treatment. J Clin Endocrinol Metab 2009; 94(4): 1162–7.

11 Crile G. Excision of cancer of the head and neck with special reference to the plan of dissection based on one hundred and thirty-two operations. JAMA 1906; 47: 1780–6.

12 Suarez O. The problem of distant lymphatic metastasis in cancer of the larynx and hypopharynx [Spanish]. Rev Otorinolaryngol Santiago 1963; 23: 83–99.

13 Bocca E, Pignataro O. A conservation technique in radical neck dissection. Ann Otol Rhinol Laryngol 1967; 76: 975–87.

14 Bocca E. Conservative neck dissection. Laryngoscope 1975; 85: 1511–15.

15 Bocca E, Pignataro O, Oldini C, Cappa C. Functional neck dissection: an evaluation and review of 843 cases. Laryngoscope 1984; 94: 942–5.

16 De Jong A, Manni J. Phrenic nerve paralysis following neck dissection. Eur Arch Otorhinolaryngol 1991; 248(3): 132–4.

17 Yaddanapudi S, Shah S. Bilateral phrenic nerve injury after neck dissection: an uncommon cause of respiratory failure. J Laryngol Otol 1996; 110(3): 281–3.

18 Teymoortash A, Hoch S, Eivazi B, Werner J. Postoperative morbidity after different types of selective neck dissection. Laryngoscope 2010; 120: 924–9.

19 Lloyd S. Accessory nerve: anatomy and surgical identification. J Laryngol Otol 2007; 121: 1118–25.

20 Tsuji T, Tanuma A, Onitsuka T, et al. Electromyographic findings after different selective neck dissections. Laryngoscope 2007; 117: 319–22.

21 Roh JL, Yoon YH, Kim S, Park C. Cervical sensory preservation during neck dissection. Oral Oncol 2007; 43: 491–8.

22 Selcuk A, Selcuk B, Bahar S, Dere H. Shoulder function in various types of neck dissection. Role of spinal accessory nerve and cervical plexus preservation. Tumori 2008; 94(1): 36–9.

23 Carr S, Bowyer D, Cox G. Upper limb dysfunction following selective neck dissection: a retrospective questionnaire study. Head Neck 2009; 31(6): 789–92.

24 Ferlito A, Rinaldo A, Silver C, et al. Elective and therapeutic selective neck dissection. Oral Oncol 2006; 42: 14–25.

25 Laverick S, Lowe D, Brown J, Vaughan E, Rogers S. The impact of neck dissection on health-related quality of life. Arch Otolaryngol Head Neck Surg 2004; 130: 149–54.

26 Smoke A, DeLegge M. Chyle leaks: consensus on management? Nutrition Clin Pract 2008; 23(5): 529–32.

27 Gregor R. Management of chyle fistulization in association with neck dissection. Otolaryngol Head Neck Surg 2000; 122: 434–9.

28 Vaiman M, Eviatar E. Lymphatic fistulae after neck dissection: the fibrin sealant treatment. J Surg Oncol 2008; 98(6): 467–71.

29 Lorenz K, Abuazab M, Sekulla C, Nguyen-Thanh P, Brauckhoff M, Dralle H. Management of lymph fistulas in thyroid surgery. Langenbeck's Arch Surg 2010; 395: 911–17.

30 Patel N, Lewandowski R, Bove M, Nemchek A, Salem R. Thoracic duct embolization: a new treatment for massive leak after neck dissection. Laryngoscope 2008; 118: 680–3.

31 Cheah W, Arici C, Ituarte P, Siperstein A, Duh QY, Clark O. Complications of neck dissection for thyroid cancer. World J Surg 2002; 26: 1013–16.

32 Porterfield J, Factor D, Grant S. Operative technique for modified radical neck dissection in papillary thyroid carcinoma. Arch Surg 2009; 144: 567–74

CHAPTER 20

Amiodarone-induced Thyrotoxicosis and Thyroid Storm

Fausto Bogazzi,[1] *Luca Tomisti,*[1] *Piero Berti*[2] *and Enio Martino*[1]

[1] Department of Endocrinology and Metabolism, University of Pisa, Pisa, Italy
[2] Department of Surgery, University of Pisa, Pisa, Italy

Introduction

Amiodarone-induced thyrotoxicosis (AIT) is a challenging complication occurring on average in 15% of patients during chronic therapy. It may develop soon after starting amiodarone or at any time during therapy and even months after drug withdrawal. Two main forms of AIT may be identified: type 1, occurring in patients with underlying thyroid diseases, and type 2 occurring in patients with normal glands. Type 1 AIT is a form of true iodine-induced hyperthyroidism triggered by excess iodine released by amiodarone metabolism unveiling a latent functional autonomy; type 2 AIT is a drug-induced destructive thyroiditis owing to the cytotoxic effect of amiodarone on thyroidal follicular cells.

Differentiation of the two types of AIT is crucial because medical therapy greatly differs: drugs which inhibit thyroid hormone synthesis are the best choice for treating patients with type 1 AIT; addition of a short course of potassium perchlorate to thionamides, favouring depletion of intrathyroidal iodine load, accelerates euthyroidism restoration. Glucocorticoids are the preferred medical therapy for type 2 AIT; increased serum thyroid hormone levels in these patients are due to the leakage from the damaged thyroid gland; hence, drugs inhibiting thyroid hormone synthesis are ineffective. Mixed forms, where destructive phenomena superimpose on increased thyroid hormone synthesis, exist and are better treated by blocking thyroid hormone synthesis and iodine recycle (using thionamides and potassium perchlorate) and reducing inflammation and thyroid hormone leakage (using glucocorticoids).

Currently, type 2 AIT is the most frequent form of AIT; type 2 AIT may spontaneously remit in a proportion of patients whereas most achieve euthyroidism during glucocorticoid therapy; however, restoration of euthyroidism may require several months, depending on the degree of thyroid damage. In addition, underlying cardiac disease may be precipitated by thyroid hormone excess and prompt control of thyrotoxicosis is then necessary. In this subset of AIT patients, total thyroidectomy is often necessary. In addition, thyroid surgery is a valid option in type 1 AIT patients because the underlying thyroid disease should be treated; this can be done, in a group of patients, after restoration of euthyroidism using a short course of iopanoic acid, when feasible. Each decision carries some risks because patients have underlying (often severe) cardiac problems: on one hand, the harmful effect of long-lasting thyroid hormone excess on the heart and on the other, the risks linked to anaesthesiological and surgical procedures. These issues will be reviewed and discussed in the next sections of this chapter; in the final section, the management of thyroid storm, a rare life-threatening condition due to untreated hyperthyroidism, will be reviewed.

Thyroid Surgery: Preventing and Managing Complications, First Edition. Edited by Paolo Miccoli, David J. Terris, Michele N. Minuto and Melanie W. Seybt.

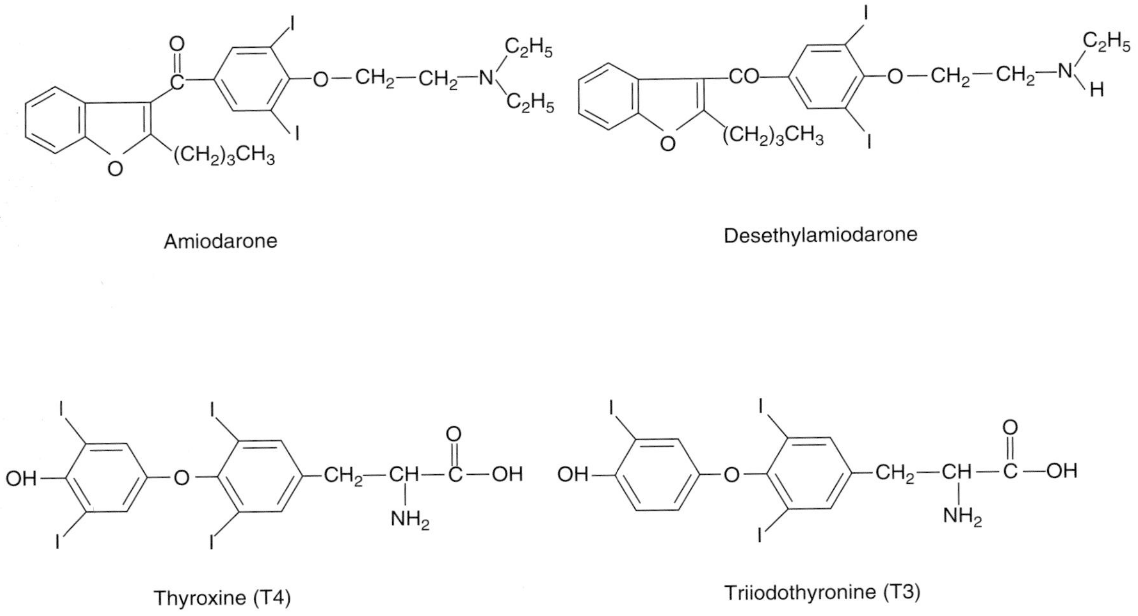

Figure 20.1 Chemical structure of amiodarone, desethylamiodarone and thyroid hormone.

Structure of amiodarone: similarity to thyroid hormone

Amiodarone is a benzofuranic iodine-rich antiarrhythmic drug, the use of which is indicated for treating various arrhythmic disturbances. Its structural formula is similar to that of thyroid hormone (Figure 20.1) and, as expected, amiodarone and its main metabolite, desethylamiodarone (DEA), have thyromimetic action. In fact, amiodarone and DEA can bind to the thyroid hormone receptor as a weak competitor, thus reducing thyroid hormone effect. These effects contribute to the peripheral hypothyroid-like condition observed in euthyroid subjects under amiodarone therapy, including the reduced expression of thyroid hormone-sensitive genes [1].

Pharmacology

Amiodarone belongs to the class III antiarrhythmic drugs; in fact, its main antiarrhythmic action is related to inhibition of myocardial Na-K ATPase activity, finally increasing the refractory period. However, amiodarone produces class I (decreasing conduction velocity, blocking Na channel), class II (antiadrenergic effect reducing β-adrenergic receptor) and class IV (suppressing calcium-mediated action potentials) effects. Owing to its multiple antiarrhythmic effects, amiodarone is used in patients with supraventricular and ventricular tachyarrhythmias and atrial fibrillation (when other therapies are ineffective) and to prevent sudden cardiac death in selected patients.

Amiodarone is highly lipophilic, which accounts for its tissue distribution and for its long-lasting storage in adipose tissue, lung and also thyroid. Amiodarone metabolism occurs mainly through N-dealkylation, leading to the main active metabolite, desethylamiodarone. Most effects are exploited by DEA, the dealkylation product of amiodarone; in addition, amiodarone may undergo deiodination and glucuroconjugation; excretion is mainly through biliary excretion. The average half-lives of amiodarone and DEA are 40 days and 57 days, respectively, thus accounting for their long-lasting effects.

Amiodarone-induced thyroid dysfunctions

A proportion of subjects under amiodarone therapy develop hypothyroidism or thyrotoxicosis. Amiodarone-induced

Table 20.1 Effects of amiodarone on thyroid function.

Mechanism	Effects	Thyroid function tests
Inhibition of type I 5'-deiodinase	Increased T4	T4 increased/high normal
	Decreased T3	T3 decreased/low normal
	Increased rT3	
Inhibition of type II 5'-deiodinase	Decreased pituitary T3 generation	Increased TSH (short term)
Inhibition of TH entry into cells	Decreased peripheral T3 production	Decreased T3/increased TSH
Interaction with TH receptor	Decreased transcription of TH-sensitive genes	Peripheral hypothyroidism
Thyroid cytotoxicity	Leakage of preformed TH	Increased T4 and T3
		Decreased TSH

TH, thyroid hormones; TSH, thyroid-stimulating hormone.

thyroid dysfunctions may occur as a consequence of excessive iodine load or the intrinsic properties of the drug.

Effects on thyroid hormones tests

Amiodarone has effects on thyroid function tests, which occur in all patients; shortly (1–2 months), after starting amiodarone therapy, a transient increase in serum thyroid-stimulating hormone (TSH) concentrations occurs owing to an inhibitory effect of amiodarone on intracellular T4 transport and pituitary D2 activity. Both effects (reduced entry of T4 into the cells and reduced metabolism of T4) lead to lower intracellular T3 content and lower T3 binding to its cognate pituitary receptor, thus reducing thyroid hormone inhibitory effect on TSH gene transcription. With chronic (>3 months) amiodarone therapy, TSH returns to the normal range, whereas serum free T4 and reverse T3 concentrations increase and serum free T3 concentrations reduce owing to the inhibitory effect of amiodarone on hepatic D1 activity. Thus, a common pattern of serum thyroid hormone in euthyroid subjects under chronic amiodarone therapy is a slight increase of T4, low to normal T3 and normal TSH [2]. This complex effect of amiodarone is known as 'peripheral hypothyroidism', mainly but not exclusively due to inhibition of deiodinase activity by amiodarone. The amiodarone effects on thyroid function tests are summarized in Table 20.1.

Effects of iodine load on normal thyroid gland

Under a standard dose of amiodarone (on average, 200 mg per day), patients are exposed to a 7 g iodine load, greatly exceeding the recommended daily allowance (150–200 μg). When exposed to a large amount of iodine, normal thyroids respond with an intrinsic autoregulatory mechanism leading to an acute block of thyroid hormone synthesis (Wolff–Chaikoff effect); as a consequence, thyroid hormone decreases or TSH increases. Usually, thyroids escape the iodine-induced block of thyroid hormone synthesis (escape from the Wolff–Chaikoff effect), reducing iodine transport; the reduced intracellular iodine concentrations are thus no longer sufficient for maintaining the Wolff–Chaikoff effect. Failure to escape the Wolff–Chaikoff effect is responsible for amiodarone-induced hypothyroidism (AIH) occurring in patients without autoimmune thyroiditis. The pathogenic role of iodine load in AIH is supported by clinical studies showing that potassium perchlorate, favouring iodine depletion of thyroid glands, restores euthyroidism in AIH patients either after stopping or continuing amiodarone therapy. In addition, amiodarone may inhibit thyroidal iodide transport by either an iodine-independent mechanism or through decrease of sodium-iodide symporter mRNA expression.

Effects of amiodarone on abnormal thyroid glands

Excessive iodine is the cause of type 1 AIT, a form of iodine-induced hyperthyroidism, in which iodine load unveils underlying thyroid autonomy or latent Graves' disease (Jod–Basedow phenomenon). In such patients iodine load triggers increased thyroid hormone synthesis in glands with potential hyperthyroidism.

Effects due to the molecular structure of amiodarone

Amiodarone and DEA have proapoptotic and cytotoxic effects on follicular epithelial cells. Thyroid cell cultures undergo increased apoptosis following amiodarone or DEA exposure through an iodine-independent cytochrome-c release mechanism. In addition, amiodarone directly induces cytotoxic effects in follicular cells, but excess iodine released by the drug may contribute to its toxic action. Histopathological studies, either in animal models or in patients with AIT who had undergone total thyroidectomy, showed disruption of thyroid structure, including follicular damage, reduced number of mitochondria, increased number of lysosomes and dilation of endoplasmic reticulum, in keeping with a drug-induced thyroid damage and similar to those occurring in subacute thyroiditis. The above mechanism is responsible for the development of type 2 AIT, which is a drug-induced destructive thyroiditis. Further evidence supporting the notion of type 2 AIT as a drug-induced destructive thyroiditis includes the self-limiting outcome, the response to glucocorticoids and the absence of any evidence of thyroid hyperfunction [2].

Epidemiology of amiodarone-induced thyroid dysfunctions

Prevalence of amiodarone-induced thyroid dysfunction is influenced by environmental iodine supply; it is well established that hypothyroidism is more frequent in iodine-sufficient areas whereas thyrotoxicosis occurs in iodine-deficient areas. Two to 12% of patients under chronic amiodarone therapy may develop thyrotoxicosis, depending on their residence in areas with high or low iodine intake. In contrast, hypothyroidism may develop in a proportion ranging from 13% to 6% from the same areas [3]. In addition, over time, the proportion of patients with type 2 AIT has increased, while that of patients developing type 1 AIT has not changed [4]. The practical consequence of this is that, currently, endocrinologists will meet mainly with amiodarone-induced destructive thyroiditis.

Predictors of amiodarone-induced thyrotoxicosis

While pre-existing autoimmune thyroiditis is a risk factor for hypothyroidism development during amiodarone therapy, nodular goitre with unrecognized functional autonomy or latent Graves' disease are risk conditions for

hyperthyroidism, which may be unveiled by iodine load due to amiodarone therapy. However, the majority of patients developing AIT have apparent normal thyroid glands, without nodules, humoral signs of autoimmunity or functional autonomy (type 2 AIT). Currently, in those subjects, identification of factors predicting AIT development is lacking.

Monitoring thyroid function during amiodarone therapy

Most patients develop AIT at unpredictable times during amiodarone therapy. In addition, thyrotoxicosis may develop months after amiodarone withdrawal. The practical consequence is that hormonal surveillance is warranted in these patients. A general approach may be drawn from the various proposed guidelines [3]: baseline evaluation, including free thyroxine (FT)4, FT3, TSH, antithyroglobulin (Ab-Tg), antithyroid peroxidase (Ab-TPO) antibodies and thyroid echography; and a follow-up assessment every 6 months measuring serum TSH (minimal evaluation) and FT4 and FT3 (complete evaluation). Measurement of antithyroid antibody is not recommended during follow-up because amiodarone therapy is not associated with development of thyroid autoimmunity.

During amiodarone therapy, the changes in thyroid function tests that may occur do not reflect thyroid abnormalities. In addition, undetectable serum TSH, suggesting subclinical thyrotoxicosis, spontaneously reverts in about half of the patients without the need for any therapy.

Pathogenesis of amiodarone-induced thyrotoxicosis

It has been recognized that amiodarone-induced thyrotoxicosis may occur in patients with underlying (often unrecognized) thyroid functional abnormalities (type 1) or in patients with normal thyroid glands (type 2). Type 1 AIT is a true form of hyperthyroidism due to iodine load (Jod–Basedow) released by amiodarone metabolism, whereas type 2 AIT is a destructive thyroiditis due to cytotoxic effects of amiodarone and DEA on follicular cells. Evidence to support this view is reported in Table 20.2.

Table 20.2 Clinical and biochemical findings of AIT types.

	Type 1	Type 2
T4/T3 ratio	Usually <4	Usually >4
ECD pattern	Increased vascularity	Normal
Thyroidal RAIU	Normal to increased	Low to suppressed
Underlying functional autonomy	Present	Absent
Spontaneous remission	No	Possible
Thionamides and KClO4	Effective	Ineffective
Glucocorticoids	Ineffective	Effective
Late hypothyroidism	–	Possible

ECD, echo colour Doppler; RAIU, radioiodine uptake.

Patients with type 1 AIT present typical features of increased thyroid hormone synthesis (a true form of hyperthyroidism): underlying thyroid disease, positive thyroid antibody (in some patients), positive TSH-receptor antibodies (TRAb) (in patients with Graves' disease), increased thyroid vascularization on colour flow Doppler sonography, normal to increased thyroidal radioactive uptake in spite of iodine load. In contrast, findings in patients with type 2 AIT are those of thyrotoxicosis without evidence of increased glandular production: absent thyroid disease, absent thyroid autoimmunity, low to suppressed thyroidal radioiodine uptake (RAIU), no increase in thyroid vascularization on colour flow Doppler sonography [1].

The fact that amiodarone and its metabolites increase apoptosis and induce cytotoxic effects on thyroid follicular cells suggests that these features may occur even in patients with underlying thyroid diseases, leading to the concept that destructive phenomena may superimpose on thyroid hormone overproduction, featuring the so-called mixed (or undefined) forms of AIT. However, so far, features of mixed forms of AIT from a clinical and biochemical perspective are still unclear. In contrast, consensus exists on the differentiation of the two main forms of AIT, which has practical consequences in terms of therapeutic options.

Clinical features of amiodarone-induced thyrotoxicosis

Overall clinical features of AIT patients are indistinguishable from those of patients with spontaneous hyperthyroidism or other forms of thyrotoxicosis. However, some special aspects should be considered.

Thyrotoxicosis may occur in older patients and apathetic hyperthyroidism may develop with atypical signs and symptoms: reduced appetite, absence of distal tremors, depression. Thyrotoxicosis may worsen underlying cardiac disease so particular attention is required when arrhythmias are no longer well controlled in older patients taking amiodarone.

Thyrotoxicosis may increase the degradation rate of vitamin-K dependent cogaulation factors so patients with atrial fibrillation on anticoagulants and amiodarone therapy with unexplained increased sensitivity to warfarin should lead physician to suspect thyrotoxicosis.

Differentiation of the two main forms of AIT is crucial, although challenging, because therapeutic options and outcome differ greatly. Currently, combination of several methods is often required to accurately differentiate type 1 and type 2 AIT, because a single method seems not sufficiently sensitive. Identification of type 1 or type 2 AIT relies on the demonstration of increased synthesis of thyroid hormone or increased leakage of thyroid hormone from a damaged gland, respectively. Increased (>4) serum T4/T3 ratio concentrations are a feature of destructive thyroiditis although not useful when applied to a single patient to distinguish AIT types. Serum thyroid autoantibodies may be found in patients with type 1 AIT due to Graves' disease [4]; however, 8% of patients with type 2 AIT may also have positive thyroid autoantibodies, owing to underlying Hashimoto's thyroiditis. The practical consequence is that a positive Ab test does not necessarily suport a type 1 AIT diagnosis, as has been suggested [5].

Thyroidal radioiodine uptake values have been reported to be low, normal or elevated in patients with AIT. However, when AIT patients were stratified according to AIT type, most patients with type 1 AIT had normal to increased RAIU values and those with type 2

	AIT type	Notes
Medical treatment		
Glucocorticoids	AIT 2	Gold standard in AIT 2
Thionamides ± potassium perchlorate	AIT 1	Gold standard in AIT 1
Iopanoic acid	AIT 2	Longer time to achieve euthyroidism Risk of recurrence
Definitive treatment		
^{131}I after rhTSH	AIT 1	Limited experience Risk of exacerbating hyperthyroidism
^{131}I after stopping amiodarone	AIT 1	–
Total thyroidectomy	AIT 1/2	Unresponsiveness to medical treatment Long predicted cure time Unstable cardiac function

Table 20.3 Different therapies proposed for AIT patients.

rhTSH, recombinant human thyroid-stimulating hormone.

AIT had low-undetectable values. Discrepancies in RAIU values in AIT patients may be due to selection of patients and other factors, including environmental iodine supply.

Silent areas of functional autonomy are not uncommon within a nodular goitre, particularly if long lasting, which may be unveiled by iodine load. However, conventional echography does not provide functional information and the presence of goitre or nodules does not necessarily mean that increased thyroid hormone synthesis is the underlying mechanism of AIT (i.e. type 1).

Colour Doppler reveals increased thyroid vascularity in most type 1 AIT patients whereas absent hypervascularity in spite of high serum thyroid hormone concentrations is almost invariably associated with type 2 AIT. Pattern 0 (i.e. normal vascularization) is shared by normal subjects, euthyroid patients under amiodarone therapy and patients with thyrotoxicosis of different origin (subacute thyroiditis, thyrotoxicosis factitia, type 2 AIT). Hence, thyroidal pattern on colour Doppler is a useful tool for differentiating forms of AIT when related to serum thyroid hormone concentrations.

The uptake of radionuclide on ^{99m}Tc-sestamibi scan was maintained in most patients classified as type 1 AIT and absent in those with type 2 AIT. Patients with persistent uptake or rapid washout were considered as having mixed forms. This diagnostic method looks promising although the limited experience and lack of a precise definition of mixed forms of AIT mean it is not currently useful for differentiating AIT types.

Thus, currently, the combination of several methods is necessary for appropriate classification of AIT type.

Therapeutic approach

Management of AIT patients is challenging, as confirmed by the results of recent surveys conducted among expert thyroidologists from Europe, North America and Latin America. Based on different pathogenic mechanisms, type 1 and type 2 AIT should be managed using different drug regimens. Classically, medical therapy of type 1 AIT is devoted to controlling increased thyroid hormone synthesis, using a combination of thionamides and, when feasible, potassium perchlorate. In contrast, the primary goal of medical therapy for type 2 AIT is to restore functional properties of damaged follicular cells using glucocorticoids.

However, type 1 AIT patients have underlying thyroid diseases, requiring a definitive therapy, while time to restore euthyroidism in some type 2 AIT patients may be exceptionally long. In both situations medical therapy might be replaced by total thyroidectomy or radioiodine therapy.

Management of AIT patient warrants strict co-operation between cardiologist and endocrinologist; in fact, AIT therapy cannot be considered apart from cardiac function, requirement of amiodarone continuation and differentiation of AIT types.

Several therapies have been proposed for AIT patients, as summarized in Table 20.3.

Patients with type 1 or 2 amiodarone-induced thyrotoxicosis who do not require amiodarone

A proportion of patients with type 2 AIT have transient thyrotoxicosis, which is self-limiting in nature, not requiring any specific treatment. Those with true thyrotoxicosis, after amiodarone withdrawal, should be treated with glucocorticoids [6]. Medical therapies in type 2 AIT are aimed at controlling effects of thyroid hormone excess (for example, reducing β-adrenergic effect, or peripheral T4 to T3 conversion) and restoring follicle integrity. Glucocorticoids are preferable to iopanoic acid. In fact, in a prospective study, it has been shown that restoration of euthyroidism occurred more rapidly with prednisone (43 ± 34 days) than with iopanoic acid (221 ± 111 days), in keeping with the effect of the two drugs on the damaged follicles or on peripheral thyroid hormone metabolism, respectively. Thionamides have no place in the medical management of type 2 AIT patients owing to their underlying pathogenic mechanism and to the results of many clinical studies, in keeping with previous reports. Baseline thyroid hormone concentrations and thyroid volume may be useful tools for predicting response time to glucocorticoids in patients with type 2 AIT. In one study, most type 2 AIT (83%) patients had stable restoration of euthyroidism after glucocorticoid therapy, whereas the remaining 17% developed permanent hypothyroidism [7]. Thus, follow-up of type 2 AIT patients after euthyroidism restoration should look for hypothyroidism.

Patients with type 1 AIT have some degree of functional autonomy unveiled by iodine load; the medical therapy of choice is thionamides associated, when feasible, with potassium perchlorate; doses of thionamides are usually greater (starting dose, 40–60 mg metimazole) than those required for spontaneous hyperthyroidism owing to the relative resistance of iodine-embedded thyroid glands. After restoration of euthyroidism, therapy of the underlying autonomous thyroid disease (nodular goitre or Graves' disease) should be considered. Options do not differ from those of patients with spontaneous hyperthyroidism, i.e. radioiodine therapy or thyroidectomy. However, owing to the long-lasting iodine load, appropriate radioiodine uptake is usually achieved several months after euthyroidism restoration. Recently, four patients with type 2 AIT and low RAIU values (<4%) treated with high RAI doses (29–80 mCi) became hypothyroid or euthyroid.

Patients with type 1 or type 2 amiodarone-induced thyrotoxicosis requiring amiodarone therapy

A single retrospective study concluded that AIT patients achieved euthyroidism independently of amiodarone

withdrawal or type AIT differentiation [8]. However, the study was retrospective and comparison of treatment encompassed groups of few patients, questioning the real significance of that observation. A very recent study [9] showed that continuation of amiodarone therapy is feasible in type 2 AIT patients treated with glucocorticoids but restoration of euthyroidism is delayed, owing to increased frequency of thyrotoxicosis recurrence. It has been reported that two patients with type 1 AIT and low RAIU values were successfully treated with radioiodine therapy after stimulation of iodine thyroidal uptake with recombinant human TSH; however, owing to the very limited experience in this subset of patients and to the exacerbation of hyperthyroidism worsening the underlying cardiac disease in reported cases, this option should be cautiously considered. Usually, AIT patients requiring amiodarone continuation have life-threatening arrhythmias; cardiac function in these patients may be rapidly worsened by thyroid hormone excess so restoration of euthyroidism should be achieved as soon as possible. AIT itself contributes to cardiac adverse effects as shown by a retrospective study [10]. In fact, AIT patients present higher rate ventricular arrhythmias (32%) compared to euthyroid patients (11%). A predictor of fatal events in AIT patients was low ejection fraction values [11].

Amiodarone-induced thyrotoxicosis patients who are candidates for total thyroidectomy

From a general point of view, AIT patients who have unstable cardiac function, which can be precipitated by thyroid hormone excess, those with extremely long predicted cure time and those who do not respond to or have thyrotoxicosis recurrence under medical therapy should be considered for total thyroidectomy [12,13]. Patients with type 2 AIT can be evaluated for the estimated cure time using a simple algorithm, bearing in mind serum thyroid hormone concentrations and the estimated thyroid volume corrected by body surface area [7]; those predicted to reach euthyroidism quickly (for example, in less than 30 days) are eligible for a short course of glucocorticoids [6]. Patients with delayed response to glucocorticoids and unstable cardiac function and those with type 1 AIT in whom radioiodine therapy is not suitable should be offered total thyroidectomy.

Studies have shown that total thyroidectomy can be easily performed in AIT patients without serious

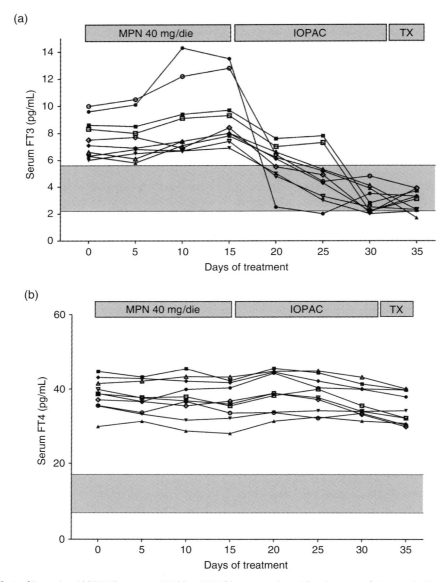

Figure 20.2 Effects of iopanoic acid (IOPAC) on serum FT3 (a) and FT4 (b) concentrations. All patients were first treated with methylprednisolone 40 mg/day. Grey area = normal range. MPN, methylprednisone; Tx, total thyroidectomy.

complications; we have extensively used iopanoic acid for 7–21 days before surgery for a rapid normalization of serum T3 concentrations (Figure 20.2). Our initial study encompassed seven AIT patients prepared with iopanoic acid and submitted to total thyroidectomy; no patients had increased bleeding, recurrent nerve injury or hypoparathyroidism, and cardiac function did not

worsen [14]. Currently, more than 20 AIT patients have undergone total thyroidectomy following the same protocol without complications (personal communication). In a pilot study, eight AIT patients with dilated cardiomyopathy or unstable rhythm disorders, after preparation with iopanoic acid, were submitted to minimally invasive total thyroidectomy under local anaesthesia without complications [15]. Whether minimally invasive total thyroidectomy under local anaesthesia is superior to a more traditional approach is still unclear.

A collaborative team of experienced endocrinologist, surgeon and anaesthetist is necessary. We believe that restoration of euthyroidism with iopanoic acid before operation and careful management of clinical conditions of AIT patients will significantly reduce the reported surgical risk [14].

Thyroid storm

Thyroid storm or thyrotoxic crisis is the extreme manifestation of hyperthyroidism/thyrotoxicosis. The boundary between severe hyperthyroidism and thyroid storm is not sharp and therefore controversial; however, prompt recognition and treatment of thyroid storm are crucial to prevent the high mortality rate associated with this disorder, which may range from 20% to 30%. Thyroid storm develops in patients with untreated or undertreated hyperthyroidism (usually Graves' disease) in whom precipitating events trigger thyroid crisis. Multisystem therapy is aimed at blocking thyroid hormone synthesis and output from the gland, blocking the peripheral effects (mainly at the heart level) of thyroid hormone excess and supporting vital functions, and should be started vigorously and without any delay.

Aetiology
The most common cause of thyroid storm is Graves' disease but toxic adenoma or toxic multinodular goitre may be other causes. Thyroid storm has also been reported in patients with rare causes of hyperthyroidism (functional metastases from differentiated follicular thyroid carcinoma, struma ovarii, TSH-secreting pituitary adenoma) and thyrotoxicosis, including thyrotoxicosis factitia, neck irradiation, cytotoxic chemotherapy, neck injury, and during other medical therapies (interferon-α, interleukin-2, amiodarone). Thyroid storm may also be triggered by several insults including trauma, myocardial infarction, diabetic ketoacidosis, infections and surgery, and sometimes toxaemia of pregnancy and parturition.

Before medical control of hyperthyroidism was introduced, surgery was the main cause of thyroid storm but appropriate preoperative preparation with iodine, thionamides and β-adrenergic receptor blockade with pro-

pranolol has dramatically reduced surgical mortality [16]. Currently, severe infections are thought to be the most common cause triggering thyroid storm.

Clinical presentation and diagnosis
Thyroid storm has an abrupt onset, triggered by a precipitating factor in an untreated thyrotoxic patient. The clinical picture is dominated by extreme symptoms of hypermetabolism, including tremors and restlessness, marked tachycardia, profuse sweating and sometimes congestive heart failure and pulmonary oedema. Fever, often extreme, is invariably present and associated with nausea, vomiting and abdominal pain. Thyrotoxic crisis may progress to apathy, stupor and coma with hypotension and multiorgan failure; such a condition, if unrecognized, is fatal.

Serum thyroid hormone concentrations did not differ in patients with thyroid storm and in those with severe thyrotoxicosis and differentiation is based mostly on clinical judgement in an untreated hyperthyroid patient with systemic illness.

Management of thyroid storm
Management of thyroid storm is based on multidrug therapy with the following goals:
• immediate cessation of thyroid hormone release from the thyroid gland
• blocking further thyroid hormone synthesis
• preventing peripheral T4 to T3 conversion
• controlling adrenergic effects
• supporting vital functions.
Iodine is the only effective drug blocking release of thyroid hormone from the gland; in most patients iodine administration may be delayed until after thionamides have been given. In such a sequence (thionamides and then iodine), a further iodine-induced increased thyroid hormone synthesis is avoided but the time delay may be harmful for the patient and some authors prefer to start iodine without any delay.

Both methimazole (80–100 mg/day) and propylthiouracil (800–1200 mg/day) are effective; propylthiouracil has the advantage of blocking peripheral T4 to T3 conversion, whereas methimazole, having a longer half-life, could administered in one or two daily doses. Both drugs may be administered rectally.

Iodine can be administered as Lugol's solution (4–8 drops every 6–8 h) or saturation solution of potassium iodide (5 drops every 6 h). Another effective source of iodine is iodinated contrast media such as iopanoic acid (1 g every 8 h for the first 24 h and then 500 mg twice daily); unfortunately, iopanoic acid is no longer available on the market.

The reduced vascular resistance due to thyroid hormone excess may lead to changes in blood supply to the heart and peripheral organs. β-Blockers are of crucial importance for controlling the adrenergic effects of thyrotoxicosis; propranolol (60–80 mg every 4 h) is central to the management of thyrotoxic crisis.

The role of glucocorticoids in the management of thyroid storm is controversial [17]; high-dose glucocorticoids (for example, hydrocortisone 100 mg intravenously every 8 h) may reduce peripheral T4 to T3 generation in addition to supportive effects.

Additional strategies, including the use of lithium carbonate, colestyramine, potassium perchlorate, reserpine and even plasmapheresis, may be used when standard protocols fail to control thyrotoxic crisis.

Supportive care, including antipyretics (acetaminophen preferred to salicylates), physical heat dispersion and hydration, is invariably necessary as well as treatment of precipitating factors.

References

1 Martino E, Bartalena L, Bogazzi F, Braverman LE. The effects of amiodarone on the thyroid. Endocr Rev 2001; 22(2): 240–54.

2 Bogazzi F, Bartalena L, Gasperi M, Braverman LE, Martino E. The various effects of amiodarone on thyroid function. Thyroid 2001; 11(5): 511–19.

3 Eskes SA, Wiersinga WM. Amiodarone and thyroid. Best Pract Res Clin Endocrinol Metab 2009; 23(6): 735–51.

4 Bogazzi F, Bartalena L, Dell'Unto E, et al. Proportion of type 1 and type 2 amiodarone-induced thyrotoxicosis has changed over a 27-year period in Italy. Clin Endocrinol (Oxf) 2007; 67(4): 533–7.

5 Franklyn JA, Gammage MD. Treatment of amiodarone-associated thyrotoxicosis. Nature Clin Pract Endocrinol Metab 2007; 3: 662–6.

6 Bogazzi F, Tomisti L, Rossi G, et al. Glucocorticoids are preferable to thionamides as first-line treatment for amiodarone-induced thyrotoxicosis due to destructive thyroiditis: a matched retrospective cohort study. J Clin Endocrinol Metab 2009; 94(10): 3757–62.

7 Bogazzi F, Bartalena L, Tomisti L, et al. Glucocorticoid response in amiodarone-induced thyrotoxicosis resulting from destructive thyroiditis is predicted by thyroid volume and serum free thyroid hormone concentrations. J Clin Endocrinol Metab 2007; 92(2): 556–62.

8 Osman F, Franklyn JA, Sheppard MC, Gammage MD. Successful treatment of amiodarone-induced thyrotoxicosis. Circulation 2002; 105(11): 1275–7.

9 Bogazzi F, Bartalena L, Tomisti L, Rossi G, Brogioni S, Martino E. Continuation of amiodarone delays restoration of euthyroidism in patients with type 2 amiodarone-induced thyrotoxicosis treated with prednisone: a pilot study. J Clin Endocrinol Metab 2011; 96(11): 3374–80.

10 Yiu KH, Jim MH, Siu CW, et al. Amiodarone-induced thyrotoxicosis is a predictor of adverse cardiovascular outcome. J Clin Endocrinol Metab 2009; 94(1): 109–14.

11 Conen D, Melly L, Kaufmann C, et al. Amiodarone-induced thyrotoxicosis: clinical course and predictors of outcome. J Am Coll Cardiol 2007; 49(24): 2350–5.

12 Farwell AP, Abend SL, Huang SK, Patwardhan NA, Braverman LE. Thyroidectomy for amiodarone-induced thyrotoxicosis. JAMA 1990; 263(11): 1526–8.

13 Franzese CB, Fan CY, Stack BC Jr. Surgical management of amiodarone-induced thyrotoxicosis. Otolaryngol Head Neck Surg 2003; 129(5): 565–70.

14 Bogazzi F, Miccoli P, Berti P, et al. Preparation with iopanoic acid rapidly controls thyrotoxicosis in patients with amiodarone-induced thyrotoxicosis before thyroidectomy. Surgery 2002; 132(6): 1114–17; discussion 1118.

15 Berti P, Materazzi G, Bogazzi F, Ambrosini CE, Martino E, Miccoli P. Combination of minimally invasive thyroid surgery and local anesthesia associated to iopanoic acid for patients with amiodarone-induced thyrotoxicosis and severe cardiac disorders: a pilot study. Langenbecks Arch Surg 2007; 392(6): 709–13.

16 Langley RW, Burch HB. Perioperative management of the thyrotoxic patient. Endocrinol Metab Clin North Am 2003; 32(2): 519–34.

17 Nayak B, Burman K. Thyrotoxicosis and thyroid storm. Endocrinol Metab Clin North Am 2006; 35(4): 663–86, vii.

PART V

Postoperative Complications Requiring Urgent Treatment

CHAPTER 21

Respiratory Failure Following Extubation

Moran Amit and Dan M. Fliss

Department of Otolaryngology, Head and Neck Surgery, and Maxillofacial Surgery,
Tel Aviv Sourasky Medical Centre, Tel Aviv, Israel

Introduction

Extubation failure is defined as the need for reinstitution of ventilatory support within 72 h of planned endotracheal tube removal. It occurs in 2–25% of all extubated patients [1]. The pathophysiological causes of extubation failure include an imbalance between respiratory muscle capacity and work of breathing, airway obstruction, neuromuscular diseases, and cardiac dysfunction. The aetiology can be either obstructive or respiratory. Obstruction is much more common and usually secondary to another complication, such as tracheomalacia, neck haematoma or bilateral vocal cord paralysis. A respiratory cause is usually the result of systemic diseases, such as myasthenia, that create respiratory muscle load and capacity imbalance. Specifically, respiratory failure is the inability of the respiratory system to oxygenate blood or eliminate carbon dioxide. In practice, it is defined as a PaO_2 value of <60 mmHg while breathing air, or a $PaCO_2$ of >50 mmHg.

The reported incidence of extubation failure after thyroidectomy is influenced by several factors, among them the institutional policy for tracheostomy in cases of questionable vocal cord integrity, hospital surgical load, expertise of staff and availability of specialized procedures, such as fibreoptic bronchoscopy, sternotomy, and postoperative mechanical ventilation [2,3]. Post-thyroidectomy respiratory failure (PTRF) is a continuation of extubation failure that usually develops within minutes to hours after thyroid surgery and is characterized by rapid deterioration. It is considered a relatively uncommon but devastating complication.

Patients who require reintubation have a higher incidence of hospital mortality, increased length of intensive care unit and hospital stay, prolonged duration of mechanical ventilation, higher hospital costs, and an increased need for tracheostomy [4]. Given the lack of established treatments for extubation failure, clinicians must be aware of the factors that predict its occurrence since a more rapid reinstitution of ventilatory support in patients who fail extubation may improve outcome. It must be borne in mind that extubation failure does not usually occur in isolation and that it is usually secondary to another, more obvious and even anticipated complication that might require the surgeon's immediate concentration and lead to delay in diagnosis. The rarity of PTRF together with its associated fatality require a high index of suspicion and intensive follow-up of patients with a possible cause for developing it.

In the following chapter we will discuss different aetiologies, preoperative risk assessment, suitable preparation and anaesthetic approach for prevention of its occurrence, and the early diagnosis and management of PTRF.

Thyroid Surgery: Preventing and Managing Complications, First Edition. Edited by Paolo Miccoli, David J. Terris,
Michele N. Minuto and Melanie W. Seybt.
© 2013 John Wiley & Sons, Ltd. Published 2013 by John Wiley & Sons, Ltd.

Aetiology

Tracheomalacia

Tracheomalacia is an extreme degree of compression of the airway, where the cross-sectional area of the trachea is reduced to less than half [5]. It results from long-standing compression by a large goitre wherein rings of the trachea may be completely damaged or considerably weakened, resulting in poor support to the trachea.

The unsupported trachea is prone to collapse after a thyroidectomy, leading to postoperative respiratory obstruction. Some authors doubt its existence, and a number of large series failed to document any clear-cut case of tracheomalacia caused by a benign goitre [6], while others have reported the incidence of tracheomalacia as being between 0.001% and 1.5% [7]. The predominant clinical feature of this condition is a progressive hypoxaemia not responding to increasing fractionated inspired oxygen concentration (FiO_2). Stridor becomes evident only when the tracheal diameter is reduced to less than 3 mm and signals critical functional obstruction [8].

There is no single criterion for confirming a diagnosis of tracheomalacia before extubation. Intraoperative diagnosis of tracheomalacia relies on the following criteria.
• A floppy trachea on palpation after gradual withdrawal of the tube for a short distance. This manoeuvre may help the surgeon in spotting the collapse of the tracheal wall.
• Obstruction of spontaneous respiration and difficulty in negotiating the suction catheter beyond the endotracheal tube (ETT) during gradual withdrawal of the ETT.
• Absence of leak on deflation of the ETT cuff, the disappearance of the volume pressure loop on the ventilator, or the appearance of respiratory stridor along with falling haemoglobin oxygen saturation (SpO_2) on pulse oximetry despite administration of increasing FiO_2 after closure of the wound.
It is also important to rule out bilateral vocal cord paralysis or glottic/subglottic oedema as a possible more common cause of stridor.

When tracheomalacia is diagnosed and other aetiologies for hypoxaemia have been ruled out, the treatment of choice is an early tracheostomy at the time of surgery, carefully choosing the most suitable tracheostomy site. Early tracheostomy also facilitates postoperative tracheal care, e.g. suctioning, and ventilatory care, if needed. Moreover, tracheostomy has been proposed to result in fibrosis around the impaired trachea, resulting in early recovery from tracheomalacia. The rates of occurrence of tracheal stenosis following tracheostomy for tracheomalacia are inconsistent and considered to be low [7], with the tracheostomy tube being removed within 10 days in most patients. Importantly, bilateral vocal cord paresis must be ruled out as a possible aetiology for obstruction before tube removal.

Other management options for tracheomalacia include prolonged intubation, trachelopexy, external splinting with Marlex mesh, and external miniplate fixation of tracheal cartilages and placement of a buttress or graft. Short-term intubation (for 48 h postoperatively) has been suggested but it is unclear how short-term intubation would convert a long-standing structurally deprived trachea that has turned significantly floppy by chronic goitre compression into an intact one [9].

Compressive haematoma

The reported incidence of compressive haematomas after thyroidectomy is about 1% [10]. This potentially life-threatening complication is unpredictable [11]. Factors such as age, pathology, type of procedure and extent of thyroidectomy, compressive symptoms and anticoagulant medications do not influence its occurrence. The majority of cases present within 6 h of the initial procedure, and almost all cases within the first 24 h [12] although late presentation of neck haematoma (beyond the first 24 h following thyroidectomy) is possible, especially in patients who are being anticoagulated. Superficial haematoma may frequently cause ecchymosis and usually does not cause respiratory distress. It has been suggested that in cases of superficial bleeding, the strap muscles work as a barrier between the haematoma and the trachea or the venous and lymphatic drainage system of the larynx and pharynx [13]. Deep haematoma from a major vessel like cricothyroid artery and the superior thyroid arteries might result in respiratory distress due to laryngeal oedema secondary to impairment of the venous return from the larynx caused by the haematoma.

There are numerous contributory factors for haematoma formation including slipping of a ligature on a major vessel, reopening of cauterized veins, retching during recovery, Valsalva manoeuvres during reversal of anaesthesia, increased blood pressure in the immediate postoperative period, and oozing from the cut edge of the thyroid gland in partial thyroidectomies. Coughing or vomiting after removal of the endotracheal tube increases venous pressure, which causes insignificant vessels that were not ligated to bleed profusely, and smooth emergence by the anaesthesiologist in such cases is crucial. Extensive dissection increases the risk of this complication [14]. Patients with Graves' disease are at risk for bleeding due to increased vascularity of the thyroid parenchyma, and it is suggested to treat them with Lugol solution or a saturated solution of potassium iodide for 10 days prior to surgery in order to reduce the vascularity of the thyroid gland [15]. Routine use of drains or pressure dressing has not been shown to significantly reduce the rate of re-peration or incidence of respiratory distress [16].

The keys to management of a postoperative neck haematoma include early detection, close observation, airway management and appropriate surgical intervention. Patients with post-thyroidectomy haematoma may present with respiratory distress, pain or a pressure sensation in the neck, or dysphagia. The signs include progressive neck swelling, suture line bleeding, dyspnoea or stridor and a significant amount of drain losses. As early recognition with immediate intervention is the key to managing this complication, the medical staff should be thoroughly aware of these signs and symptoms. Immediate intubation should be performed in the case of respiratory distress from airway obstruction. Emergency treatment requires immediate removal of surgical clips or sutures, evacuation of haematoma and establishment of an airway by reintubation. Decompression of the wound is the key factor for providing relief from hypoxia and the resulting cardiovascular instability. A conservative approach may be considered in selected patients with minimal haematoma and no progression.

Recurrent laryngeal nerve paresis/ paralysis

Recurrent laryngeal nerve palsy bears the most serious consequenses in thyroid surgery. While unilateral palsy or paresis might result in significant impairment of the quality of life, bilateral palsy might be lethal. The incidence of RLNP varies from 0% to 4% and has been related to the extent of thyroidectomy, the presence of Graves' disease, thyroid carcinoma and the need for reoperation [17]. Most cases of RLNP are transient and the occurrence of permanent RLNP is in less than 1% of cases. Routine visual nerve identification and preservation have been shown to significantly reduce RLNP rates [18].

Extensive resections, preoperative diagnosis of thyroid malignancy and recurrent goitre were identified as significant independent risk factors for RLNP [19].

Causes of nerve palsy include damage to the nerve's anatomical integrity; thermal lesions; excessive nerve skeletization; axon damage caused by excessive strain, oedema, haematoma and difficult tracheal intubation; and neuritis caused by scar tissue and viral neuritis. Unusual causes such as neuromuscular diseases, cerebrovascular accidents, diabetics with RLN neuropathy, and viral aetiology in cases of idiopathic vocal fold paralysis might lead to preoperative RLN paresis. In such cases meticulous preoperative assessment of vocal cord mobility must be done.

Clinically, unilateral RLN injury presents as dysphonia. While in bilateral vocal fold paralysis voice quality is typically good, airway patency is jeopardized by the paramedian position of the vocal folds. Vocal cord paralysis is present preoperatively in 2–4% of cases. Since symptomatic assessment of voice does not correlate with objective findings in goitre patients [20], preoperative laryngoscopy is recommended for all patients who undergo thyroid surgery [21]. Another entity that might mimic RLN injury is arytenoid dislocation or subluxation. Although rare, it happens usually after upper airway instrumentation and presents in a similar way. Clinical presentation usually includes hoarseness, breathy voice quality, vocal fatigue up to aphonia. Dysphagia, odynophagia, sore throat and cough are less common. A thorough laryngeal examination should be performed using a laryngeal mirror, flexible fibreoptic laryngoscope or rigid telescope. Reduced vocal fold mobility and arytenoid oedema with loss of arytenoid symmetry are physical signs that suggest acute AS. Poor glottic closure, posterior glottic chink and malalignment of the true vocal folds are often noted.

Bilateral RLN might lead to respiratory failure or negative pressure pulmonary oedema, discussed next, and a tracheotomy may be required acutely, followed by surgery to improve the size of the glottic airway. RLN injury is discussed in detail in Chapter 13.

Negative pressure pulmonary oedema

Negative pressure pulmonary oedema is a rare diagnostic entity [22]. There are two types of negative pressure pulmonary oedema. Type 1 follows a sudden upper airway obstruction, such as in the case of tracheomalacia or bilateral vocal cord paralysis, while type 2 develops after surgical relief of chronic upper airway obstruction attributable, for example, to a large compressive goitre. The pathophysiology of negative pressure pulmonary oedema is incompletely understood and is likely to be multifactorial. In type 1, upper airway obstruction initially leads to the generation of markedly negative intrathoracic pressures. Intrathoracic pressure normally varies during inspiration between $-2\,cm$ and $-12\,cmH_2O$, and it falls to as low as $-50\,cmH_2O$ when there is airway obstruction [22]. The excess pressure generated in response to obstruction produces mechanical stress and direct capillary injury, increasing permeability and leakage into the interstitium [23]. Movement of fluid into the interstitium is promoted by falling intrapleural pressures and impaired pulmonary capillary integrity, leading to pulmonary oedema. The onset of symptomatic negative pressure pulmonary oedema following upper airway obstruction ranges from 3 to 150 min [24]. Type 2 is associated with the loss of long-standing auto-positive end-expiratory pressure (PEEP) due to obstruction by the lesion. It has been suggested that unresolved altered permeability and pre-existing occult interstitial fluid result in interstitial fluid transduction and pulmonary oedema upon the sudden loss of PEEP.

Suspicion should be raised clinically by any patient presenting with radiographic evidence of pulmonary oedema together with respiratory distress associated with stridor, hypoxaemia or hypercapnia. The diagnosis of negative pressure pulmonary oedema requires this high index of suspicion since the patient's age, symptoms, electrocardiogram and chest X-ray are most suggestive of cardiogenic pulmonary oedema in the majority of cases. Typically, negative pressure pulmonary oedema is self-limited, with clinical and radiographic improvement within 12–48 h. Delayed recognition and treatment are associated with longer recovery times [24].

Once identified, the initial treatment of negative pressure pulmonary oedema is relief of the airway obstruction. Most cases resolve with a short-acting muscle relaxant, such as succinylcholine, and reintubation but surgical tracheostomy is sometimes unavoidable [25]. Type 2 cases that developed after resection of a giant goitre and the release of tracheal stenosis have been described. Although many patients with negative pressure pulmonary oedema have a good prognosis and improvement is seen within 36 h, some patients require

prolonged continuous positive airway pressure (cPAP) or 3-day PEEP mechanical ventilation [26]. Non-invasive positive pressure ventilation is a method that triggers the beginning of inspiration and assists respiration under bi-level PAP using a nasal device or a sealed facemask. It secures the airway by expiratory PAP (ePAP). Non-invasive positive pressure ventilation in place of intubation and mechanical ventilation shortens the length of hospitalization in the intensive care unit and reduces the risk for hospital-acquired, ventilation-associated pneumonia that increases the mortality rate in patients with acute respiratory distress syndrome (ARDS). At present, non-invasive positive pressure ventilation is often used in patients with early-stage ARDS whose background disease may be improved by this intervention. It is thought that preoperative induction of non-invasive positive pressure ventilation in patients with chronic upper airway stenosis may contribute to a reduction in the incidence of postoperative pulmonary oedema.

Respiratory insufficiency

A respiratory aetiology is less common than an obstructive one and usually occurs in patients with either diagnosed or undiagnosed neurological disease, such as multiple sclerosis, amyotrophic lateral sclerosis, syringomyelia, myasthenia gravis (MG), Guillain–Barré and Parkinson disease, undergoing thyroid surgery. These pathologies create respiratory muscle load and capacity imbalance, that might be aggravated by obstructive goitre, bilateral RLN palsy or tracheomalacia, leading to respiratory failure.

Epidemiological studies have shown that although autoimmune thyroid diseases occur in 5–10% of patients with MG, it is relatively uncommon in patients with autoimmune thyroid disease [27]. Myasthenic crisis may be the presenting manifestation of MG. Most cases of crisis are provoked by infection, surgery, stress and certain drugs. Notably, the onset of crisis may be preceded by several days of respiratory difficulty. Sputum retention has been identified as a contributory factor. Unilateral vocal cord palsy increases respiratory muscle work and leads to exertion which, in turn, induces the attack of crisis. However, surgical stress itself may precipitate a crisis, while no predisposing factor can be found in some patients. When a crisis does occur, there should be a low threshold for endotracheal intubation and ventilatory support because weakness increases with repeated muscle use. Early recognition is of paramount importance, although arriving at the final diagnosis may not be possible until full-blown features of MG have been demonstrated. MG crisis should be included in the differential diagnosis of post-thyroidectomy respiratory failure. Awareness of this combination may help early identification, prompt intervention and, if possible, prevention of an impending crisis.

Preoperative assessment

The surgeon's preoperative assessment of the patient for possible post-thyroidectomy respiratory failure is crucial, in spite of the fact that screening tests are of limited value. An otolaryngologist must perform a thorough laryngeal examination using a flexible fibreoptic laryngoscope, including the presence of oedema, deviation and vocal cord mobility.

Shortness of breath has a low sensitivity for tracheal deviation or compression but substernal extension was highly associated with both entities. The presence of dysphagia, dyspnoea, orthopnoea, hoarseness and a positive Pemberton sign is not predictive for postoperative airway complications, nor is the duration of symptoms, radiological finding of tracheal deviation or extent of thyroid resection [3]. Flow volume loops can detect tracheal stenosis when the tracheal diameter is reduced to 5 mm but they may not be affected in less severely involved airways and do not correlate with goitre size [28]. In contrast, older patients and patients with large tumours (>200 g) were found to be more likely to have postoperative airway complications [3]. Axial computed tomographic scanning assessment of tracheal calibre was found to be sensitive and significantly ($p < 0.0001$) to airway compromise [2].

The preoperative physical exam should also include airway assessment by experienced anaesthesia personnel. It should include jaw and tongue size, the determination of an anteriorly positioned larynx and the available degree of head extension.

Anesthesia considerations

Airway management

Transoral intubation is appropriate in the majority of cases, and awake fibreoptic intubation is a reasonable option if there is any question about the adequacy of a mask ventilation, given the size and location of a goitre. An emergency tracheotomy through the mass is typically not a viable option. Newer video laryngoscopes (GlideScope) are also an excellent adjunct for intubation in such patients. An experienced anaesthesiologist should be notified of the patient's characteristics prior to operation and should be prepared to perform awake fibreoptic intubation if necessary [3]. In the setting of a large, longstanding cervical goitre, the larynx very likely has reduced venous and lymphatic drainage and so it might develop significant and long-lasting oedema if there are multiple traumatic intubation attempts [29]. Other risk factors for glottic or subglottic narrowing include excessive cuff pressure and tracheal infection.

Emergence from anaesthesia

Coughing and vomiting during emergence from general anaesthesia after surgery may lead to a number of potentially dangerous sequelae, including laryngospasm, detrimental haemodynamic changes and increased intraocular and intracranial pressure. Severe coughing may cause post-thyroidectomy bleeding, resulting in acute airway obstruction or the need for reoperation [13]. Intravenous opioids delivered at the end of surgery may enable smooth emergence by reducing coughing, agitation and deleterious haemodynamic changes [30]. However, these agents can also cause depression of ventilation and delay awakening. Deliverance of short-acting opioids (e.g. remifentanil) may be maintained during emergence from anaesthesia due to their rapid onset and offset of action. Their usage during emergence from sevoflurane-remifentanil anaesthesia has been shown to suppress coughing without serious adverse events in patients undergoing elective thyroidectomy [31].

Extubation

Monitoring of respiratory rate, oxygen saturation, blood pressure, heart rate and blood gases and evidence of hypoxaemia or hypercapnia have a sensitivity of only up to 50% for detecting early signs of load–capacity imbalance. Assessment of airway patency before tube removal is complicated, the positive predictive value of the quantitative cuff leak test (i.e. the absence of air leak after deflation of the endotracheal tube balloon) is low, and there is a high rate of false-positive results [32]. In addition, deciding the management of patients with a positive cuff leak test result must take into account that fewer than 50% of patients with postextubation stridor require reintubation, and those that do have reasonably favourable outcomes [33,34].

In summary, the best predictor of extubation success depends on preoperative findings together with respiratory parameters, spontaneous breathing trials at the end of surgery, the presence of an adequate cough, the absence of excessive respiratory secretions and a patent upper airway.

References

1 Rothaar RC, Epstein SK. Extubation failure: magnitude of the problem, impact on outcomes, and prevention. Curr Opin Crit Care 2003; 9(1): 59–66.

2 Shin JJ, Grillo HC, Mathisen D, et al. The surgical management of goiter: Part I. Preoperative evaluation. Laryngoscope; 121(1): 60–7.

3 Shen WT, Kebebew E, Duh QY, Clark OH. Predictors of airway complications after thyroidectomy for substernal goiter. Arch Surg 2004; 139(6): 656–9; discussion 9–60.

4 Rady MY, Ryan T. Perioperative predictors of extubation failure and the effect on clinical outcome after cardiac surgery. Crit Care Med 1999; 27(2): 340–7.

5 Jokinen K, Palva T, Sutinen S, Nuutinen J. Acquired tracheobronchomalacia. Ann Clin Res 1977; 9(2): 52–7.

6 Mackle T, Meaney J, Timon C. Tracheoesophageal compression associated with substernal goitre. Correlation of symptoms with cross-sectional imaging findings. J Laryngol Otol 2007; 121(4): 358–61.

7 Green WE, Shepperd HW, Stevenson HM, Wilson W. Tracheal collapse after thyroidectomy. Br J Surg 1979; 66(8): 554–7.

8 Mohamed SA, Thrush S, Scott-Coombes DM. Acute stridor secondary to recurrent multinodular goitre after previous subtotal thyroidectomy: compartment syndrome of the neck. Eur J Surg 2002; 168(6): 372–3.

9 Agarwal A, Mishra AK, Gupta SK, Arshad F, Tripathi M, Singh PK. High incidence of tracheomalacia in longstanding goiters: experience from an endemic goiter region. World J Surg 2007; 31(4): 832–7.

10 Shaha AR, Jaffe BM. Practical management of post-thyroidectomy hematoma. J Surg Oncol 1994; 57(4): 235–8.

11 Burkey SH, van Heerden JA, Thompson GB, Grant CS, Schleck CD, Farley DR. Reexploration for symptomatic hematomas after cervical exploration. Surgery 2001; 130(6): 914–20.

12 Rosenbaum MA, Haridas M, McHenry CR. Life-threatening neck hematoma complicating thyroid and parathyroid surgery. Am J Surg 2008; 195(3): 339–43; discussion 43.

13 Lee HS, Lee BJ, Kim SW, et al. Patterns of post-thyroidectomy hemorrhage. Clin Exp Otorhinolaryngol 2009; 2(2): 72–7.

14 Prim MP, de Diego JI, Hardisson D, Madero R, Gavilan J. Factors related to nerve injury and hypocalcemia in thyroid gland surgery. Otolaryngol Head Neck Surg 2001; 124(1): 111–14.

15 Mittendorf EA, McHenry CR. Complications and sequelae of thyroidectomy and an analysis of surgeon experience and outcome. Surg Technol Int 2004; 12: 152–7.

16 Samraj K, Gurusamy KS. Wound drains following thyroid surgery. Cochrane Database Syst Rev 2007; 4: CD006099.

17 Ku CF, Lo CY, Chan WF, Kung AW, Lam KS. Total thyroidectomy replaces subtotal thyroidectomy as the preferred surgical treatment for Graves' disease. ANZ J Surg 2005; 75(7): 528–31.

18 Chiang FY, Wang LF, Huang YF, Lee KW, Kuo WR. Recurrent laryngeal nerve palsy after thyroidectomy with routine identification of the recurrent laryngeal nerve. Surgery 2005; 137(3): 342–7.

19 Erbil Y, Barbaros U, Issever H, et al. Predictive factors for recurrent laryngeal nerve palsy and hypoparathyroidism after thyroid surgery. Clin Otolaryngol 2007; 32(1): 32–7.

20 Michel LA. Surgery of substernal goiter. Acta Otorhinolaryngol Belg 1987; 41(5): 863–80.

21 Randolph GW, Kamani D. The importance of preoperative laryngoscopy in patients undergoing thyroidectomy: voice, vocal cord function, and the preoperative detection of invasive thyroid malignancy. Surgery 2006; 139(3): 357–62.

22 Sharma ML, Beckett N, Gormley P. Negative pressure pulmonary edema following thyroidectomy. Can J Anaesth 2002; 49(2): 215.

23 Oswalt CE, Gates GA, Holmstrom MG. Pulmonary edema as a complication of acute airway obstruction. JAMA 1977; 238(17): 1833–5.

24 Van Kooy MA, Gargiulo RF. Postobstructive pulmonary edema. Am Fam Physician 2000; 62(2): 401–4.

25 Koh MS, Hsu AA, Eng P. Negative pressure pulmonary oedema in the medical intensive care unit. Intensive Care Med 2003; 29(9): 1601–4.

26 Ikeda H, Asato R, Chin K, et al. Negative-pressure pulmonary edema after resection of mediastinum thyroid goiter. Acta Otolaryngol 2006; 126(8): 886–8.

27 Cheng SP, Liu SC, Chou CL, Liu HC, Lee JJ. An uncommon cause of postthyroidectomy respiratory failure. Thyroid 2009; 19(10): 1129–30.

28 Miller MR, Pincock AC, Oates GD, Wilkinson R, Skene-Smith H. Upper airway obstruction due to goitre: detection, prevalence and results of surgical management. Q J Med 1990; 74(274): 177–88.

29 Reeve TS, Delbridge L, Brady P, Crummer P, Smyth C. Secondary thyroidectomy: a twenty-year experience. World J Surg 1988; 12(4): 449–53.

30 Mendel P, Fredman B, White PF. Alfentanil suppresses coughing and agitation during emergence from isoflurane anesthesia. J Clin Anesth 1995; 7(2): 114–18.

31 Jun NH, Lee JW, Song JW, Koh JC, Park WS, Shim YH. Optimal effect-site concentration of remifentanil for preventing cough during emergence from sevoflurane-remifentanil anaesthesia. Anaesthesia 2010; 65(9): 930–5.

32 Engoren M. Evaluation of the cuff-leak test in a cardiac surgery population. Chest 1999; 116(4): 1029–31.

33 Epstein SK, Ciubotaru RL. Independent effects of etiology of failure and time to reintubation on outcome for patients failing extubation. Am J Respir Crit Care Med 1998; 158(2): 489–93.

34 Darmon JY, Rauss A, Dreyfuss D, et al. Evaluation of risk factors for laryngeal edema after tracheal extubation in adults and its prevention by dexamethasone. A placebo-controlled, double-blind, multicenter study. Anesthesiology 1992; 77(2): 245–51.

CHAPTER 22

Postoperative Bleeding

Richelle T. Williams and Peter Angelos
Department of Surgery, University of Chicago Medical Center, Chicago, IL, USA

Can the thyroid gland, when in a state of enlargement, be removed with a reasonable hope of saving the patient? Experience emphatically answers, no... If a surgeon should be so adventurous or foolhardy as to undertake the enterprise... every stroke of his knife will be followed by a torrent of blood, and lucky will it be for him if his victim live long enough to enable him to finish his horrid butchery. Should the patient survive...death will be almost certain to overtake him from secondary haemorrhage... No honest and sensible surgeon would ever engage in it.

Samuel D. Gross, 1866[1]

Introduction

Bleeding has been one of the most dreaded complications of thyroid surgery since the first documented procedure in approximately 1000 AD. During the 1800 s, the mortality rate after thyroid surgery was about 40%, with the majority of deaths due to either bleeding or infection. Through meticulous surgical technique, Billroth, Kocher and Halsted (among others) advanced thyroid surgery to the procedure we know today, reducing mortality rates to <1% by the 1930s [2]. Meticulous haemostasis remains one of the essential objectives of thyroid surgery, not only because it prevents potentially life-threatening postoperative haemorrhage but also because it minimizes the risk of complications like laryngeal nerve and parathyroid gland injury. Intraoperative bleeding stains the tissues, which may obscure these important structures and

increase the risk of inadvertent injury. In comparison, postoperative bleeding may lead to an expanding haematoma in the closed paratracheal space, resulting in potentially fatal respiratory compromise.

The reported incidence of bleeding after thyroidectomy varies. Postoperative bleeding has been inconsistently defined, with some authors including all haematomas while others including only those requiring surgical intervention. Depending on the definition utilized, estimates of the incidence of post-thyroidectomy bleeding range from 0.3% to 4.2% [3–11]. In most series, however, the risk of clinically significant haemorrhage after thyroid surgery is 1% or less.

Timing, risk factors and implications

Timing

The length of time after thyroidectomy during which bleeding occurs is quite variable. Most patients (~50–75%) with significant bleeding present within 6–8 h after surgery, but there have been reports describing patients with delayed bleeding occurring days after thyroidectomy [4,5,9]. Overall, approximately 80–97% of patients with bleeding complications present within the first 24 h [3,4, 9,11–13]. As discussed below, this has implications for the practice of outpatient thyroid surgery.

Risk factors

Several studies have attempted to identify factors that increase the risk of postoperative haemorrhage following thyroidectomy, but results so far are conflicting. For any

Thyroid Surgery: Preventing and Managing Complications, First Edition. Edited by Paolo Miccoli, David J. Terris, Michele N. Minuto and Melanie W. Seybt.
© 2013 John Wiley & Sons, Ltd. Published 2013 by John Wiley & Sons, Ltd.

given study showing a significant association between the risk of postoperative bleeding and a certain factor, there are multiple studies that find no relationship. This is likely related to the fact that bleeding is such a rare complication that many of these studies are underpowered to detect statistically significant differences. With that caveat in mind, potential risk factors may be classified into one of two broad categories: patient-related factors or surgery-related factors (Box 22.1). Patient-related risk factors may be further subdivided into demographic factors (age, gender), factors related to co-morbid disease (inherited bleeding disorders such as haemophilia or von Willebrand's disease, therapeutic anticoagulation, use of aspirin or other antiplatelet medications, steroid use, cirrhosis, chronic renal failure) and factors related to the underlying thyroid pathology (malignancy, hyperthyroidism). Surgery-related risk factors include extent of surgery, reoperative surgery, intraoperative bleeding, surgical techniques for access and closure, and anaesthesia-related factors (coughing or retching during extubation, postoperative nausea/vomiting, hypertension due to postoperative pain).

Regarding the demographic patient risk factors, multiple large series have demonstrated that men seem to be at increased risk of postoperative haematoma [10, 11, 13]. Men are about 1.5–2 times as likely to develop haematomas as women. While two of these studies also found that older patients were more likely to develop postoperative haematomas, age was not a significant risk factor in the analysis done by Leyre *et al.* [13]. In one study the relative risk of bleeding in patients 50 years or older was 1.5 times

the risk in patients younger than 50 [11]. In the second study, Bergenfelz *et al.* observed that patients with bleeding had a median age of 60 compared to a median age of 48 in patients without bleeding, which was a statistically significant difference [10].

For co-morbid disease, patients with any bleeding diathesis, inherited or acquired, have traditionally been considered a high-risk group with respect to postoperative bleeding. While there is some supporting evidence in the form of reports that cite coagulopathy as the underlying cause in patients with bleeding [5], the best studies specifically examining this issue have found no difference comparing patients with haematomas to matched controls [4,13]. Even so, few would disagree with the need for perioperative optimization in this patient population to minimize the risk of both intraoperative and postoperative bleeding. For example, patients with haemophilia should have clotting factors repleted to recommended levels perioperatively, those with von Willebrand's disease should be treated with desmopressin or factor concentrates as needed, and those on therapeutic anticoagulation or antiplatelet medications should have these held perioperatively if possible. For patients with platelet dysfunction in the setting of chronic renal failure, coagulopathy from cirrhosis or other conditions that may be associated with bleeding, optimization should be tailored to the specific condition.

Finally, the underlying thyroid pathology has been reported to play a role in the likelihood of postoperative bleeding. In their series of 230 haematomas among 5490

Box 22.1 Risk factors for post-thyroidectomy bleeding

Patient-related factors	Surgery-related factors
Demographics	***Extent of surgery*** (bilateral)
Age (older)	***Reoperative surgery***
Gender (male)	***Intraoperative blood loss***
Co-morbid disease	***Technique for access and closure***
Bleeding disorder (haemophilia, von Willebrand's disease)	Division of strap muscles
Therapeutic anticoagulation (e.g. coumadin)	Longitudinal closure of strap muscles (anterior jugular vein injury)
Aspirin or other antiplatelet drugs	***Anaesthesia-related***
Steroid use	Coughing or retching during extubation
Cirrhosis	Postoperative nausea and vomiting
Chronic renal failure	Postoperative hypertension
Thyroid pathology	
Malignancy	
Hyperthyroidism	

patients, Godballe *et al.* showed malignant histology to be an independent risk factor for post-thyroidectomy haemorrhage [11]. In contrast, Burkey *et al.* examined 42 haematomas out of 13,817 patients and found no association between malignant histology and bleeding [4]. However, only nine of the 42 patients with haematomas also had malignant disease, so this latter study was likely underpowered to detect a difference. Similarly, patients with hyperthyroidism have long been thought to harbour a greater risk of bleeding due to increased vascularity of the thyroid gland. In fact, several institutions treat these patients with potassium iodide (Lugol's solution) preoperatively to decrease thyroid parenchymal blood flow [14,15]. Menegaux *et al.* observed rates of post-thyroidectomy bleeding of 15% among patients with hyperthyroidism compared to 1.6% among euthyroid patients, which was a statistically significant difference [16]. Once again, though, despite this well-documented hypervascularity and reports of increased postoperative bleeding in patients with hyperthyroidism [3,7,16], there are also multiple large series that have not found a significant association [4,11,13,17].

In terms of surgery-related risk factors, much of the supporting evidence is also inconsistent. Extent of surgery (meaning bilateral versus unilateral thyroidectomy) and reoperative surgery have both been identified as risk factors for bleeding complications in some series, but not others. A large Danish study identified bilateral procedures as an independent risk factor for bleeding while reoperative surgery was not significant [11]. In contrast, another study showed significantly different rates of postoperative haematoma comparing primary and reoperative thyroid surgery patients (0.7% and 2.5% respectively) [16]. Yet another study found neither extent of surgery nor reoperative surgery to be a significant predictor of postoperative bleeding [4].

Next, the amount of intraoperative bleeding is thought to correlate with the risk of postoperative bleeding and is often one of the determinants of whether a drain is placed by surgeons who use them selectively. This may explain why drains seem to increase the likelihood of bleeding in some series. The idea that intraoperative bleeding begets postoperative bleeding is also part of the rationale for the use of Lugol's solution in patients with hyperthyroidism, which has been shown to decrease intraoperative bleeding [15]. While there are no studies specifically examining the effect of Lugol's solution on the incidence of

postoperative bleeding, there are studies that find no difference in the rate of postoperative haematoma on the basis of intraoperative blood loss [4]. On the other hand, Godballe *et al.* found intraoperative bleeding to be a significant predictor of postoperative haematoma on univariate analysis, although it was no longer statistically significant after multivariate analysis [11].

Surgical techniques for access and closure of the wound are also postulated to affect the risk of bleeding. If the strap muscles are transected instead of simply separated in the midline and retracted, then the muscle itself is a potential source of bleeding. It is not always possible to avoid cutting the strap muscles, however, particularly in cases where there is significant inflammation with adhesions or when there is malignant invasion of the muscle requiring resection for negative margins. There can also be injury to the anterior jugular veins during vertical closure of the strap muscles, yielding another potential source of bleeding. While these make intuitive sense as potential risk factors, there is little evidence to support them beyond finding muscle and jugular vein sources with some frequency at the time of reoperation for postoperative bleeding [4,8].

Lastly, anaesthesia-related factors may play a role in bleeding risk. The most frequently cited factors are retching during extubation, postoperative coughing or vomiting, and postoperative hypertension due to pain. The common underlying mechanism for these factors is a sudden increase in venous and/or arterial pressure. Rosenbaum *et al.* [9] and Shaha & Jaffe [3] both describe patients who developed instant haematomas during postoperative episodes of coughing/vomiting and hypertension. For this reason, many advocate a deep extubation that avoids significant coughing or retching, liberal use of antiemetics, and effective pain control that limits the use of narcotics, which may precipitate nausea and vomiting.

Implications

Taken together with the timing of bleeding events, the inability to identify reliable risk factors and consequently to define a high-risk patient subgroup has implications for the practice of outpatient thyroid surgery. Proponents of outpatient surgery argue that most patients with clinically significant bleeding will manifest within the 6–8-h postoperative observation period prior to discharge from the postanaesthesia care unit. Furthermore, if there is more than expected neck swelling or other cause for concern, the patient will be admitted overnight for observation. Since bleeding is a rare complication to begin with, affecting only ~1% of patients, the other 99% of patients undergoing thyroid surgery can be safely discharged, leading to increased patient satisfaction and decreased hospital costs [18–20].

In contrast, there are thyroid surgeons who advocate hospitalizing all patients for overnight observation following thyroidectomy. Along with concerns about pain control and hypoparathyroidism, supporters of this practice cite the potentially devastating outcomes of out-of-hospital post-thyroidectomy haemorrhage. An unwitnessed event or significant delays in getting to the hospital carry a high probability of death or permanent disability. Because only ~50–75% of haematomas manifest within 6–8 h while 80–97% occur within 24 h, overnight admission will reduce the risk of haemorrhage in the outpatient setting from 25–50% to 3–20%. Furthermore, they argue that the additional cost of an overnight stay relative to 6–8 h of observation in the recovery unit is small and certainly not worth the potential lives lost [5,13,19]. Through decision analysis, Schwartz *et al.* estimated that about 94 haemorrhage-related deaths per 100,000 thyroid operations could be prevented by a 24-h versus a 6-h observation period [19].

There are still other authors who recommend an intermediate approach where patients undergoing thyroid lobectomy are routinely scheduled for discharge after a period of observation as long as there are no complications, while patients treated with subtotal or total thyroidectomies are admitted for overnight observation [9].

There are good arguments for all three approaches as long as there has been serious consideration of the relevant issues. There is clearly a need for better identification of the subset of patients most at risk for suffering this life-threatening complication. Until then, given the varied length of the interval between the initial operation and haematoma development, patient factors and practice realities all need to be taken into account when establishing outpatient thyroidectomy guidelines. Relevant patient factors to consider include proximity to the hospital, patient reliability, availability of caregivers who know the signs/symptoms to look for, and whether or not the patient has co-morbidities that increase the likelihood of a bad outcome. For example, patients with disabilities or cognitive dysfunction may not recognize or alert others to symptoms as quickly and require close observation.

Specific practice considerations may include the ability to perform operations early enough to allow sufficient time for 6–8 h of observation in the recovery room, a mechanism in place to ensure careful examination of patients prior to discharge, and a way to maintain regular communication with the patient following discharge [8,19–21].

Diagnosis and management

Diagnosis

Since post-thyroidectomy bleeding is potentially fatal, rapid diagnosis and management are imperative. Haematomas most often present as a firm area of anterior or lateral neck swelling beneath the incision. A certain amount of swelling following thyroid surgery is not uncommon and is related to soft tissue oedema. However, more than normal or rapidly enlarging neck swelling, particularly in the first few hours after surgery, should raise concern for bleeding. Patients typically display one or more of a limited number of signs and symptoms (Table 22.1). These include respiratory distress such as dyspnoea and/or stridor (~50%), neck pain or pressure (25–50%), wound drainage (10–15%), dysphagia (6–20%), and agitation/confusion and sweating (5%) [4, 22]. If a drain was left in place another sign might be high drain output, but the caveat is there may still be significant bleeding despite low or no drain output if the drain is blocked.

Management

The first step in management of a patient with a suspected haematoma is to assess the patient's airway (Figure 22.1). If there is severe respiratory distress with impending airway compromise, the wound should be reopened at the bedside. Because the goal is evacuation

Table 22.1 Presenting signs and symptoms of post-thyroidectomy bleeding.

Sign/symptom	Frequency
Respiratory distress	50%
Neck pain/pressure	25–50%
Wound drainage	10–15%
Dysphagia	6–20%
Agitation/confusion	5%

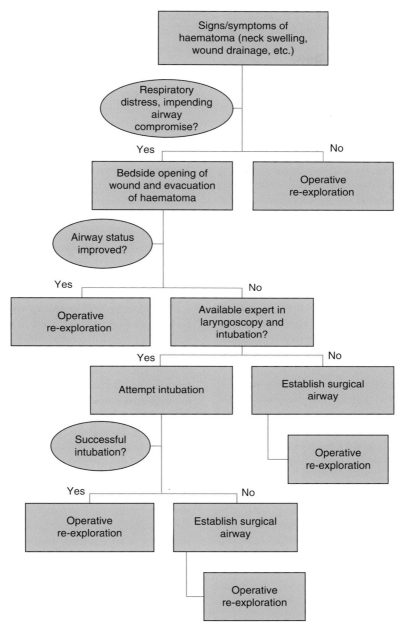

Figure 22.1 Algorithm for management of post-thyroidectomy bleeding.

of the haematoma, it is not enough to just remove skin sutures or those closing the platysma. The strap muscles must be opened as well. If there is significant improvement in the patient's status following opening of the wound, then the patient is transferred urgently to the operating room for re-exploration. If, however, the patient remains in distress following evacuation of the haematoma, the airway must be secured prior to transfer. If there is an expert in laryngoscopy and endotracheal intubation readily available, an attempt at intubation is reasonable. If there is no expert or the attempt fails then a surgical airway should be established. Not long ago all thyroid surgery patients had emergency tracheostomy trays available at the bedside for this very reason. Patients who do not have severe respiratory distress on initial assessment should be brought to the operating room and the wound explored after a controlled intubation. Once again, a senior person should perform the intubation since there is frequently significant laryngeal oedema from venous congestion as a result of the haematoma [3]. A trial of non-operative management may be reasonable in an asymptomatic patient with a small, non-expanding haematoma as long as the patient is observed closely [17,19].

The goal of operative re-exploration is to identify and control any bleeding sources. All remaining haematoma is removed and the wound irrigated, being extremely careful not to injure the parathyroid glands or laryngeal nerves. Causes of bleeding include slipping of the ligature on a major blood vessel, reopening of veins that had previously been cauterized, and oozing from the cut edge of thyroid or muscle and other soft tissue [3]. Deep haematomas are more likely to require operative intervention than are superficial ones [4,17]. Among the 42 patients who required re-exploration for symptomatic haematoma, Burkey and colleagues identified four superficial and 38 deep haematomas. The bleeding source was arterial in 26% with an equal frequency of superior and inferior vessels, venous in 19%, remnant thyroid in 19%, soft tissue in 12%, and unidentified in 24% [4]. Once all bleeding sources are controlled the wound is closed. Many surgeons routinely leave drains after a re-exploration to facilitate prompt evacuation of serous fluid. Patients typically remain intubated for at least 24 h after the operation to allow the airway oedema to subside prior to extubation. Steroids are sometimes used to aid this process. Occasionally, patients have difficulty weaning from the ventilator due to persistent airway obstruction and require a formal tracheostomy. In this situation one should perform laryngoscopy to check for vocal cord paresis due to nerve injury. Finally, there have been instances where patients develop recurrent haematomas so a certain level of vigilance is still necessary following reoperation [3].

Prevention

The old saying 'prevention is better than cure' definitely applies to post-thyroidectomy bleeding, and many strategies have been utilized in attempts to minimize the risk of bleeding or to mitigate its effects. The following is an overview of some of these strategies.

Perioperative techniques

Careful haemostasis is, of course, the key principle in thyroid surgery. To ensure haemostasis, several authors recommend performance of a Valsalva manoeuvre by the anaesthesiologist prior to closure. This increases venous pressure, which may highlight bleeding sources to be controlled before closing [3,7,12]. Reeve & Thompson also advocate re-evaluation of haemostasis once the shoulder roll has been removed and the neck flexed because the decreased tension on blood vessels may reveal additional bleeding sites [12].

The technique for closure of the strap muscles has also been emphasized. Partial closure is preferred, since this is believed to allow decompression of blood into the subcutaneous tissue. This theoretically results in earlier development of visible neck swelling to indicate a haematoma and also increases the volume of blood needed to produce respiratory compromise [3,12,19]. One possible disadvantage is adhesion of the trachea to the overlying skin, leading to decreased cosmesis and a potentially difficult reoperation should the patient require one [19].

Gentle application of manual pressure in line with the incision until after extubation is thought to help avoid the rise in pressure at the wound associated with coughing that frequently occurs at the time of extubation [12]. It should be noted that these practices are largely empiric, and there is only anecdotal evidence to indicate a decrease in the rate of postoperative bleeding when they are utilized. The key for any surgeon is to adopt a system that they are most comfortable with and that achieves optimal results in their hands.

Drains

Historically, drains were used routinely with the thought that this would evacuate blood from the paratracheal space, thereby decreasing the risk of airway compromise due to haematoma. Also, a high drain output could indicate excessive bleeding and trigger reoperation. However, over time drains have been used more and more selectively as mounting observational data suggested no effect on bleeding complications. Frequently, the drains were clogged at the time of reoperation for a symptomatic haematoma [3,17]. A randomized controlled trial of 100 patients by Ahluwalia *et al.* in 2007 comparing suction drain to no drain found no difference in postoperative fluid collections and a prolonged hospital stay in the group with drains. In addition, all three patients who developed haematomas in this study were in the suction drain group [23]. A Cochrane meta-analysis performed that same year by Samraj and Gurusamy combined the results of 13 randomized controlled trials comparing drainage with no drainage. They found no difference in reoperation rates, rates of respiratory distress, rates of wound infection, or incidence of fluid collection, but did note a significantly longer hospital stay (+1.18 days) and more pain in the group with drains [24]. The studies examined excluded patients with lateral neck dissection, coagulation disorders, Graves' disease and large substernal goitres so the results do not necessarily apply to these groups. For all other patients undergoing thyroid surgery, however, the evidence does not support routine use of drains.

Haemostatic devices and agents

In many cases a problem with haemostasis is identified at the time of reoperation for bleeding (e.g. failed ligation of a vessel). In addition, achieving complete haemostasis can be quite time consuming, so there is ongoing demand for devices and agents that can be used to optimize intraoperative haemostasis. We briefly explore some of the most commonly utilized haemostatic devices and agents in thyroid surgery below.

The Harmonic™ Scalpel (Ethicon Endo-Surgery, Cincinnati, OH) and electrothermal bipolar vessel-sealing system (LigaSure™, Valleylab, Boulder, CO) are the two most widely used haemostatic devices in thyroid surgery. The Harmonic Scalpel takes advantage of high-frequency (~55.5 kHz) vibration to simultaneously cut and coagulate tissue. In comparison with standard electrosurgical devices, this ultrasonic coagulation and dissection is reported to result in less lateral thermal injury (1–3 mm, which is about half that of bipolar devices), does not use any electrical energy and does not cause neuromuscular stimulation [25,26]. The Harmonic can be used to seal vessels up to 5 mm in diameter. Studies comparing the

Harmonic to conventional haemostasis (clamp and tie techniques) have consistently found a statistically significant decrease in operative time using the Harmonic, although the absolute magnitude of decrease varies anywhere from about 7 to 40 min [25–29]. Some studies have also shown decreases in pain, transient hypocalcaemia, wound drainage and length of stay (LOS), but there are no studies demonstrating a difference in the rate of postoperative bleeding [27,29,30].

In comparison, the LigaSure uses high current (4 A) and low voltage (<200 V) to achieve vessel sealing and division. Collagen and elastin in the vessel wall are denatured while the pressure applied by the scissors allows formation of a seal [31]. The device can be used to seal vessels up to 7 mm in diameter. Similar to the Harmonic Scalpel, the only consistent finding across studies comparing LigaSure to conventional haemostasis has been a reduction in operative time [30–32]. Again, there was no difference in the rate of postoperative bleeding complications [31,32]. In a single-institution, retrospective study comparing the Harmonic to LigaSure among 231 patients, operative time and LOS were shorter with the Harmonic (by 7–15 min and 0.2 days respectively), but there was no difference in complication rates, including postoperative haematoma [30]. A randomized, controlled trial comparing LigaSure, Harmonic and conventional haemostasis also found no difference in postoperative bleeding [29]. Thus, overall there is no difference in post-thyroidectomy haemorrhage using these devices and possibly a slight advantage of the Harmonic with respect to operative time and length of stay. Given the cost, the decision to use one or other of these devices depends on surgeon preference in combination with the individual institution's evaluation of the cost-effectiveness.

Absorbable haemostatic agents like oxidized regenerated cellulose (e.g. Surgicel™, Ethicon,), gelatin compressed sponge (e.g. Gelfoam™, Pfizer, New York), topical thrombin (e.g. Floseal™, Baxter Healthcare Corporation, Deerfield, IL) and fibrin sealants (e.g. Tisseel™, Baxter Healthcare Corporation) are also utilized with some frequency. Unfortunately, they are often used without careful consideration of the mechanism of action of the particular agent, which dictates the effectiveness in a given patient. Oxidized regenerated cellulose is derived from plants. It acts both by mechanical tissue pressure as well as contact activation of the intrinsic pathway. In this way it promotes blood cells to form a coagulum within the interstices of the cellulose. Since it works proximally in the clotting cascade, the patient needs to have functioning clotting factors in order to achieve haemostasis. Gelatin sponge or Gelfoam is made from purified porcine skin gelatin. It is also believed to promote haemostasis through both mechanical pressure and contact activation of the intrinsic pathway. Therefore, Gelfoam also requires the patient to have adequate clotting factors.

Floseal is a combination of topical thrombin and a gelatin matrix derived from cross-linking bovine collagen. It acts in the common pathway where thrombin directly activates fibrinogen, converting it to fibrin, bypassing the other clotting factors. It does, however, require the patient to have functional fibrinogen in order to work. In a prospective, randomized controlled trial comparing Floseal, oxidized cellulose and haemostasis without these agents, Testini *et al.* found the Floseal group had shorter operative times, shorter time to drain removal and decreased LOS compared to the other two groups. However, there was no difference in postoperative complications, including bleeding, among the three groups [33].

Finally, fibrin sealants come in several forms. They are typically a combination of fibrinogen, thrombin and sometimes an antifibrinolytic agent to help stabilize the clot. Fibrin sealants thus act at the same point in the cascade as topical thrombin agents like Floseal, but they come with their own fibrinogen. They have been shown to decrease wound drainage but not specifically postoperative bleeding complications after thyroidectomy [34].

All the studies of these agents in thyroid surgery have been relatively small so it would be difficult to detect a difference in postoperative bleeding even if one does actually exist. They do seem to help with intraoperative haemostasis, although it is important to reiterate that they are not a substitute for meticulous technique.

Conclusion

Bleeding occurs about 1% of the time in patients undergoing thyroid surgery. The timing of this complication and lack of irrefutable risk factors have implications for the practice of outpatient thyroid surgery. It is a potentially life-threatening complication and thus requires vigilance and prompt action once identified. Treatment for a postoperative haematoma is relatively standardized, with the key principles being securing the airway and operative re-exploration. Perioperative techniques for prevention may be helpful for surgeons who consistently use them with good results although no data support their use. Routine drains are not indicated. Devices like the electrothermal bipolar vessel-sealing system and Harmonic Scalpel can be used to increase the efficiency of obtaining haemostasis, but the cost–benefit analysis is left up to the individual surgeons and institutions. No device has shown a change in postoperative haemorrhage rates. Similarly, haemostatic agents can be used to decrease bleeding intraoperatively and play a role when used in accordance with their mechanism of action. However, no agent has been shown to decrease rates of postoperative haemorrhage.

Postoperative bleeding after thyroidectomy continues to be a source of morbidity and mortality. Since this complication occurs infrequently and other than known bleeding diatheses, no specific risk factors have been agreed upon, surgeons must remain vigilant to assure haemostasis intraoperatively so that the risk of postoperative haemorrhage is made as low as possible.

References

1 Halsted WS. The operative story of goiter. Johns Hopkins Hosp Rep 1929; 19: 84.

2 Hegner CF. A history of thyroid surgery. Ann Surg 1932; 95(4): 481–92.

3 Shaha AR, Jaffe BM. Practical management of post-thyroidectomy hematoma. J Surg Oncol 1994; 57(4): 235–8.

4 Burkey SH, van Heerden JA, Thompson GB, Grant CS, Schleck CD, Farley DR. Reexploration for symptomatic hematomas after cervical exploration. Surgery 2001; 130(6): 914–20.

5 Abbas G, Dubner S, Heller KS. Re-operation for bleeding after thyroidectomy and parathyroidectomy. Head Neck 2001; 23(7): 544–6.

6 Bhattacharyya N, Fried MP. Assessment of the morbidity and complications of total thyroidectomy. Arch Otolaryngol Head Neck Surg 2002; 128(4): 389–92.

7 Rosato L, Avenia N, Bernante P, *et al.* Complications of thyroid surgery: analysis of a multicentric study on 14,934 patients operated on in Italy over 5 years. World J Surg 2004; 28(3): 271–6.

8 Spanknebel K, Chabot JA, DiGiorgi M, *et al.* Thyroidectomy using local anesthesia: a report of 1,025 cases over 16 years. J Am Coll Surg 2005; 201(3): 375–85.

9 Rosenbaum MA, Haridas M, McHenry CR. Life-threatening neck hematoma complicating thyroid and parathyroid surgery. Am J Surg 2008; 195(3): 339–43.

10 Bergenfelz A, Jansson S, Kristoffersson A, *et al.* Complications to thyroid surgery: results as reported in a database from a multicenter audit comprising 3,660 patients. Langenbecks Arch Surg 2008; 393(5): 667–73.

11 Godballe C, Madsen AR, Pedersen HB, *et al.* Post-thyroidectomy hemorrhage: a national study of patients treated at the Danish departments of ENT Head and Neck Surgery. Eur Arch Otorhinolaryngol 2009; 266(12): 1945–52.

12 Reeve T, Thompson NW. Complications of thyroid surgery: how to avoid them, how to manage them, and observations on their possible effect on the whole patient. World J Surg 2000; 24(8): 971–5.

13 Leyre P, Desurmont T, Lacoste L, *et al.* Does the risk of compressive hematoma after thyroidectomy authorize 1-day surgery? Langenbecks Arch Surg 2008; 393(5): 733–7.

14 Ansaldo GL, Pretolesi F, Varaldo E, *et al.* Doppler evaluation of intrathyroid arterial resistances during preoperative treatment with Lugol's iodide solution in patients with diffuse toxic goiter. J Am Coll Surg 2000; 191(6): 607–12.

15 Erbil Y, Ozluk Y, Giriş M, *et al.* Effect of lugol solution on thyroid gland blood flow and microvessel density in the patients with Graves' disease. J Clin Endocrinol Metab 2007; 92(6): 2182–9.

16 Menegaux F, Turpin G, Dahman M, *et al.* Secondary thyroidectomy in patients with prior thyroid surgery for benign disease: a study of 203 cases. Surgery 1999; 126(3): 479–83.

17 Bergamaschi R, Becouarn G, Ronceray J, Arnaud JP. Morbidity of thyroid surgery. Am J Surg 1998; 176(1): 71–5.

18 Mowschenson PM, Hodin RA. Outpatient thyroid and parathyroid surgery: a prospective study of feasibility, safety, and costs. Surgery 1995; 118(6): 1051–3.

19 Schwartz AE, Clark OH, Ituarte P, Lo Gerfo P. Therapeutic controversy: thyroid surgery – the choice. Clin Endocrinol Metab 1998; 83(4): 1097–105.

20 Inabnet WB, Shifrin A, Ahmed L, Sinha P. Safety of same day discharge in patients undergoing sutureless thyroidectomy: a comparison of local and general anesthesia. Thyroid 2008; 18(1): 57–61.

21 Lo Gerfo P. Local/regional anesthesia for thyroidectomy: evaluation as an outpatient procedure. Surgery 1998; 124(6): 975–8.

22 Palestini N, Tulletti V, Cestino L, *et al.* Post-thyroidectomy cervical hematoma. Minerva Chir 2005; 60(1): 37–46.

23 Ahluwalia S, Hannan SA, Mehrzad H, Crofton M, Tolley NS. A randomised controlled trial of routine suction drainage after elective thyroid and parathyroid surgery with ultrasound evaluation of fluid collection. Clin Otolaryngol 2007; 32(1): 28–31.

24 Samraj K, Gurusamy KS. Wound drains following thyroid surgery. Cochrane Database Syst Rev 2007; 4: CD006099.

25 Siperstein AE, Berber E, Morkoyun E. The use of the harmonic scalpel vs conventional knot tying for vessel ligation in thyroid surgery. Arch Surg 2002; 137(2): 137–42.

26 Miccoli P, Berti P, Dionigi G, d'Agostino J, Orlandini C, Donatini G. Randomized controlled trial of harmonic scalpel use during thyroidectomy. Arch Otolaryngol Head Neck Surg 2006; 132(10): 1069–73.

27 Koh YW, Park JH, Lee SW, Choi EC. The harmonic scalpel technique without supplementary ligation in total thyroidectomy with central neck dissection: a prospective randomized study. Ann Surg 2008; 247(6): 945–9.

28 Shemen L. Thyroidectomy using the harmonic scalpel: analysis of 105 consecutive cases. Otolaryngol Head Neck Surg 2002; 127(4): 284–8.

29 Manouras A, Markogiannakis H, Koutras AS, *et al.* Thyroid surgery: comparison between the electrothermal bipolar vessel sealing system, harmonic scalpel, and classic suture ligation. Am J Surg 2008; 195(1): 48–52.

30 Zarebczan B, Mohanty D, Chen H. A Comparison of the LigaSure and harmonic scalpel in thyroid surgery: a single institution review. Ann Surg Oncol 2011; 18(1): 214–18.

31 Saint Marc O, Cogliandolo A, Piquard A, Famà F, Pidoto RR. LigaSure vs clamp-and-tie technique to achieve hemostasis in total thyroidectomy for benign multinodular goiter: a prospective randomized study. Arch Surg 2007; 142(2): 150–6.

32 Yao HS, Wang Q, Wang WJ, Ruan CP. Prospective clinical trials of thyroidectomy with LigaSure vs conventional vessel ligation: a systematic review and meta-analysis. Arch Surg 2009; 144(12): 1167–74.

33 Testini M, Marzaioli R, Lissidini G, *et al.* The effectiveness of FloSeal matrix hemostatic agent in thyroid surgery: a prospective, randomized, control study. Langenbecks Arch Surg 2009; 394(5): 837–42.

34 Uwiera TC, Uwiera RR, Seikaly H, Harris JR. Tisseel and its effects on wound drainage post-thyroidectomy: prospective, randomized, blinded, controlled study. J Otolaryngol 2005; 34(6): 374–8.

CHAPTER 23

The Occurrence and Management of Pneumothorax in Thyroid Surgery

Kamran Samakar, Jason Wallen and Alfred Simental

Department of Surgery, Loma Linda University School of Medicine, Loma Linda, CA, USA

Introduction

Pneumothorax is defined by the presence of air or gas in the pleural space between the lung and the chest wall. Pneumothorax can be classified as spontaneous, traumatic or iatrogenic [1]. Spontaneous pneumothoraces are further subdivided into primary and secondary subtypes. A primary spontaneous pneumothorax (PSP) presents in an otherwise healthy person without underlying pulmonary disease while a secondary pneumothorax complicates pre-existing lung disease with underlying blebs. The majority of pneumothoraces are classified as traumatic pneumothoraces resulting from blunt or sharp force injury. These include the class of complications resulting from iatrogenic injury during either diagnostic or therapeutic interventions such as central venous access and percutaneous lung biopsy. The following chapter focuses on clinical manifestations and management of iatrogenic pneumothoraces in the setting of thyroid surgery.

Pathophysiology

Pneumothorax and pneumomediastinum are rare but known complications of thyroid surgery. Multiple mechanisms for this cause–effect relationship have been

hypothesized. In thyroid surgery, these entities are usually associated with dissection toward the pleura or superior mediastinum in cases of mediastinal goitre and extensive thyroid malignancy. Air may gain access to the mediastinal and pleural space through direct extension from full-thickness perforations into the trachea or oesophagus. Perforations in the trachea usually occur at the fibrous septations between the tracheal rings, especially when extensive tracheal deformation has occurred. Unrecognized oesophageal perforations usually occur in the setting of thyroid malignancy where the surgical planes may be obscured and result in leakage of air and oesophageal fluids into the paratracheal region and subsequently into the pleural spaces. Air may also track directly along the fascial planes of the neck as a result of surgical dissection. The pleura may be inadvertently violated during dissection, allowing for entry of air, especially when dissecting under the clavicle in cases of thyroid malignancy or goitre. Injury to the pleura in the form a pleural rent should be distinguished from direct parenchymal injury since the subsequent course of the corresponding pneumothoraces may differ greatly. Pneumothorax has also been known to result from underlying lung disease, including metastatic thyroid carcinoma [2,3]. Lastly, pneumothorax may occur as a result of positive pressure ventilation during surgery in patients with or without underlying lung disease [4].

Thyroid Surgery: Preventing and Managing Complications, First Edition. Edited by Paolo Miccoli, David J. Terris, Michele N. Minuto and Melanie W. Seybt.

Pneumothorax resulting from thyroid surgery has limited reports in the literature, possibly due to the undesired stigma of reporting unusual iatrogenic complications. Wilson and Page reported incidents of pneumothorax following thyroidectomy as far back as 1947 [5,6]. Lee et al. reported a pneumothorax after right thyroidectomy with left neck dissection without any obvious signs of injury to the pleura or the chest [7]. Similarly, Taniguchi et al. reported bilateral pneumothorax following total thyroidectomy and radical neck dissection [8].

The risk of pleural injury is likely highest when neck dissection extends below the level of the clavicles or in cases of substernal extension of goitres. Several authors reported the risk of pneumothorax associated with thyroid surgery extending into the mediastinum [9,10]. Central and low neck dissections have also been reported as playing a role in the formation of pneumothorax. Lee et al. reported bilateral pneumothorax and pneumomediastinum after total thyroidectomy and central neck dissection in a patient who had a known tracheal perforation [11]. Eltzschig et al. reported five cases of pneumothorax in a study of 363 patients undergoing thyroid surgery enrolled in a study investigating intraoperative monitoring of recurrent laryngeal nerve function [12]. Two of these cases were associated with internal jugular node dissections which extended below the level of the clavicles. Reported cases of pneumothorax associated with thyroid surgery identify neck dissection below the level of the clavicles, mediastinal extension and extensive neck dissection as risk factors for the formation of pneumothorax. Wu et al. reported three cases of pneumothorax in a series of 24 patients with mediastinal invasion by thyroid carcinomas [9]. Similarly, Irabor reported a pneumothorax after delivery of a massive retrosternal goitre which was managed with tube thoracostomy [10]. Slater & Inabnet reported a case of pneumothorax following minimally invasive parathyroidectomy which they hypothesized to be due to proximity of the adenoma to the mediastinum [4].

Tracheal injury can be directly attributed to the formation of pneumothorax after thyroid surgery. Tracheal injury may create a point of egress for air that can directly track down into the mediastinum. However, the causative effect of direct pleural injury in the setting of neck dissection is not present in the mechanism associated with tracheal injury. Lee et al. define the risk of tracheal injury as highest when freeing the isthmus from the trachea and during dissection of the lateral and posterior aspect of the trachea close to the area where the recurrent laryngeal nerve enters the tracheal cartilage. Fortunately, the risk of tracheal injury remains relatively low in thyroid surgery. Gosnell et al. identified tracheal perforation as exceedingly rare during thyroid surgery and described less than one in every 1000 thyroid surgeries in a review of 11,917 operations [13]. While tracheal injury provides a mechanism for the escape of air, deep cervical dissection with inadvertent pleural injury allows for air to directly enter the pleural space, creating a pneumothorax. Without pleural violation, the sequelae of tracheal injury would be mostly limited to subcutaneous emphysema and pneumomediastinum. Fortunately, subcutaneous emphysema and pneumomediastinum in the setting of thyroid surgery usually resolve spontaneously in non-intubated patients.

Fewins et al. concluded that pneumothoraces and pneumomediastinum after thyroid and parathyroid surgery result from air tracking through cervical fascial planes under low pressure or direct violation of the pleura in their review of complications of thyroid and parathyroid surgery [14]. While we agree that air can track through cervical fascial planes, it is important to acknowledge that injury to the pleura is usually necessary for the production of clinically relevant pneumothorax. There are no 'tissue planes' that communicate directly with the pleural space. Noppen & Keukeleire, in their review of pneumothorax, suggested that one of three events must occur for air to be present in the pleural space: communication between alveoli and the pleura, communication between the atmosphere and the pleural space, or the presence of gas-producing organisms in the pleural space [15]. Communication between the atmosphere and pleural space likely happens through inadvertent violation of the pleura during deep dissection and plays the central role in formation of pneumothorax in the setting of thyroid surgery.

Clinical manifestations

Clinical symptoms of pneumothorax may be subtle but characteristically include pleuritic chest pain, shortness of breath and palpitations. The associated signs of pneumothorax include diminished or absent breath sounds, decreased ipsilateral chest excursion and hyper-resonant percussion. Tachycardia, tachypnoea and hypotension may be indicative of tension pneumothorax and require immediate recognition and intervention. Intervention may take the form of simple intercostal needle decompression or formal chest tube placement. While hypoxaemia secondary to shunting is common, hypercapnia is rare in the setting of adequate ventilation of the contralateral lung. This is due to the rapid diffusion of CO_2, being approximately 40 times greater than the oxygen diffusion capacity in the non-pathogenic lung. Arterial blood gas measurements are not routinely indicated if oxygen saturations remain normal (>92%), but typically reveal acute respiratory alkalosis.

Pneumothorax as an intraoperative complication during thyroid surgery may be the result of direct injury from surgical dissection or from alveolar rupture due to positive airway pressure from assisted ventilation [16]. Symptoms of pneumothorax during general anaesthesia are tachycardia, hypotension, hypercapnia and hypoxia. Mechanical ventilation creates the potential for progression of a simple pneumothorax to tension pneumothorax, as a result of the positive pressure ventilation. Tension pneumothorax may cause cardiovascular collapse as the mediastinum is displaced, the contralateral lung is compressed and venous return into the right atrium is diminished. Patients with underlying lung disease, particularly chronic obstructive lung disease or emphysematous changes, should warrant heightened vigilance because of their increased susceptibility to pneumothorax.

Diagnosis

The presence of a pneumothorax is established by identifying a visceral pleural line found displaced from the chest wall on a chest radiograph (x-ray). Ideally, chest x-rays should be obtained in the upright posterior-anterior (PA) fashion. Inspiratory and expiratory radiographs have equal sensitivity in detecting pneumothoraces [17–19]. Lateral and supine x-rays are generally less sensitive than PA x-rays for the diagnosis of pneumothorax [20,21]. Limitations of standard x-rays have been well documented and include difficulty in accurately identifying pneumothorax size [22]. Still, the upright PA x-ray remains the mainstay of clinical practice in the setting of suspected pneumothorax. While computed tomography (CT) remains the 'gold standard' in the detection and measurement of pneumothoraces, it is generally not indicated for uncomplicated pneumothoraces. CT imaging

may be helpful for identifying underlying lung disease and/or aberrant chest tube placement [23].

Management

Iatrogenic pneumothorax after thyroid surgery is by definition classified as a subgroup of traumatic pneumothoraces. The majority of these likely result from small pleural violations as a result of inadvertent electrocautery or blunt dissection. Deep penetrating violations of the thoracic cavity are unlikely and should be treated differently as the risk of lung injury and subsequent course of pneumothorax will vary. Pleural rents resulting from thyroid surgery will cause pneumothoraces that behave in large part as PSPs. The majority of these will act similar to rupture of a pleural bleb with subsequent spontaneous sealing. Central to their management will be determination of ongoing air leak and progression of pneumothorax. Treatment of pneumothorax after thyroid surgery will be framed in similar fashion to treatment of PSP. The clinician, however, must be aware of subtle differences and the potential for ongoing air leak, haemothorax and a variable course consistent with a true traumatic injury.

Management of pneumothorax resulting from thyroid surgery depends on the clinical significance of the pneumothorax as well as the unique patient characteristics. Initial treatment options for pneumothorax include observation, supplemental oxygen, needle- or catheter-based aspiration, tube thoracostomy, persistent neck drains and possible thoracoscopy. The goals of treatment are elimination of the intrapleural air collection, facilitation of pleural healing and prevention of recurrence. Defining a management strategy relies more on the clinical significance of the pneumothorax than the size. For instance, shortness of breath in the context of a known pneumothorax requires active intervention regardless of size. Importantly, though, size of the pneumothorax determines the rate of resolution/reabsorption which has been previously described as somewhere between 1.25% and 2.2% of volume of the hemithorax per day [24,25]. Assuming the most recent estimate of 2.2% per day as accurate, a large pneumothorax may take several weeks to resolve spontaneously.

Consensus guidelines generally agree that clinically stable patients with a small primary pneumothorax, defined as less then 15% percent of the hemithorax or less than 2–3 cm between the lung and chest wall on chest x-ray, may be candidates for observation and supplemental oxygen therapy [26–28]. The American College of Chest Physicians (ACCP) defines small pneumothorax as <3 cm apex-to-cupola distance while the British Thoracic Society (BTS) uses a visible rim of <2 cm between the lung and chest wall as its definition. At the authors' institution, a measurement of 2–3 cm is judged alongside the clinical significance of a pneumothorax to weigh management options. Regardless of the size, supplemental oxygen should be applied in most patients to increase the rate of resorption approximately fourfold [29]. The authors believe that a small pneumothorax resulting from thyroid surgery in the clinically stable patient can generally be treated as a primary spontaneous pneumothorax.

Conservative management of small pneumothoraces with a combination of observation and supplemental oxygen has been shown to be safe and effective. Clinically stable patients with small pneumothoraces can be discharged home after 4–6 h of observation if a repeat chest radiograph excludes progression of the pneumothorax. Patients should be admitted for observation if they live an unacceptable distance from emergency medical services, are deemed generally unreliable or upon discretion of the practising clinician. Patients discharged home should be advised against high-risk activities such as flying, diving and trips to higher elevations. Moreover, specific discharge instructions as well as follow-up arrangements within 48 h should be made for follow-up chest x-ray and evaluation.

Patients with a pneumothorax larger than 3 cm or greater than 15% of the hemithorax, signs of clinically instability (e.g. hypoxia, tachycardia), or evidence of progression of the pneumothorax should have some form of pleural intervention. The goals of drainage are fivefold: re-expansion of the lung, prevention of additional injury, minimization of hospital stay, pleura-to-pleural apposition and prevention of recurrence. Once the decision to drain the pleural space has been made, one must make three more decisions. The surgeon must decide on an access point, the type of access and the drainage collection system. Numerous commercial devices are available to drain air from the pleural space. Selection and management of such devices should be tailored by the surgeon's comfort level, the availability of expert consultation and the patient's unique considerations.

Simple aspiration has received contrary recommendations from two reputable sources for the management of pneumothorax. The current ACCP consensus guidelines found aspiration to be rarely appropriate in any clinical circumstance. In contrast, the most recent BTS guidelines for the management of spontaneous pneumothorax recommend aspiration as the first-line treatment for all pneumothoraces requiring intervention. A recent Cochrane review comparing simple aspiration versus intercostal tube drainage for PSP in adults found no significant difference between the two interventions regarding immediate success rate or 1-year success rate (i.e. recurrence of pneumothorax at 1 year) [30]. Moreover, simple aspiration resulted in a significant reduction in proportion of patients hospitalized but no difference was noted in the duration of hospitalization [31].

The BTS guidelines recommend the use of 14–16 G needle aspiration as first-line therapy for PSP. They advise that needle aspiration should cease after 2.5 L of air has been aspirated since the likelihood of further lung re-expansion is limited by the likely presence of an air leak. While needle aspiration may be less painful and equally efficacious to catheter placement, failure will often require a second procedure. Repeat needle aspiration is not generally recommended. In contrast, the ACCP recommends intervention using a small-bore catheter (≤14 F) or placement of a 16 F to 22 F chest tube as first-line management of clinically stable patients with large pneumothoraces. Catheters and chest tubes may be attached to a Heimlich valve or to a water seal device and left in place until lung re-expansion and exclusion of ongoing air leak. The role of suction, in conjunction with a water seal system, will be discussed later in this chapter.

Simple aspiration

Simple aspiration may be accomplished using a variety of commercial kits or readily available equipment. Typically, an 16–18 gauge needle with a small-bore (7–14 F) catheter is inserted into the pleural space and the air is manually removed once the needle has been withdrawn. Access through the second intercostal space at the midclavicular line is the preferred entry site at our institution. A three-way stopcock is attached to the angiocatheter. Air is aspirated until no more can be withdrawn, keeping track of the volume, syringe by syringe, throughout the process. Various criteria for successful aspiration have been reported in the literature, including tactile resistance to aspiration and demonstration of resolution on follow-up chest radiograph 6 h after aspiration. Absence of resistance to aspiration after 2–3 L is suggestive of an air leak that should prompt thoracic surgery consultation for consideration of further intervention.

After successful aspiration, several options exist for management of the catheter, including immediate withdrawal. Conversion from simple aspiration to placement of a chest tube by the attachment of a water seal device or one-way valve allows for continued observation, greater safety and the potential to avoid further intervention should the pneumothorax reaccumulate. At our institution, we find little utility in simple aspiration and catheter withdrawal, preferring instead to place the catheter to one-way Heimlich valve or water seal device until convincing clinical and radiographic evidence dictates removal of the tube.

Pleural drain or chest tube placement

Placement of pleural drains and chest tubes is an acceptable treatment of pneumothoraces. The two most common sites for placement of pleural drains and aspiration of pneumothorax are the fourth or fifth intercostal space in the mid- or anterior axillary line and the second intercostal space in the midclavicular line. At the authors' institution, the anterior approach is favoured for simple pneumothoraces, since air tends to accumulate in the anterior apex of the pleural space. Generally, this is managed with a small-bore catheter, directed towards the apex of the pleural space. Large-bore catheters can be placed bluntly in this location as well, but we have found that the indications for this are limited. While many types of commercial pleural drain system have become available, no randomized controlled trials exist comparing the various systems.

Selection of the type of tube depends on the clinical picture and the patient profile. Clinically stable patients with a small, uncomplicated pneumothorax can be managed successfully with a small chest tube (< 22 F) or catheter (< 14 F) in most instances [32,33]. Unstable patients or patients with large pneumothorax should be considered for larger size chest tubes, depending on the several factors including likelihood of air leak and presence of active intrathoracic haemorrhage. Since flow through the tube is a function of the tube's radius, small increases in tube radius lead to large changes in the volume of air the tube can accommodate. Patients at risk of large air leak, those suspected of having an accompanying haemothorax or mechanically ventilated patients should be treated with a large-bore tube (≥ 24 F) [34].

Seldinger technique

The Seldinger technique should be used for pleural drain placement [35]. At our institution we use the general outline described here. Prior to placement drain, close radiographic inspection should be done to ensure separation of the parietal and visceral pleura.

1 Local anaesthetic should be administered along with conscious sedation at the discretion of the practising clinician.

2 Selection of access site depends on the goal of pleural drain placement. Drains for evacuation of pneumothorax are placed in the second intercostal space at the midclavicular line at our institution. Traditionally, the fourth or fifth intercostal space at the mid- or anterior axillary line has been used as well. Drains for effusions should be placed in the latter position for greater access to fluid collections.

3 The patient should be placed in the supine position with the arm extended over the head if lateral chest wall access is being performed. For anterior chest wall access, the patient may alternatively be placed in a semi-recumbent position to allow for air in the pleural space to collect in the apex of the hemithorax.

4 Prepare the skin with chlorhexidine and sterile drapes.

5 Ultrasound guidance should be performed at this time for confirmation of entry site.

6 Insert the introducer needle into the pleural space, immediately above the rib, with aspiration of air or fluid.

7 Insert the guidewire through the introducer needle and remove needle. The guidewire should be directed apically for a pneumothorax.

8 Make a small skin incision allowing for passage of the catheter at the entry point of the guidewire.

9 Pass graduated dilators over the guidewire to create a tract for the catheter.

10 Pass the catheter into place and remove guidewire.

11 Aspirate through the pleural drain until resistance is met, with subsequent placement of a one-way flutter valve or pleural drain system.

12 Secure the pleural drain with an interrupted suture and apply the appropriate dressing.

13 Perform chest x-ray following placement of the catheter.

Standard blunt dissection chest tube placement

Standard chest tube placement using blunt dissection may proceed as follows.

1 Local anaesthetic should be administered along with conscious sedation at the discretion of the clinician. At our institution we prefer to do an intercostal nerve block.

2 Make a 2 cm skin incision parallel to the intercostal space and carry it down through subcutaneous tissue. Additional local anaesthetic may be administered into the surrounding tissues at this time.

3 Using Kelly forceps, blunt dissection should proceed in a tunnelling manner from the incision toward the intercostal space the tube will enter, aiming to pass the tube just above the rib in order to avoid injury to the neurovascular bundle.

4 A closed Kelly clamp should be pushed into the rib space and through the parietal pleura into the pleura space. The intercostal muscles should then be spread apart.

5 Insert a finger into the pleural space to confirm position and absence of adhesions. Significant adhesions should not be disrupted as they may lead to significant bleeding or worsened air leak.

6 The chest tube should be clamped by a Kelly and inserted into the pleural cavity aimed apically for a pneumothorax.

7 Once the chest tube has been positioned and the Kelly removed, visual confirmation of condensation within the tube during respiration along with drainage of fluid can aid in confirmation of placement. The tube should be advanced until the last (sentinel) hole is within the pleural cavity.

8 The skin incision should be closed with an interrupted or mattress suture that may be used to close the site upon removal. For small catheters, < 16 F, a 2-0 suture is recommended while larger tubes will require a 0-0 silk suture.

9 The site should be covered with gauze and secure tape to prevent inadvertent removal.

10 The chest tube should be placed to the pleural draining system and all connections should be examined and secured.

11 A postplacement chest x-ray should be obtained after the procedure.

Drainage system/water seal/suction

Once a pleural catheter or chest tube is in place, the clinician must decide on the role of suction and drainage systems. The use of a unidirectional flutter valve (i.e. Heimlich valve) has been shown to be a safe method of managing small-bore catheters in clinically stable patients [36]. The role of water seal devices and suctioning has been widely discussed in the literature with little in the way of a consensus. The decision algorithm largely depends on the clinical picture and the course of the pneumothorax. According to the ACCP guidelines, patients with large air leaks or requiring positive pressure ventilation should be managed with a water seal device without suction initially. Those patients whose lungs fail to re-expand with water seal drainage should have suction applied. Similarly, patients initially treated with a Heimlich valve whose lungs fail to re-expand should also be treated with a water seal device and suction.

The role of suctioning is thought to affect apposition of the visceral and parietal pleura by suctioning of the air in the pleural cavity at a rate that exceeds egress of air through the violation in the visceral pleura. Optimal suction has been suggested as between −10 to −20 cmH$_2$O [37]. Guidelines from the BTS recommend against routine use of suction, instead deferring suction for cases of failed lung re-expansion with the use of preliminary measures such as one-way valves and water seal devices. At our institution, water seal devices are initially employed when a chest tube is initially placed. The authors find that the use of Heimlich valves is a safe means of managing simple pneumothorax and suction should be initially avoided unless there are concerns for a large persistent air leak or with use of mechanical ventilation.

Air leaks

The management of air leaks should be informed by a systematic approach to diagnosis and classification. First, the clinician must ensure that the air leak originates from the lung rather than the chest tube and drainage system. Close inspection of the tubing, all attachment sites, the chest access point and any potential alternative site for air leakage should be performed. Second, it is important to differentiate commonly referenced 'broncho-pleural fistula' from the much more common peripheral air leaks referred to as alveolar-pleural fistulas. Broncho-pleural fistula results from disruption of a 'named' airway, such as the segmental, lobar or mainstem bronchus. Broncho-pleural fistulas typically lead to large and continuous leaks and are most commonly seen after pneumonectomies, lobectomy or segmentectomy [38]. Alveolar-pleural fistulas are not as severe a physiological disruption and are likely to resolve spontaneously while broncho-pleural fistulas usually require operative repair.

Alveolar-pleural fistulas can be classified by their size and timing within the respiratory cycle. These leaks typically present during the expiratory phase or during forced expiration (coughing) [39]. Grading can be done with specially designed graded water seal chambers allowing for assessment of the severity and likelihood of spontaneous resolution. In the absence of such information, the role of the clinician is to monitor the progression of pneumothorax versus lung re-expansion. Persistent air leaks may present with varying degrees of lung re-expansion. The literature is not clear on absolute indications for surgical intervention. Studies on patients with primary pneumothorax found that 75% of air leaks resolve after 7 days of drainage, while one study reported that there was a lower likelihood of resolution of air leaks lasting longer than 2 days [40].

Multiple strategies have been employed in the management of persistent air leaks. Some proponents advocate watchful observation for a period lasting between 2 and 14 days in the hope that the injury will heal and resolve without intervention [41]. Common interventions include infusion of autologous blood into the pleural space, pleurodesis, placement of a one-way valve, and video-assisted thoracoscopy with oversewing of the affected area [42,43]. In cases of persistent air leak or failure of the lung to re-expand after 3–5 days, thoracic surgical consultation should be obtained.

The role of daily chest x-rays

The overwhelming majority of clinicians order daily chest x-rays on patients with a chest tube in place without clear evidence suggesting this need. Some proponents argue that if pleural-pleural apposition is present upon initial chest x-ray after chest tube placement, in the absence of an air leak, daily chest x-rays serve little role in ongoing management strategies. At our institution, chest x-rays are ordered at the discretion of the clinician, typically at the time of placement, post placement and at the time of removal. In our opinion, routine chest x-rays in the management of a clinically stable patient with a simple pneumothorax are not indicated.

Complications

Complications of chest tube placement and needle aspiration include chest tube malposition, lung injury, diaphragmatic perforation, subcutaneous placement, intercostal artery bleeding, recurrence and empyema.

Reports in the literature include injury to the abdominal organs, perforation of the heart and lungs, contralateral pneumothorax, cardiogenic shock and mediastinal perforation. Although rare, serious complications can occur and the emphasis should be placed on proper supervision and expert consultation during both procedural and maintenance aspects of thoracic interventions. With regard to infection control, trials have failed to show a benefit from prophylactic antibiotics during chest tube insertion and while the chest tube is in place. Limited benefit has been demonstrated in the trauma population where traumatic injury is thought to increase the risk of pleural infection and empyema [44].

Chest tube malposition is the most common complication of tube thoracostomy. Malposition was detected in up to a quarter of patients in one study of chest tubes placed as an emergency [45]. Importantly, chest tube malposition has been associated with persistent pneumothorax. At our institution, clinical or radiographic suspicion prompts CT evaluation of chest tube position and subsequent repositioning or replacement as indicated.

Removal guidelines

Chest tube removal should be performed in a manner that ensures resolution of the pneumothorax and minimizes risk of recurrence. Many clinicians prefer to perform removal in a stepwise fashion, initially removing suction, followed by a trial of water seal, repeat x-ray and removal. Regardless of clinician preference, most experts would agree that the first stage in chest tube removal includes radiographic evidence for the resolution of pneumothorax in the absence of air leak. In cases of fluid drainage, both the quantity and quality of output affect the decision for drain removal. In the setting of thyroid surgery, excessive fluid drainage should prompt thoracic surgical consultation. Generally, daily fluid output should be less than 100–200 mL/day prior to chest tube removal.

Opinion is divided as to the utility of clamping the chest tube prior to removal. Proponents of this approach contend that 4–6 h of clamping prior to removal will identify small air leaks that would otherwise go undetected. At our institution, a period of water seal without evidence of air leak, along with radiographic evidence of lung re-expansion, suffices for chest tube removal. Expert opinion on removal of chest tubes placed for pneumothorax in a patient receiving mechanical ventilation is mixed. The authors prefer to leave drains in place during the course of positive pressure ventilation as long as the patient requires mechanical ventilation.

Removal of the chest tube should be done in a standardized fashion. Prior to removal, supplies should be situated within reach and include a petroleum gauze dressing, gauze covering and tape. Sutures anchoring the chest tube should be freed and if a mattress suture was placed at the incision site at the time of original placement, it should be prepared for closure upon removal. Our preference is for the patient to inspire and perform a Valsalva manoeuvre while the clinician simultaneously and quickly removes the tube and covers the opening with gauze dressing. There are no clear guidelines on postremoval chest x-ray. At our institution, we obtain a postpull chest x-ray 4–6 h after removal of the chest tube unless otherwise indicated. Recurrent pneumothorax after chest tube removal should prompt thoracic surgery consultation for further evaluation.

Discharge and follow-up

All patients treated for pneumothorax should be given clear instructions for return to the nearest emergency medical services should they experience recurrent symptoms. Patients should be advised against high-risk activities such as scuba diving, flying, mountain or other high-elevation activities until further evaluated by their physician. Some experts recommend that patients should abstain from highly strenuous activity until evaluated at the initial follow-up visit. Follow-up should be arranged in advance and chest x-ray obtained for review at that visit. Patients treated with chest tube, pleural drain or needle aspiration should have a repeat chest x-ray and follow-up generally within 1 week, if not sooner.

Conclusion

Pneumothorax in the setting of thyroid surgery is a rare but known complication. The practising surgeon should be knowledgeable about the risks and aware of the clinical signs should an occult pneumothorax present itself. Management strategies should be tailored to the unique patient characteristics as well as the clinical presentation. General guidelines for the management of pneumothorax have been discussed. While these guidelines serve as a basis for treatment, the decision-making process must be informed by the clinician's experience, expertise and

comfort level. Thoracic surgical consultation should be considered at the discretion of the practising surgeon.

References

1 Sahn SA, Heffner JE. Spontaneous pneumothorax. N Engl J Med 2000; 324(12): 868–74.

2 Lee MJ, Kim EK, Kim JM, *et al.* Spontaneous pneumothorax in metastatic thyroid papillary carcinoma. J Clin Oncol 2007; 25; 2616–18.

3 Nenkov R, Rader R, Christosov K, *et al.* Hurthle cell carcinoma of the thyroid with bilateral pneumothorax. Thyroid 2005; 15: 627–8.

4 Slater B, Inabnet WB. Pneumothorax: an uncommon complication of minimally invasive parathyroidectomy. Surg Laparosc Endosc Percutan Tech 2005; 15: 38–40.

5 Page AP. Pneumothorax after thyroidectomy. Lancet 1947; 2: 150.

6 Wilson E. Pneumothorax after thyroidectomy. Lancet 1947; 2: 70.

7 Lee SJ, Lee DJ, Kim MC, *et al.* Pneumothorax in a postanesthetic care unit after right thyroidectomy with left neck dissection – a case report. Korean J Anesthesiol 2010; 59: 429–32.

8 Taniguchi K, Noguchi T, Oda S, *et al.* Bilateral pneumothorax following total thyroidectomy and radical neck resection. Masui 1985; 34: 112–14.

9 Wu Y, Wang J, Wang Z. [Cancer of the thyroid gland with mediastinal extension.] In French. Chirurgie 1998; 123: 74–7.

10 Irabor DO. A giant retrosternal goiter with severe tracheal compression and superior vena cava syndrome: an operative experience. Ethiop Med J 2003; 41: 63–8.

11 Lee SW, Cho SH, Lee JD, *et al.* Bilateral pneumothorax and pneumomediastinum following total thyroidectomy with central neck dissection. Clin Exp Otorhinolaryngol 2008; 1: 49–51.

12 Eltzschig HK, Posner M, Moore FD. The use of readily available equipment in a simple method for intraoperative monitoring of recurrent laryngeal nerve function during thyroid surgery. Arch Surg 2002: 137: 452–7.

13 Gosnell JE, Campbell P, Sidhu S, *et al.* Inadvertent tracheal perforation during thyroidectomy. Br J Surg 2006; 93: 55–6.

14 Fewins J, Simpson CB, Miller FR. Complications of thyroid and parathyroid surgery. Otolaryngol Clin North Am 2003; 36: 189–206.

15 Noppen M, Keukeleire TD. Pneumothorax. Respiration 2008; 76: 121–7.

16 MacIntyre NR. Assist-control mechanical ventilation. In: Fink MP, Abraham E, Vincent JL, Kochanek PM (eds) Textbook of Critical Care, 5th edn. Philadelphia: Elsevier Saunders, 2005: 500–1.

17 Schramel FM, Golding RP, Haakman CD, *et al.* Expiratory chest radiographs do not improve visibility of small apical pneumothoraces by enhanced contrast. Eur Respir J 1996; 9: 406–9.

18 Seow A, Kazerooni EA, Cascade PN, *et al.* Comparison of upright inspiratory and expiratory chest radiographs for detecting pneumothoraces. AJR 1996; 166: 313–16.

19 Schramel FM, Wagenaar M, Sutedja TG, *et al.* Diagnosis of pneumothorax not improved by additional roentgen pictures of the thorax in the expiratory phase. Ned Tijdschr Geneeskd 1995; 139: 131–3.

20 Beres RA, Goodman LR. Pneumothorax: detection with upright versus decubitus radiography. Radiology 1993; 186: 19–26.

21 Tocino IM, Miller MH, Fairfax WR. Distribution of pneumothorax in the supine and semirecumbent critically ill adult. AJR 1985; 144: 901–5.

22 Engdahl O, Toft T, Boe J. Chest radiograph – a poor method for determining the size of a pneumothorax. Chest 1993; 103: 26–9.

23 Light RW. Primary spontaneous pneumothorax in adults. In: Sahn SA (ed) UpToDate. Waltham, MA: UpToDate, 2011.

24 Kircher LT, Swartzel RL. Spontaneous pneumothorax and its treatment. JAMA 1954; 155: 24–9.

25 Kelly AM, Loy J, Tsang AYL, *et al.* Estimating the rate of re-expansion of spontaneous pneumothorax by a formula derived from computed tomography volumetry studies. Emerg Med J 2006; 23: 780–2.

26 De Leyn P, Lismonde M, Ninana V, *et al.* Belgian Society of Pulmonology: guidelines on the management of spontaneous pneumothorax. Acta Chir Belg 2005; 105: 265–7.

27 Baumann MH, Strange C, Heffner JE, *et al.* Management of spontaneous pneumothorax: an American College of Chest Physicians Delphi consensus statement. Chest 2001; 119: 590–602.

28 MacDuff A, Arnold A, Harvey J, BTS Pleural Disease Guideline Group. Management of spontaneous pneumothorax: British Thoracic Society pleural disease guideline 2010. Thorax 2010; 65(Suppl 2): ii18–ii31.

29 Northfield TC. Oxygen therapy for spontaneous pneumothorax. BMJ 1971; 4: 86–8.

30 Wakai A, O'Sullivan RG, McCabe G. Simple aspiration versus intercostal tube drainage for primary spontaneous pneumothorax in adults. Cochrane Database Syst Rev 2007; 1: CD004479.

31 Devanand A, Koh MS, Ong TH, *et al.* Simple aspiration versus chest-tube insertion in the management of primary spontaneous pneumothorax: a systematic review. Respir Med 2004; 98(7): 579–90.

32 Benton IJ, Benfield GF. Comparison of a large and small-calibre tube drain for managing spontaneous pneumothoraces. Respir Med 2009; 103(10): 1436–40.

33 Fysh ETH, Smith NA, Lee YCG. Optimal chest drain size: the rise of the small-bore pleural catheter. Semin Respir Crit Care Med 2010; 31: 760–8.

34 Baumann MH. Treatment of spontaneous pneumothorax. Curr Opin Pulmon Med 2000; 6: 275–80.

35 Doelken, P. Tube thoracostomy. In: Sahn SA, Hilary S, Wolfson AB (eds) UpToDate. Waltham, MA: , UpToDate, 2011.

36 Hassani B, Foote J, Borgundvaag B. Outpatient management of primary spontaneous pneumothorax in the emergency department of a community hospital using a small-bore catheter and a Heimlich valve. Acad Emerg Med 2009; 16(6): 513–18.

37 Munnell ER. Thoracic drainage. Ann Thorac Surg 1997; 63: 1497–502.

38 Cerfolio RJ, Tummala RP, Holman WL, *et al.* A prospective algorithm for the management of air leaks after pulmonary resection. Ann Thorac Surg 1998; 66: 1726–31.

39 Cerfolio RJ, Bryant AS. The management of chest tubes after pulmonary resection. Thorac Surg Clin 2010; 20: 399–405.

40 Schoenenberger RA, Haefeli WE, Weiss P, *et al.* Timing of invasive procedures in therapy for primary and secondary spontaneous pneumothorax. Arch Surg 1991; 126: 764–6.

41 Chee CB, Abisheganaden J, Yeo JK, *et al.* Persistent air-leak in spontaneous pneumothorax – clinical course and outcome. Respir Med 1998; 92: 757–61.

42 Oliveira FH, Cataneo DC, Ruiz RL, *et al.* Persistent pleuropulmonary air leak treated with autologous blood: results from a university hospital and review of literature. Respiration 2010; 79(4): 302–6.

43 Ozpolat B. Autologous blood patch pleurodesis in the management of prolonged air leak. Thorac Cardiovasc Surg 2010; 58(1): 52–4.

44 Gonzalez RP, Holevar MR. Role of prophylactic antibiotics for tube thoracostomy in chest trauma. Am Surg 1998; 64: 617.

45 Baldt MM, Bankier AA, German PS, *et al.* Complications after emergency tube thoracostomy: assessment with CT. Radiology 1995; 195: 539.

PART VI

Postoperative Complications

CHAPTER 24

The Recurrent Laryngeal Nerve

Michele P. Morrison[1] and Gregory N. Postma[2]

[1] Department of Otolaryngology – Head and Neck Surgery, Naval Medical Center Portsmouth, Portsmouth, VA, USA

[2] Department of Otolaryngology, Georgia Health Sciences University, Augusta, GA, USA

Introduction

Recurrent laryngeal nerve (RLN) damage is a well-recognized complication after thyroidectomy. The incidence of permanent RLN paralysis from thyroid surgery varies from 0% to 3.5% [1]. The risk is higher after surgery for a thyroid malignancy [2]. Most studies advocate routine identification of the RLN during thyroid surgery to prevent injury [3]. Documentation of pre- and postoperative vocal fold mobility via flexible laryngoscopy is always recommended [2,4].

Unilateral vocal fold immobility or paresis can lead to a variety of problems including aspiration, dysphonia, vocal fatigue and dyspnoea. If a patient has bilateral vocal fold immobility, they will have dyspnoea with exertion and often at rest, which can result in an airway emergency.

Pathophysiology

The concepts of neural injury and regeneration are essential to understanding functional patient outcomes. Neurapraxia involves a temporary blockage in nerve conduction but complete recovery of function usually occurs within several weeks. Axonotmesis involves disruption of the myelin sheath with an intact nerve resulting in retrograde degeneration and then spontaneous regrowth. This can lead to decreased muscle function and poor vocal quality. Neurotmesis involves disruption of the endoneurial, perineurial and/or epineurial sheath, which leads to regrowth via alternative pathways, causing synkinesis. Vocal fold synkinesis is caused by misdirected reinnervation leading to a vocal fold with muscle tone but which remains immobile on adductory and/or abductory tasks. Axonal regrowth is a slow process and, depending on the location of nerve injury, may take up to 12 months before considered complete [1].

Evaluation of vocal fold hypomobility

Patients suspected of having RLN injury should undergo laryngoscopy with stroboscopy. Findings consistent with vocal fold hypomobility include increased amplitude or an asymmetrical 'chasing' mucosal wave on stroboscopy, decreased lateral movement of vocal fold with the 'ee-sniff' manoeuvre (performed by asking the patient to alternately sniff and then say 'ee' repetitively), glottic gap, bowing of affected vocal fold and altered height of the vocal fold. Vocal fold positioning in patients with RLN injury is variable; the vocal fold may be median, paramedian or lateral (cadaveric). Vocal fold position does *not* correlate with neural injury [5,6].

Aerodynamic measures such as maximal phonation time exist; however, results vary based on who is administering the test and patient effort, and are therefore unreliable. Although outside the scope of this chapter, it should be mentioned that several validated indices are

Thyroid Surgery: Preventing and Managing Complications, First Edition. Edited by Paolo Miccoli, David J. Terris, Michele N. Minuto and Melanie W. Seybt.

available to measure the degree to which a patient is affected by their vocal complaints. These include the Voice Handicap Index (VHI), the VHI-10 and the Glottal Function Index (GFI) [7–9].

Laryngeal electromyography (LEMG) can be used to help determine prognosis for recovery of RLN function. LEMG is usually performed jointly by a laryngologist (who positions the needle) and an electromyographer. Electromyographic responses include insertional activity and recruitment. Insertional activity is the burst of electrical activity exhibited as motor unit action potentials (MUAPs) upon insertion of the EMG needle. This response is present in normal and partially denervated muscle. Recruitment is tested by having the patient phonate to activate the muscle; normally a brisk recruitment pattern is seen [10]. Fibrillations, which are spontaneous muscle fibre action potentials at rest, are evidence of denervation. Fibrillations can be preceded by positive sharp waves, which also indicate acute denervation. Large polyphasic MUAPs on LEMG indicate reinnervation [10]. LEMG is most predictive if performed 6–7 weeks after injury.

Munin *et al.* used the presence or absence of recruitment and spontaneous activity as criteria to determine RLN recovery. They looked at 31 cases of vocal fold paralysis that underwent LEMG between 3 weeks to 6 months after symptom onset. The presence or absence of recruitment and spontaneous activity were their principal criteria. Good prognosis required normal recruitment and no spontaneous activity, and prognosis declined with declining recruitment. RLN function returned in four of six patients (67%) with good prognosis and failed to return in 20 of 25 patients (80%) with fair or poor prognosis, yielding sensitivity of 91% and specificity of 44% [11]. LEMG remains somewhat subjective, especially in quantifying neural damage and degree of recovery; further research still needs to be performed in this area [10,11].

Treatment options

When considering the various treatment options for vocal fold hypomobility, it is critical to ascertain a patient's vocal needs (i.e. are they a singer, teacher, etc.?) [12,13].

Treatment of unilateral vocal fold paralysis (UVFP) can be subdivided into several categories:
• No treatment.

• Observation for 12 months – intervention if continued dysphonia at that time.
• Speech pathology referral for vocal exercises and compensatory manoeuvres.
• Surgical intervention:
  – temporary: injection augmentation
  – permanent: medialization laryngoplasty, arytenoid adduction, laryngeal reinnervation, and possibly injection augmentation with selected substances.

In a patient with low vocal demands and no aspiration symptoms, observation may be appropriate. Some patients may not desire any surgical intervention once it is explained to them that the likelihood of recovery is high and may decide to pursue speech therapy. Of course, all of these therapies overlap. Someone who has a high vocal demand or is aspirating is a good candidate for temporary injection augmentation to get them through the first 3 months and then re-evaluate for improvement or compensation. The perfect injectable would be inexpensive, inert, ready off the shelf and biocompatible. Temporary injectables include bovine gelatin, collagen-based products, carboxymethylcellulose and hyaluronic acid gel. Injections can be performed in the office setting under local anaesthesia or in the operating room under general anaesthesia. Benefits of in-office injection include immediate voicing to know if injecting enough material, patient convenience, decreased cost and no risk of general anaesthesia. In-office techniques include per oral, percutaneous via translaryngeal, cricothyroid membrane or via the thyrohyoid membrane. All of these techniques are well tolerated by patients [12–14].

Injections under general anaesthesia allow for more precise injection and are performed through a laryngoscope using either binocular microscopy or a 0° Hopkins telescope. It is crucial that injection is not superficial – the ideal injection is at a point where a transverse line from the tip of the vocal process laterally intersects the superior arcuate line (Figure 24.1). The depth of injection is usually 3–5 mm. Overinjection is recommended for most injectable substances due to absorption of carrier. Patients may undergo a repeat injection augmentation if still symptomatic [12,14].

If no neural recovery occurs, patients may opt to undergo a more 'permanent' injection of either calcium hydroxyapatite or autologous fat. Calcium hydroxyapatite has been shown to last up to 18 months while fat, after initial absorption, lasts years [15]. The patient must

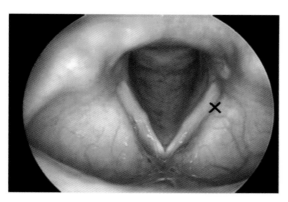

Figure 24.1 Correct injection site for vocal fold augmentation.

be under general anaesthesia for autologous fat harvest and injection, otherwise techniques are the same as above [16].

Patients could also opt for a medialization laryngoplasty. This surgery is performed under conscious sedation and involves an external neck incision. A thyroid cartilage window is made and an implant is placed to medialize the affected vocal fold, having the patient phonate while endoscopically visualizing the vocal fold to determine correct implant placement. Common implant materials include silastic, silicone and Gore-Tex [17,18]. Arytenoid adduction may also need to be performed at the same setting if there is a significant posterior glottal gap after laryngoplasty is performed [18].

Laryngeal reinnervation should also be considered if there are no signs of reinnervation after a period of 6–12 months. This technique can prevent the loss of thyroarytenoid muscle tone and bulk over time which can affect the long-term results seen with the previously mentioned laryngoplasty techniques. It is also a technically simple procedure. The disadvantages include requirement for general anaesthesia, prolonged time to voice improvement and requirement of intact donor and recipient nerve. The most commonly used donor nerve is the ansa cervicalis. Lorenz *et al.* performed this procedure on 46 patients, all of whom had improved vocal roughness, breathiness and vocal strain. They also had improvement in glottic closure and supraglottic compensatory effort [19]. Wang *et al.* found similar results in their 56 patients with UVFP who underwent laryngeal reinnervation with the contralateral ansa cervicalis nerve [20]. Improvement is usually seen by 4 months [21].

Treatment of bilateral vocal fold paralysis includes:
- tracheotomy
- endoscopic suture lateralization
- posterior transverse cordotomy
- medial arytenoidectomy
- total arytenoidectomy
- Botox injection
- arytenoid abduction
- laryngeal pacing.

Thyroidectomy is the leading cause of bilateral vocal fold immobility (BVFI) in adults (57%). Often BVFI necessitates emergency intubation or tracheotomy. Tracheotomy can be life saving; however, due to the decreased quality of life, many patients will opt for a laryngeal airway surgical enlargement procedure to relieve the airway obstruction caused by BVFI [22]. Goals of treatment include achieving a safe and adequate airway, preservation of voice quality, functional swallow and laryngeal competence [23]. Surgical approaches usually sacrifice voice quality in exchange for an improvement in breathing [22].

In early cases of BVFI when nerve recovery is expected, a temporizing method is the endoscopic suture lateralization technique. This involves general anaesthesia and either jet ventilation or a small endotracheal tube. Under laryngoscopic guidance, lateral fixation sutures are pushed through the larynx below the posterior third of the vocal fold and another suture is placed above the posterior third of the vocal fold. A second suture is placed in a similar fashion 2 mm anterior to the first suture. An incision is made between the two sutures after they have been pushed through the thyroid cartilage and neck skin in order to bury the suture or they can be tied over a button. If nerve function returns, the sutures can be removed and patients recover their normal voices. If nerve function does not return or if LEMG demonstrates poor prognosis, patients will likely require a more permanent procedure [24].

Posterior transverse cordotomy is a permanent procedure to enlarge the posterior glottis. This surgery is performed under general anaesthesia either with jet ventilation or a laser-safe endotracheal tube. The larynx is exposed with a laryngoscope and the CO_2 laser is used to make an incision anterior to the vocal process (avoiding exposure of cartilage). The vocal fold is separated from the vocal process and the cut is often extended into the false vocal fold tissue (usually 4 mm) [22,23].

Medial arytenoidectomy is performed with a similar set-up as mentioned for posterior transverse cordotomy. The medial portion of the arytenoid cartilage is ablated with the CO_2 laser (approximately 3 mm in width), preserving the vocal process. One must be careful not to violate the interarytenoid area to prevent posterior glottic stenosis. If further enlargement of the posterior glottis is necessary, this can progress to a total arytenoidectomy by removing arytenoid tissue until the operative defect is flush with the wall of the cricoid ring posteriorly and laterally. Voice results and aspiration risk tend to be better with posterior transverse cordotomy and medial arytenoidectomy than total arytenoidectomy [22,25,26]. Bosley et al. compared transverse cordotomy and medial arytenoidectomy for treatment of BVFI and found that both are equally effective in improving laryngeal airway restriction symptoms and both have a low incidence of postoperative voice and swallowing complications [22].

Botulinum toxin (Botox) causes a temporary loss of muscle tone by blocking neurotransmission. Its first reported use in the larynx was for the management of focal laryngeal dystonias. Ekbom et al. performed a retrospective chart review looking at patients with longstanding BVFI who had been treated with Botox injection into both the thyroarytenoid (TA) and lateral cricoarytenoid (LCA) muscles under electromyographic guidance. They had 11 patients in the study, six of whom had bilateral RLN injury from prior thyroidectomy. Overall, the average dose of Botox injected into each vocal fold was 2.5 units. The average time period for improved inspiration after injection was 11 weeks. Ten of the 11 patients reported improved inspiration after injection and pursued repeat injections. The exact mechanism is unknown but it is hypothesized that the chemical denervation of the TA/LCA complex produces a somewhat flaccid vocal fold, allowing the reinnervated abductor fibres to have an unopposed affect on vocal fold position. This treatment option is usually used to allow patients to consider their treatment options and wait for potential functional recovery. It may be continued in patients who refuse other treatment options [27].

Arytenoid abduction can also be considered to relieve airway obstruction. This technique is performed under general anaesthesia through a neck incision exposing the posterior border of the thyroid cartilage. The inferior constrictor muscle and pyriform sinus are separated from the thyroid cartilage, thus exposing the muscular process

of the arytenoid cartilage. A multi-stranded permanent suture is placed through the muscular process and tied securely. Direct laryngoscopy is performed to ensure abduction of the vocal fold with inferior traction on the suture. The suture is then secured to the inferior cornu of the thyroid cartilage and the incision is closed. It is reversible but technically more challenging than the endoscopic procedures described previously [28].

A discussion regarding treatment of BVFI would not be complete without mentioning laryngeal pacing. This technique involves electrical stimulation of the posterior cricoarytenoid muscle during inspiration, leading to abduction of the vocal folds. The concept of using functional neuromuscular stimulation to reanimate the laryngeal muscles was introduced by Zealear & Dedo [29]. Zealear et al. described the first attempt to electrically pace a paralysed human larynx in 1996. An electrode was implanted into the posterior cricoarytenoid muscle, which was then connected to an external pacemaker device. The pacemaker co-ordinated stimulation with inspiration, causing abduction of the vocal folds with inspiration. The authors found the degree of abduction was sufficient to improve ventilation [30]. This technique is still not widespread and studies are ongoing.

Conclusion

Various methods can be used to treat unilateral or bilateral RLN injury. The key point to remember is that treatment needs to be tailored to each patient's unique vocal and airway needs.

References

1 Hartl DM, Travagli JP, Leboulleux S, et al. Clinical review: current concepts in the management of unilateral recurrent laryngeal nerve paralysis after thyroid surgery. J Clin Endocrinol Metab 2005; 90: 3084–8.

2 Prim MP, de Diego JI, Hardisson D, Madero R, et al. Factors related to nerve injury and hypocalcemia in thyroid gland surgery. Otolaryngol Head Neck Surg 2001; 124: 111–14.

3 O'Neill JP, Fenton JE. The recurrent laryngeal nerve in thyroid surgery. Surgeon 2008; 6: 373–7.

4 Herranz-Gonzalez J, Gavilan J, Matinez-Vidal J et al. Complications following thyroid surgery. Arch Otolaryngol Head Neck Surg 1991; 117: 516–18.

5 Koufman JA, Walker FO, Joharji GM. The cricothyroid muscle does not influence vocal fold position in laryngeal paralysis. Laryngoscope 1995; 105: 368–72.

6 Woodson GE. Configuration of the glottis in laryngeal paralysis. II: Animal experiments. Laryngoscope 1993; 103: 1235–41.

7 Jacobson B, Johson A, Grywalsky C, et al. The Voice Handicap Index (VHI): development and validation. Am J Speech Lang Pathol 1997; 6: 66–70.

8 Rosen CA, Lee AS, Osborne J, et al. Development and validation of the Voice Handicap Index–10. Laryngoscope 2004; 114: 1549–56.

9 Bach KK, Belafsky PC, Wasylik K, et al. Validity and reliability of the glottal function index. Arch Otolaryngol Head Neck Surg 2005; 131(11): 961–4.

10 Sulica L, Blitzer A. Electromyography and the immobile vocal fold. Otolaryngol Clin North Am 2004; 37: 59–74.

11 Munin MC, Rosen CA, Zullo T. Utility of laryngeal electromyography in predicting recovery after vocal fold paralysis. Arch Phys Med Rehabil 2003; 84: 1150–3.

12 Rosen CA. Phonosurgical vocal fold injection: indications and techniques. Oper Tech Otolaryngol Head Neck Surg 1998; 9: 203–9.

13 Sulica L, Rosen CA, Postma GN, et al. Current practice in injection augmentation of the vocal folds: indications, treatment principles, techniques, and complications. Laryngoscope 2010; 120(2): 319–25.

14 Simpson CB, Amin MR. Office-based procedures for the voice. Ear Nose Throat J 2004; 83(Suppl): 6–9.

15 Rosen C, Garner-Schmidt J, Casiano R, et al. Vocal fold augmentation with calcium hydroxylapatite (CaHA). Otolaryngol Head Neck Surg 2007; 136: 198–204.

16 Brandenburg JH. Vocal cord augmentation with autogenous fat. Laryngoscope 1992; 102: 485–500.

17 Netterville JL, Stone RE, Luken ES, et al. Silastic medialization and arytenoids adduction: the Vanderbilt experience. A review of 116 phonosurgical procedures. Ann Otol Rhinol Laryngol 1993; 102: 413–24.

18 Cohen JT, Bates DD, Postma GN. Revision Gore-Tex medialization laryngoplasty. Otolaryngol Head Neck Surg 2004; 131: 236–40.

19 Lorenz RR, Esclamado RM, Teker AM, et al. Ansa cervicalis-to-recurrent laryngeal nerve anastomosis for unilateral vocal fold paralysis: experience of a single institution. Ann Otol Rhinol Laryngol 2008; 117(1): 40–5.

20 Wang W, Chen S, Chen D, et al. Contralateral ansa cervicalis-to-recurrent laryngeal nerve anastomosis for unilateral vocal fold paralysis: a long-term outcome analysis of 56 cases. Laryngoscope 2011; 121: 1027–34.

21 Lee WT, Milstein C, Hicks D, et al. Results of ansa to recurrent laryngeal nerve reinnervation. Otolaryngol Head Neck Surg 2007; 136: 450–4.

22 Bosley B, Rosen CA, Simpson CB, et al. Medial arytenoidectomy versus transverse cordotomy as a treatment for bilateral vocal fold paralysis. Ann Otol Rhinol Laryngol 2005; 114: 922–6.

23 Dennis DP, Kashima H. Carbon dioxide laser posterior cordectomy for treatment of bilateral vocal cord paralysis. Ann Otol Rhinol Laryngol 1989; 98: 930–4.

24 Lichtenberger G. Reversible lateralization of the paralyzed vocal cord without tracheostomy. Ann Otol Rhinol Laryngol 2002; 111: 21–6.

25 Crumley RL. Endoscopic laser medial arytenoidectomy for airway management in bilateral laryngeal paralysis. Ann Otol Rhinol Laryngol 1993; 102: 81–4.

26 Hillel AD, Benninger M, Blitzer A, et al. Evaluation and management of bilateral vocal cord immobility. Otolaryngol Head Neck Surg 1999; 121: 760–5.

27 Ekbom DC, Garrett CG, Yung KC, et al. Botulinum toxin injections for new onset bilateral vocal fold motion impairment in adults. Laryngoscope 2010; 120: 758–63.

28 Woodson G, Weiss T. Arytenoid abduction for dynamic rehabilitation of bilateral laryngeal paralysis. Ann Otol Rhinol Laryngol 2007; 116(7): 483–90.

29 Zealear DL, Dedo HH. Control of paralyzed axial muscles by electrical stimulation. Acta Otolaryngol 1977; 83: 514–27.

30 Zealear DL, Rainey CL, Netterville JL, et al. Electrical pacing of the paralyzed human larynx. Ann Otol Rhinol Laryngol 1996; 105: 689–93.

CHAPTER 25

The Parathyroids

Claudio Marcocci and Luisella Cianferotti

Department of Endocrinology, Unit of Endocrinology and Bone Metabolism, University of Pisa, Pisa, Italy

Introduction

The parathyroids are four small endocrine glands which lie on the posterolateral capsule of the thyroid lobes. Their number and location may vary among normal individuals [1]. The position of the upper parathyroids is relatively constant, while the lower glands can migrate during development along a line from the lateral neck regions down to the mediastinum. Because of their location, the parathyroids and the thyroid share the same blood supply. About 90–95% of lower parathyroid arteries and 80% of upper parathyroid arteries originate from the inferior thyroid artery. In the remaining cases, the superior parathyroid artery can receive some to all supply from the superior thyroid artery or from anastomotic branches between the inferior and the superior thyroid arteries.

The particular position of the parathyroids, their size and delicate blood supply make injury to the parathyroid glands one of the major complications of thyroid surgery. The preservation of parathyroid glands is a key event during thyroid surgery. First, the glands have to be identified at the time of thyroidectomy. Then, in order to maintain their blood supply, it is important to ligate thyroid arteries as close to the thyroid gland as possible, distal to the origin of parathyroid vessels. If parathyroid glands are accidentally devascularized, removed or simply nicked, various grades of parathyroid insufficiency may develop [2].

Parathyroid physiology and calcium metabolism

The parathyroid glands secrete parathyroid hormone (PTH), one of the major hormones involved in the control of mineral ion homeostasis [3]. The main task of PTH is to maintain calcium within a narrow range in the extracellular compartment. Calcium in the blood is in part bound to plasma proteins (45%, mainly albumin), in part complexed to small anions (10%, such as phosphate, bicarbonate), and in part ionized or free (45%). Only the ionized calcium is able to shift between different compartments, enter into the intracellular space and activate cellular processes. Ionized calcium concentration is sensed by the calcium-sensing receptor on the parathyroid glands and controls PTH secretion. A rise in ionized calcium will be followed by a decrease in PTH synthesis and secretion. The opposite occurs when there is a drop in the ionized calcium. Although ionized calcium (Ca^{++}, reference range 1.13–1.32 mmol/L or 4.5–5.3 mg/dL) is the metabolically active form, total calcium (reference range 2.05–2.55 mmol/L, 8.2–10.2 mg/dL), rather than the ionized fraction, is commonly measured in clinical practice. Since almost half of the total calcium is bound to albumin, albumin concentration may affect serum calcium levels. For a better estimate of the effective serum calcium

Thyroid Surgery: Preventing and Managing Complications, First Edition. Edited by Paolo Miccoli, David J. Terris, Michele N. Minuto and Melanie W. Seybt.

concentration, calcaemia should be corrected by means of the following formula:

Corrected total calcium =
Total calcium[a] + [0.8 × (4 − Serum albumin[b])]

[a] Calcium expressed as mg/dL; [b] serum albumin expressed as g/dL.

Thus, hypoalbuminaemia observed in patients with several chronic illnesses, malnourished or hospitalized may be responsible for a reduction in total serum calcium concentration.

PTH increases total calcium levels by means of direct and indirect mechanisms. PTH directly promotes renal tubular calcium reabsorption and bone resorption. Moreover, it induces the renal 1α-hydroxylase, responsible for synthesis of the biologically active form of vitamin D (1,25(OH)$_2$D) which, in turn, increases intestinal active calcium absorption. Since PTH also increases renal phosphate excretion, low PTH levels will result in hypocalcaemia and hyperphosphataemia or high-normal serum phosphate [4].

Surgical hypoparathyroidism: definition, causes and classification

Hypoparathyroidism (HPT) is the combination of symptoms due to inadequate production of PTH leading to hypocalcaemia. It rarely occurs as a spontaneous condition. In the majority of cases it is due to unintentional damage or removal of parathyroid glands at the time of neck surgery (mainly thyroid and parathyroid surgery), and usually manifests within a few days after the operation. Postsurgical HPT is the most common cause of acquired HPT. During thyroid surgery, parathyroid glands can be devascularized by ligation of thyroid arteries proximal to the origin of parathyroid arteries (i.e. proximal ligation of vascular pedicles), thermally damaged by accidental electrocoagulation by heat induction using an electric scalpel, and, rarely, inadvertently removed, damaged or simply nicked [4,5].

Postsurgical HPT can be transient (t-HPT) or permanent (p-HPT). t-HPT is usually due to reversible parathyroid ischaemia and commonly resolves within a few weeks, but may persist up to 6 months after surgery. p-HPT is defined as insufficient PTH to maintain normocalcaemia, which persists 6 months after surgery.

The occurrence of either t- or p-HPT varies according to the experience of the thyroid surgeon and the number of total thyroidectomies performed annually [6,7]. Surgeons are 'experienced' when they have a prior personal performance of at least 100 total thyroidectomies [8,9]. Longitudinal and retrospective studies indicate that the rates of t- and p-HPT after thyroidectomy in tertiary referral endocrine centres with experienced surgeons can be as low as 5.4–9.6% and 0.5–1.7%, respectively [9–14]. In a recent multicentre, register-based retrospective Scandinavian study assessing the rate of complications after thyroid surgery, t-HPT occurred in 5.5% of patients and p-HPT in 4.4% [15].

Transient HPT can be asymptomatic. Thus, its prevalence can be underestimated when serum calcium is not routinely assessed, and only measured if hypocalcaemic symptoms are present.

Besides surgical experience, the rate and duration of postoperative HPT depend also on the degree of thyroid resection and underlying thyroid pathology. The risk for postoperative HPT is higher following thyroidectomy for retrosternal goitres, Graves' disease, thyroid cancer and radical neck lymph node dissections [2].

Hypoparathyroidism develops when less than one parathyroid gland is functioning and significant damage has occurred, given the large parathyroid reserve. Therefore, lobectomy rarely causes hypoparathyroidism. Conversely, subtotal, near-total or total thyroidectomy and repeated neck surgery for recurrent or persistent disease are associated with a higher risk for HPT, since all four parathyroid glands are potentially placed at risk of injury.

Other factors, such as low 25-hydroxyvitamin D levels, magnesium depletion and high bone turnover state, due to preoperative severe hyperthyroidism or hyperparathyroidism, may contribute to development of postoperative symptomatic hypocalcaemia. In the latter case, also called 'hungry bone syndrome', surgical cure of the underlying disease leads to a rapid normalization of bone resorption, while a relatively increased rate of bone formation persists for several weeks. This will account for a persistently increased calcium influx into bone, leading to a long-lasting drop in serum calcium levels [16,17]. Thus, the hungry bone syndrome is characterized by prolonged symptomatic hypocalcaemia and mild decrease of serum phosphate. It may occur even in the presence of a normal parathyroid function.

Hypoparathyroidism: evaluation and clinical manifestations

The clinical manifestations of postoperative HPT are directly related to the severity and speed of onset of hypocalcaemia. Postoperative hypocalcaemia can range from asymptomatic, if the decrease in serum calcium is mild, to a severe, life-threatening condition that requires rapid and intensive treatment.

Biochemical and hormonal evaluation

Postsurgical HPT typically develops within a few days after thyroidectomy. Usually, patients become hypocalcaemic on the first postoperative day but calcium levels may reach the lowest value even 3 days after surgery. Thus hypocalcaemia can become clinically manifest even 3–4 days after the operation in patients who were almost asymptomatic before [18]. Patients with t-HPT may be asymptomatic. Therefore, all patients who have had total or subtotal thyroidectomy should have their serum calcium measured, independently from the presence of symptoms.

The measurement of albumin-corrected serum calcium or ionized calcium, where available, in the perioperative period is a reliable method of excluding or confirming postsurgical HPT. Additional biochemical measurements, which are not mandatory, include the assessment of intact PTH and phosphate levels to confirm the diagnosis. PTH levels are low or inappropriately normal in the setting of hypocalcaemia. In this regard, a recent study describes eight patients with p-HPT, who had PTH levels in the low-normal range. This finding is likely explained by the inability of the residual functioning parathyroid tissue to secrete sufficient PTH to restore calcium homeostasis [19]. The authors conclude that it is better to use the term *parathyroid insufficiency* instead of HPT to define postoperative hypocalcaemia. Serum phosphate is high or in the high-normal range because of the lack of the phosphaturic action of PTH. The finding of low postoperative phosphate and high PTH in the setting of hypocalcaemia points to a hungry bone syndrome.

Measurements of serum magnesium and 25-hydroxyvitamin D levels can be considered as second-level diagnostic tests [20]. Co-existing hypomagnesaemia can further decrease PTH secretion and induce peripheral PTH resistance, thus exacerbating and prolonging hypocalcaemic symptoms.

Symptoms and signs

Hypocalcaemia causes neuromuscular irritability, neurological and electrocardiographic alterations. Symptoms of neuromuscular irritability are most common in the setting of acute hypocalcaemia. They vary from numbness and tingling in the fingertips, toes and circumoral region in mild hypocalcaemia to paraesthesias of the upper and lower extremities in moderate hypocalcaemia. In the most severe forms tetanic muscle cramps can occur in the form of carpal spasms or diffuse tetany. Some patients can experience bronchospam and laryngospasm with acute respiratory failure. Neurological symptoms such as confusion, disorientation, delirium or seizure can also occur. Cardiac abnormalities of hypocalcaemia consist of prolonged QT interval on electrocardiogram, arrhythmias and congestive heart failure in the most severe cases [21].

On physical examination, the Chvostek and Trousseau signs,which are related to neuromuscular irritability (Figure 25.1), may unveil a latent tetany [21]. The Chvostek sign consists of a contraction of ipsilateral facial muscles evoked by tapping the facial nerve anterior to the external auditory meatus (Figure 25.1a,b). It has low sensitivity and specificity; it has been reported that 29% of confirmed hypoparathyroid patients display a negative Chvostek sign. Moreover, the Chvostek sign is present in up to 10–15% of normal individuals. Thus it is important to assess this sign preoperatively. The Trousseau sign consists of a carpal spasm (extension of the wrist, extension of interphalangeal joints, adduction of the thumb) generated by inflation of a sphygmomanometer 20 mmHg above systolic blood pressure for 3–5 min (Figure 25.1c). Hyperventilation can be used to increase the sensitivity of this manoeuvre. Hyperventilation causes a metabolic alkalosis that, in turn, will increase the binding of calcium to albumin, decreasing the available ionized calcium.

Clinical signs often related to congenital or chronic hypocalcaemic syndromes, such as brain calcifications, electroencephalogram alterations, ectodermal changes and dysmorphic abnormalities are typically absent in postsurgical HPT, also in the permanent forms.

Predictive factors of postsurgical hypoparathyroidism

Various attempts have been made to select perioperative factors to identify patients at risk for postoperative

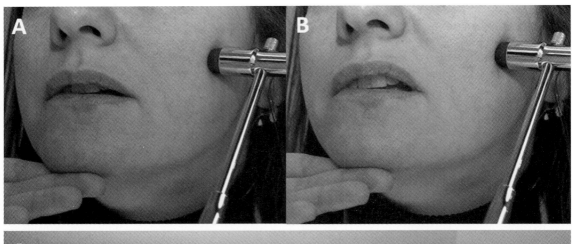

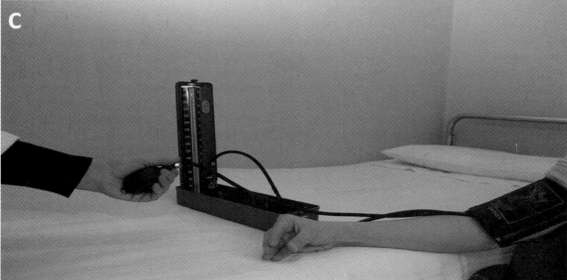

Figure 25.1 (a,b) Chvostek sign and (c) Trousseau sign evoking latent tetany.

hypocalcaemia. An early diagnosis of postsurgical HPT would allow prompt management. Several approaches have been proposed to predict the occurrence of postsurgical HPT. However, there is a lack of consensus about a standard protocol to be used for predicting hypocalcaemia after thyroid surgery. As stated above, hypocalcaemia usually presents on the first day after surgery. Thus, serum calcium level 1 day after surgery is a reliable index of postoperative parathyroid status [22]. However, hypocalcaemia can occasionally develop or worsen a few days after surgery. For this reason, albumin-corrected

serum calcium levels should also be assessed on day 3–4 after surgery. Conversely, plasma PTH promptly decreases soon after surgery because of its short half-life [18].

The rise in serum calcium levels in samples obtained 6 and 12 h after thyroidectomy was a strong predictor (predictive value of 100%) of normocalcaemia in a retrospective study [23]. In those patients in whom calcium did not increase, values ≥ 8 mg/dL 12 h after surgery excluded further development of hypocalcaemia. The authors proposed that these patients could be safely discharged from hospital 12 h after surgery.

Other authors have evaluated the possibility of predicting hypocalcaemia by means of PTH values on the first postoperative day, in combination with serum calcium levels on the second postoperative day [14]. Serum PTH levels less than 15 pg/mL together with serum calcium levels less than 1.9 mmol/L were associated with an increased risk of developing hypocalcaemia after thyroidectomy.

Several studies suggest that measurement of PTH levels intraoperatively or immediately after surgery can be used as a clue to predict HPT, either alone or in combination with postoperative calcium levels [24–26]. Intact PTH values less than 10 pg/mL early in the postoperative period (i.e. 1 h after surgery) predicted the decrease in serum calcium as measured 1 day after thyroidectomy. In other studies, PTH less than 10 pg/mL 1–4 h after surgery or a drop of PTH greater than 75% intraoperatively or 65% 6 h after surgery was used to predict hypocalcaemia [27–31], with high sensitivity (92.3–100%) and specificity (72–99%). In a recent meta-analysis, a drop of PTH greater than 65% after thyroidectomy displayed high sensitivity (96.4%) and specificity (91.4%) in detecting postoperative hypocalcaemia [32]. Therefore, these authors suggested that measurement of PTH in the immediate postoperative period could be used to recognize patients at risk for hypocalcaemia and initiate appropriate treatment, thus preventing hypocalcaemic crisis.

Prevention of postsurgical hypoparathyroidism

Prevention of postoperative HPT is important since hypocalcaemia can delay discharge from hospital and increase morbidity after thyroidectomy.

The best way to preserve parathyroid gland function is to identify the glands and maintain their blood supply during surgery [10]. As already stated, it is particularly relevant to select an experienced thyroid surgeon. In addition, other factors can be assessed preoperatively and appropriately corrected to prevent or limit the development of symptomatic hypocalcaemia. Factors such as poor vitamin D status (as measured by 25-hydroxyvitamin D levels) and magnesium deficiency can worsen postsurgical hypocalcaemia. Thus, it is advisable to check vitamin D status and magnesium concentration before surgery,

particularly when the risk of postsurgical HPT is high (extensive neck surgery, total thyroidectomy or reintervention) [5]. If the level of 25-hydroxyvitamin D is lower than 20 ng/mL, which according to the recent consensus [33] is necessary to maintain a normal mineral ion homeostasis, appropriate supplementation with cholecalciferol (vitamin D3), ergocalciferol (vitamin D2) or calcifediol (25-hydroxyvitamin D) would be needed.

The prevalence of hypomagnesaemia (2% in a primary care cohort) can be as high as 65% in intensive care units, mainly in the case of protracted diarrhoea, poor nutrition in the case of chronic alcohol abuse, use of diuretics or chemotherapeutics [20,21]. A concomitant hypomagnesaemia can delay recognition of hypocalcaemia and make it difficult to correct. Thus, it is important to optimize magnesium reserve before surgery.

When the risk of postoperative HPT is high, preventive therapy with calcitriol should be administered prior to surgery and maintained afterwards to prevent symptomatic hypocalcaemia.

Management of postsurgical hypoparathyroidism

Formal guidelines for the management of HPT are not available. However, some common procedures exist in clinical practice and depend upon the severity and speed of onset of hypocalcaemia.

Medical treatment of acute hypoparathyroidism

Symptomatic HPT is an endocrine emergency and requires prompt treatment with calcium and active vitamin D metabolites (Figure 25.2). According to the degree and speed of onset of hypocalcaemia and the severity of symptoms, intravenous (IV) calcium may be needed until an oral regimen can be established [2]. No guidelines on the management of postsurgical HPT are available. Our personal approach is depicted in Figure 25.2.

Severe hypocalcaemia (serum calcium less than 1.75 mmol/L or 7 mg/dL) with overt neuromuscular irritability (with severe tetany, laryngospasm, bronchospasm, mental confusion) usually requires treatment in hospital, aggressively administering IV calcium [2]. However, latent tetany, as unveiled by signs of hypocalcaemia and/or serum calcium values less than 1.9 mmol/L (or

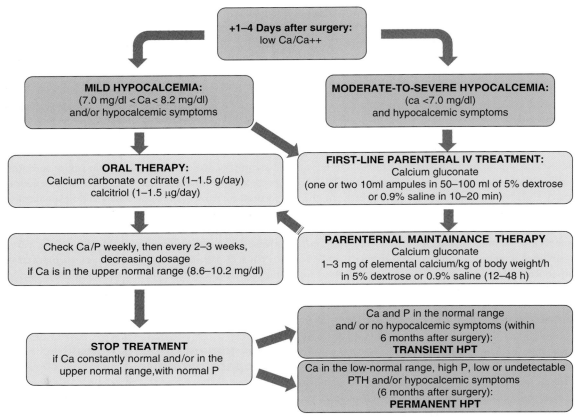

Figure 25.2 Suggested acute HPT management/monitoring. In the presence of mild hypocalcaemia and/or mild hypocalcaemic symptoms (positive Chvostek and Trousseau signs), oral therapy should be initiated. In patients with mild hypocalcaemia and relevant hypocalcaemic symptoms, IV calcium therapy could be also considered. In the setting of moderate-to-severe hypocalcaemia and/or severe symptoms, IV treatment with calcium gluconate should be established. While parenteral treatment is maintained, an oral regimen with calcium salts and active vitamin D metabolites should be established, further adjusting the dose (see text and Table 25.1). t-HPT, which typically resolves within 6 months after surgery, should be excluded if serum albumin-corrected calcium (Ca)/ionized calcium (Ca++) and phosphate (P) are persistently normal, gradually tapering down or stopping the treatment. For conversion of Ca from mg/dL to mmol/L, multiply by 0.2495.

7.6 mg/dL), requires prompt therapy that brings immediate relief [2,21]. Calcium gluconate is the preferred form to be infused, since calcium chloride can cause tissue necrosis in the case of extravasation. One or two 10 mL ampoules of 10% calcium gluconate (93 or 186 mg of elemental calcium, respectively) in 50–100 mL of 5% dextrose can be infused rapidly over a period of 10–20 min in the case of hypocalcaemic crisis, or more slowly in less severe cases. Since the effect of this infusion usually lasts up to 2–4 h, in the majority of cases it has to be followed by a slow infusion of calcium gluconate in 1 L of 5% dextrose or 0.9% saline, administered over several hours, at a rate of

1–3 mg of elemental calcium/kg body weight/h [4] (see Figure 25.2). Since arrhythmias can occur if the correction of hypocalcaemia is too rapid, electrocardiographic and clinical monitoring is required, especially during rapid calcium infusions and in patients taking digoxin. Ionized calcium or corrected serum calcium should be checked initially every 1–2 h and every 4–6 h afterwards [2,4,5].

The goal of therapy is to control hypocalcaemic symptoms and achieve and maintain a serum calcium level within the lower normal range (8–8.5 mg/dL). Subsequently, especially if the patient is still symptomatic or hypocalcaemia persists or recurs, the infusion can be

Table 25.1 Oral vitamin D metabolites commonly used in postoperative HPT

| | $1,25(OH)_2D_3$ | $1\alpha OHD_3$ | DHT |
	calcitriol	alfacalcidiol	dihydrotachysterol
Daily dose	0.5–2 µg	0.5–3 µg	0.2–1 mg
Time to correct hypocalcaemia	1–2 days	1–2 days	4–7 days
Washout time	2–3 days	5–7 days	7–21 days
Pharmaceutical formulation	Capsules	Drops	Drops

prolonged up to 12–48 h, the dose can be adjusted and the infusion can be slowed down and terminated as symptoms resolve and calcium is normalized (see Figure 25.2). Meanwhile, an oral regimen with calcium salts (1–2 g daily) and calcitriol (1–1.5 µg daily) is initiated. Oral supplementation with calcium (1–1.5 g/ day) and calcitriol (0.5–1.5 µg/day), as described in the next paragraph, can be the first approach in the case of mild/moderate forms of hypocalcaemia or in the case of asymptomatic hypocalcaemia.

The oral dose of calcium and calcitriol or other vitamin D metabolites should be individually tailored by checking serum calcium and phosphate initially every week, and then every 2–3 weeks or monthly. Once stable normocalcaemia is achieved and serum phosphate normalizes, therapy can be gradually reduced, decreasing the dose of calcium salt (500 mg every week) and calcitriol (0.25 µg every 2–3 weeks). If hypocalcaemia develops during tapering down oral calcium and calcitriol, the previous effective dose should be resumed. Alternatively, treatment can be stopped suddenly, checking serum calcium and phosphate after 1 week.

Postoperative symptomatic hypocalcaemia does not necessarily mean permanent hypoparathyroidism, even when IV calcium has been initially required. Moreover, t-HPT should always be excluded by gradual withdrawal of treatment even in patients who have been continuously treated for several weeks.

Medical treatment of chronic hypoparathyroidism

The goal of therapy is to control hypocalcaemic symptoms while maintaining serum calcium levels in the low-normal range and normal serum phosphate, providing the minimal amount of calcium and vitamin D metabolites. This will minimize complications of treatment, such as hypercalcaemia, hypercalciuria (urinary calcium

>300 mg/24 h), nephrolithiasis and nephrocalcinosis, which may occur even in the face of normocalcaemia [2].

Chronic treatment of parathyroid insufficiency requires oral calcium and active or partially active vitamin D metabolites (Table 25.1) not requiring renal hydroxylation, which is impaired because of the lack of PTH stimulus. Vitamin D metabolites are essential to increase calcium absorption. In the long term some patients may be kept eucalcaemic only by taking calcitriol.

Calcium carbonate and calcium citrate are the most common available forms of oral calcium, containing 40% and 21% of elemental calcium, respectively. Calcium carbonate requires an acidic environment to be absorbed, so its availability is decreased if proton pump inhibitors are taken or in the case of atrophic gastritis. In these cases, calcium citrate is the preferred form, where available. In patients not tolerating these supplements, other calcium preparations, such as calcium lactate or calcium gluconate, can be used [4].

Calcitriol is the biologically active form of vitamin D, which does not require any hydroxylation. Calcitriol is rapidly absorbed and promptly increases intestinal calcium absorption in a few hours, with a maximal effect at about 10 h and duration of action of 2–3 days. Starting doses of calcitriol are 0.25–2 µg/day given in split doses two or three times per day, because of the short half-life (see Table 25.1).

Alfacalcidiol (1α-hydroxyvitamin D3 or 1α-OHD$_3$) requires a further hepatic hydroxylation to be fully activated. The rapidity of action and clinical effectiveness are comparable to calcitriol, but the duration of action is longer because of the longer half-life (see Table 25.1).

Dihydrotachysterol (DHT) is a vitamin D analogue not requiring renal hydroxylation. It increases calcium absorption within several hours. Because of the longer half-life, its effect lasts for 7–21 days. In the case of intoxication with this analogue, hypercalcaemia can take up to

21 days to resolve (see Table 25.1). For this reason it is rarely used [4].

Cholecalciferol, ergocalciferol and calcifediol should not be used to increase calcium absorption in HPT since they require renal hydroxylation to be fully activated.

It is worth noting that treatment with active vitamin D analogues does not correct a poor vitamin D status, if present. As previously stated, cholecalciferol or ergocalciferol should be employed to correct a poor vitamin D status either before or after surgery, regardless of calcitriol treatment for hypocalcaemia.

Follow-up in chronic hypoparathyroidism

The aim of therapy with calcium and vitamin D metabolites is to relieve hypocalcaemic symptoms, maintaining albumin-corrected serum calcium concentration in the lower normal range (8–8.5 mg/dL), a calcium phosphate product below 55 and urinary calcium below 250–300 mg/24 h. The complications of overtreatment (vitamin D intoxication) are hypercalcaemia, hyperphosphataemia and hypercalciuria, which in the long term could cause nephrolithiasis and calcifications of soft tissues, such nephrocalcinosis and cataract. Hypoparathyroid patients themselves are prone to develop hypercalciuria because of the lack of PTH-mediated calcium reabsorption in the renal distal tubule [2].

Careful monitoring during long-term treatment of HPT is mandatory. Hypercalcaemia should be suspected in patients who, under calcium and calcitriol treatment, develop gastrointestinal symptoms (nausea, dyspepsia, vomiting), alteration of mental status and fatigue. If hypercalcaemia occurs, treatment with active vitamin D metabolites should be discontinued. Since the hypercalcaemic effect can persist for several days to weeks when vitamin D metabolites with long half-lives are used, parenteral saline hydration and/or oral glucocorticoids can be required [2].

Albumin-corrected serum calcium, phosphate, calciuria and creatinine should be checked periodically (every 6–12 months), even in asymptomatic patients, once a stable regimen is established. If urinary calcium is greater than 250–300 mg/24 h, a thiazide diuretic should be given in order to decrease hypercalciuria and maintain normocalcaemia. Excessive sodium intake should be avoided since it increases urinary calcium excretion. Since the risk for soft tissue calcification is high when

calcium phosphate product is >55, hyperphosphataemia should be corrected by means of a low-phosphorus diet and/or a phosphate binder [4].

Although therapy with calcium and calcitriol is effective in preventing hypocalcaemic symptoms in p-HPT, it does not restore physiological mineral homeostasis and bone microstructure [34]. In fact, p-HPT patients on calcium and calcitriol therapy display high rates of cataract and nephrolithiasis (44% and 8%, respectively) and an overall altered quality of life compared to control subjects with intact parathyroid function.

Parathyroid hormone replacement therapy in chronic hypoparathyroidism

Parathyroid insufficiency is one of the few endocrinopathies for which replacement of the missing hormone is not currently employed. As already mentioned, calcium homeostasis and quality of life are not fully restored by treatment with calcium and vitamin D metabolites [35]. For this reason, an alternative approach with teriparatide (PTH 1-34) [36–39] and intact PTH(1-84) [40] administered subcutaneously has been tested in these patients. In a 3-year randomized trial [37], PTH(1-34) twice daily has proven to be as effective as calcitriol in maintaining calcium levels in the low-normal range or slightly below. However, urinary calcium excretion was significantly lower in the PTH(1-34)-treated group compared to the calcium/calcitriol-treated group. There were no changes in bone mineral density, bone mineral content in adults or bone structure in children, although, as expected, bone markers were increased during PTH(1-34) treatment compared to the chronic treatment with calcitriol.

In a 2-year open-label trial [40], 100 μg of PTH (1-84) administered every other day decreased daily requirement for calcium and vitamin D, without any effect on urinary calcium excretion. A modest increase in bone mineral density at the lumbar spine (rich in trabecular bone) and a slight decrease in bone mineral density at the distal radius (rich in cortical bone) were observed.

Data on quality of life, physical endurance and long-term effects on bone metabolism and the rate of complications during treatment with PTH(1-34) or PTH(1-84) have not yet been assessed. Neither PTH(1-34) nor PTH(1-84) is approved by the US Food and Drug Administration for replacement therapy in HPT, yet.

Parathyroid autotransplantation

Parathyroid autotransplantation is not routinely performed but it has been used in some centres in patients at high risk of developing postoperative HPT. In a large prospective study of 5846 patients who underwent bilateral thyroid surgery, none of those who received parathyroid graft (7.5%) developed definitive HPT [11]. A recent multicentre study has assessed the rate of successful reimplantation and function of cryopreserved parathyroid glands [41]. Only 1.6% of the total cryopreserved glands had been reimplanted and a minority (10%) of the successfully reimplanted glands were fully functional at 2-year follow-up. The success rate depended upon the experience of the surgical centre.

Conclusion

Postoperative parathyroid insufficiency is the most common complication of thyroid surgery and represents significant morbidity. The rate of HPT mainly depends on surgeon experience and the extent of neck surgery. Serum calcium should be checked routinely at 1–4 days after surgery, even in asymptomatic patients. Perioperative PTH measurement can be an additional predictive parameter. Calcium and vitamin D metabolites or analogues are the therapy of choice. Treatment should be carefully monitored and modulated in each patient. Overtreatment and subsequent complications are common in the long term. In addition, hypoparathyroid patients taking appropriate calcium and calcitriol display altered calcium/phosphate homeostasis and poorer quality of life compared to age- and sex-matched subjects with intact parathyroid function. Thus, replacement with the missing hormone itself would be desirable. Treatment with PTH (1-34 or 1-84) is still under investigation. The use of parathyroid autografting is still limited and, when used, its success is strictly dependent on the technical experience of the surgical centre.

References

1 Livolsi VA. Parathyroids: morphology and pathology. In: Bilezikian JP, Marcus R, Levine MA (eds) The Parathyroids: Basic and Clinical Concepts, 2nd edn. San Diego, CA: Academic Press, 2001: 1–15.

2 Shoback D. Clinical practice. Hypoparathyroidism. N Engl J Med 2008; 359: 391–403.

3 Favus MJ, Goltzman D. Regulation of calcium and magnesium. In: Primer on the Metabolic Bone Diseases and Disorders of Mineral Metabolism. Section III: Mineral Homeostasis, 7th edn. Washington, DC: American Society for Bone and Mineral Research, 2009: 104–7.

4 Walker Harris V, Jan de Beur S. Postoperative HPT: medical and surgical therapeutic options. Thyroid 2009; 19: 967–73.

5 Khan MI, Waguespack SG, Hu MI. Medical management of postsurgical HPT. Endocr Pract 2011; 17(Suppl 1): 18–25.

6 Zarnegar R, Brunaud L, Clark OH. Prevention, evaluation, and management of complications following thyroidectomy for thyroid carcinoma. Endocrinol Metab Clin North Am 2003; 32: 483–502.

7 Udelsman R. Experience counts. Ann Surg 2004; 240: 26–7.

8 Sosa JA, Bowman HM, Tielsch JM, Powe NR, Gordon TA, Udelsman R. The importance of surgeon experience for clinical and economic outcomes from thyroidectomy. Ann Surg 1998; 228: 320–30.

9 Zambudio AR, Rodríguez J, Riquelme J, Soria T, Canteras M, Parrilla P. Prospective study of postoperative complications after total thyroidectomy for multinodular goiters by surgeons with experience in endocrine surgery. Ann Surg 2004; 240: 18–25.

10 Pattou F, Combemale F, Fabre S, et al. Hypocalcemia following thyroid surgery: incidence and prediction of outcome. World J Surg 1998; 22: 718–24.

11 Thomusch O, Machens A, Sekulla C, Ukkat J, Brauckhoff M, Dralle H. The impact of surgical technique on postoperative HPT in bilateral thyroid surgery: a multivariate analysis of 5846 consecutive patients. Surgery 2003; 133: 180–5.

12 Rosato L, Avenia N, Bernante P, et al. Complications of thyroid surgery: analysis of a multicentric study on 14,934 patients operated on in Italy over 5 years. World J Surg 2004; 28: 271–6.

13 Page C, Strunski V. Parathyroid risk in total thyroidectomy for bilateral, benign, multinodular goitre: report of 351 surgical cases. J Laryngol Otol 2007; 121: 237–41.

14 Asari R, Passler C, Kaczirek K, Scheuba C, Niederle B. HPT after total thyroidectomy: a prospective study. Arch Surg 2008; 143: 132–7.

15 Bergenfelz A, Jansson S, Kristoffersson A, et al. Complications to thyroid surgery: results as reported in a database from a multicenter audit comprising 3,660 patients. Langenbecks Arch Surg 2008; 393: 667–73.

16 Michie W, Duncan T, Hamer-Hodges DW, et al. Mechanism of hypocalcemia after thyroidectomy for thyrotoxicosis. Lancet 1971; 1: 508–14.

17 See AC, Soo KC. Hypocalcaemia following thyroidectomy for thyrotoxicosis. Br J Surg 1997; 84: 95–7.

18 Hermann M, Ott J, Promberger R, Kober F, Karik M, Freissmuth. Kinetics of serum parathyroid hormone during and after thyroid surgery. Br J Surg 2008; 95: 1480–7.

19 Promberger R, Ott J, Kober F, Karik M, Freissmuth M, Hermann M. Normal parathyroid hormone levels do not exclude permanent HPT after thyroidectomy. Thyroid 2011; 21: 145–50.

20 Wilson RB, Erskine C, Crowe PJ. Hypomagnesemia and hypocalcemia after thyroidectomy: prospective study. World J Surg 2000; 24: 722–6.

21 Cooper MS, Gittoes NJ. Diagnosis and management of hypocalcaemia. BMJ 2008; 336: 1298–302.

22 Bentrem DJ, Rademaker A, Angelos P. Evaluation of serum calcium levels in predicting HPT after total/near-total thyroidectomy or parathyroidectomy. Am Surg 2001; 67: 249–51.

23 Nahas ZS, Farrag TY, Lin FR, Belin RM, Tufano RP. A safe and cost-effective short hospital stay protocol to identify patients at low risk for the development of significant hypocalcemia after total thyroidectomy. Laryngoscope 2006; 116: 906–10.

24 Lindblom P, Westerdahl J, Bergenfelz A. Low parathyroid hormone levels after thyroid surgery: a feasible predictor of hypocalcemia. Surgery 2002; 131: 515–20.

25 Wong C, Price S, Scott-Coombes D. Hypocalcaemia and parathyroid hormone assay following total thyroidectomy: predicting the future. World J Surg 2006; 30: 825–32.

26 Miccoli P, Minuto MN, Panicucci E, et al. The impact of thyroidectomy on parathyroid glands: a biochemical and clinical profile. J Endocrinol Invest 2007; 30: 666–71.

27 Soon PS, Magarey CJ, Campbell P, Jalaludin B. Serum intact parathyroid hormone as a predictor of hypocalcaemia after total thyroidectomy. ANZ J Surg 2005; 75: 977–80.

28 Quiros RM, Pesce CE, Wilhelm SM, Djuricin G, Prinz RA. Intraoperative parathyroid hormone levels in thyroid surgery are predictive of postoperative HPT and need for vitamin D supplementation. Am J Surg 2005; 189: 306–9.

29 Barczyński M, Cichoń S, Konturek A. Which criterion of intraoperative iPTH assay is the most accurate in prediction of true serum calcium levels after thyroid surgery? Langenbecks Arch Surg 2007; 392: 693–8.

30 Grodski S, Lundgren CI, Sidhu S, Sywak M, Delbridge L. Postoperative PTH measurement facilitates day 1 discharge after total thyroidectomy. Clin Endocrinol (Oxf) 2009; 70: 322–5.

31 Grodski S, Serpell J. Evidence for the role of perioperative PTH measurement after total thyroidectomy as a predictor of hypocalcemia. World J Surg 2008; 32: 1367–73.

32 Noordzij JP, Lee SL, Bernet VJ, et al. Early prediction of hypocalcemia after thyroidectomy using parathyroid hormone: an analysis of pooled individual patient data from nine observational studies. J Am Coll Surg 2007; 205: 748–54.

33 Ross AC, Manson JE, Abrams SA, et al. The 2011 report on dietary reference intakes for calcium and vitamin D from the Institute of Medicine: what clinicians need to know. J Clin Endocrinol Metab 2011; 96: 53–8.

34 Rubin MR, Bilezikian JP. HPT: clinical features, skeletal microstructure and parathyroid hormone replacement. Arq Bras Endocrinol Metabol 2010; 54: 220–6.

35 Arlt W, Fremerey C, Callies F, et al. Well-being, mood and calcium homeostasis in patients with HPT receiving standard treatment with calcium and vitamin D. Eur J Endocrinol 2002; 146: 215–22.

36 Winer KK, Yanovski JA, Cutler GB Jr. Synthetic human parathyroid hormone 1-34 vs calcitriol and calcium in the treatment of HPT. JAMA 1996; 276: 631–6.

37 Winer KK, Ko CW, Reynolds JC, et al. Long-term treatment of HPT: a randomized controlled study comparing parathyroid hormone (1-34) versus calcitriol and calcium. J Clin Endocrinol Metab 2003; 88: 4214–20.

38 Winer KK, Sinaii N, Peterson D, Sainz B Jr, Cutler GB Jr. Effects of once versus twice-daily parathyroid hormone 1-34 therapy in children with HPT. J Clin Endocrinol Metab 2008; 93: 3389–95.

39 Winer KK, Sinaii N, Reynolds J, Peterson D, Dowdy K, Cutler GB Jr. Long-term treatment of 12 children with chronic HPT: a randomized trial comparing synthetic human parathyroid hormone 1-34 versus calcitriol and calcium. J Clin Endocrinol Metab 2010; 95: 2680–8.

40 Rubin MR, Sliney J Jr, MMahon DJ, Silverberg SJ, Bilezikian JP. Therapy of HPT with intact parathyroid hormone. Osteoporos Int 2010; 21: 1927–34.

41 Borot S, Lapierre V, Carnaille B, Goudet P, Penfornis A. Results of cryopreserved parathyroid autografts: a retrospective multicenter study. Surgery 2010; 147: 529–35.

CHAPTER 26

The Rare Ones: Horner's Syndrome, Complications from Surgical Positioning and Post-sternotomy Complications

Lukas H. Kus and Jeremy L. Freeman

Department of Otolaryngology – Head and Neck Surgery, University of Toronto, Toronto, Canada

Introduction

In the course of their career, every endocrine surgeon will encounter rare thyroid surgery complications which are important to recognize. This chapter describes several such complications. Horner's syndrome is a defect of the sympathetic nervous system that causes ipsilateral eyelid ptosis, pupillary constriction and anhidrosis. It has been reported as an iatrogenic injury after thyroidectomy. Injuries related to patient positioning consist primarily of pressure ulcers and peripheral nerve injuries, which can result from prolonged ischaemia. Neck extension during thyroidectomy and other head and neck procedures have also been reported to cause neurologic complications. Sternotomy is the division of the sternum in order to gain surgical access to the mediastinum. In thyroid surgery, it can be performed for selected cases of retrosternal goitre and thoracic thyroid cancer metastases. Related complications include sternal dehiscence, deep wound infection and rib fractures. We will describe each of these complications and their clinical presentations, present aetiologies, highlight important diagnostic modalities, provide information regarding prognoses and suggest treatments.

Horner's syndrome

Horner's syndrome, also known as oculosympathoparesis or Bernard–Horner syndrome, is a constellation of neurologic findings first described in 1852 by the French physiologist Claude Bernard and then in 1869 by the Swiss ophthalmologist Johann Friedrich Horner. It is characterized by ipsilateral blepharoptosis, pupillary miosis and facial anhidrosis (Figure 26.1). The syndrome occurs as a result of injury to any portion of the sympathetic pathway that supplies the head, eye and neck [1] and has been reported as a complication of thyroidectomy [2–7].

Knowledge of sympathetic nervous system anatomy is essential for understanding the aetiology of Horner's syndrome (Figure 26.2). The sympathetic system that innervates the eye consists of a three-neuron pathway originating in the central nervous system. First-order (central) neurons originate from the posterolateral hypothalamus and descend caudally through the brainstem to synapse in the intermediolateral columns of the cervical spinal cord at the levels of C8–T2 [1]. From here, second-order (preganglionic) neurons exit the spinal cord at the T1 level in the white ramus communicans and travel through the brachial plexus over the lung apex [2]. They ascend the sympathetic trunk to synapse in the superior

Thyroid Surgery: Preventing and Managing Complications, First Edition. Edited by Paolo Miccoli, David J. Terris, Michele N. Minuto and Melanie W. Seybt.

cervical ganglion, located between the internal jugular vein and the internal carotid artery [8]. Third-order (postganglionic) neurons then ascend cephalad, forming a plexus around the internal carotid artery. Sudomotor fibres responsible for facial sweating and piloerection follow the external carotid artery while other sympathetics travel with the internal carotid artery, entering the skull base through the carotid canal and coursing through the middle cranial fossa and cavernous sinus [9]. Oculosympathetic fibres travel with the intracavernous abducens nerve before joining the ophthalmic division (V_1) of the trigeminal nerve. Sympathetic fibres follow the nasociliary nerve through the superior orbital fissure

to innervate the dilator pupillae muscle, the smooth superior tarsal muscle (Müller's muscle) in the upper eyelid and its unnamed lower eyelid analogue, the lacrimal gland and orbital vasomotor fibres [1].

Loss of sympathetic innervation in Horner's syndrome may produce only a subtle ptosis, although a loss of the upper eyelid crease may be distinguishable [1]. Paresis of the smooth muscle supporting the lower eyelid causes lower eyelid elevation, or *inverse ptosis*. Together, these defects narrow the palpebral fissure and produce an apparent enophthalmos [10]. Blepharoptosis is thought to be present in 88% of Horner's syndrome cases [11].

Pupil size is regulated by a balance between the sympathetically activated iris dilator muscle and parasympathetically activated iris constrictor muscle. With sympathetic denervation, unopposed iris constrictor activity produces pupillary miosis and anisocoria that is more pronounced in dim illumination. Miosis is found in 98% of Horner's patients [11]. Pupillary dilation in the affected eye becomes slower, as it is only a passive process resulting from constrictor relaxation [10]. This sign is known as *dilation lag*. Conjunctival hyperaemia may be transient in acute Horner's syndrome and results from loss of sympathetic vasoconstrive effects [10].

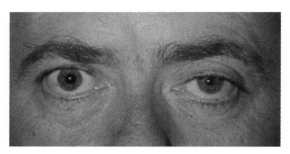

Figure 26.1 Horner's syndrome with left ptosis and miosis.

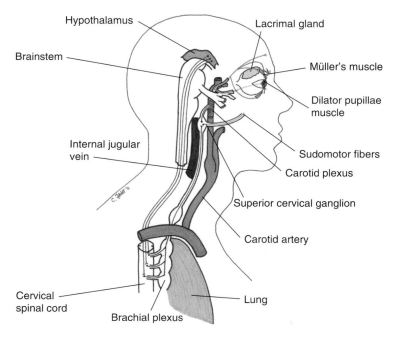

Figure 26.2 Anatomy of the sympathetic nervous system.

Anhidrosis results from sympathetic denervation of the facial sweat glands. Sudomotor sympathetics innervating the medial forehead branch off with the postganglionic fibres while those that supply the rest of the face branch off from the sympathetic chain more proximally. As a result, hemifacial anhidrosis indicates central or preganglionic lesions while anhidrosis limited to the medial forehead signifies a postganglionic lesion [1]. Anhidrosis is frequently not apparent to patients or clinicians and is reported in only 4% of cases [11].

The patient's associated neurologic signs and symptoms provide clues as to the location of the lesion. Diplopia, ataxia or vertigo suggest a brainstem aetiology while features such as muscle weakness, sensory deficits, bowel incontinence or urinary retention point to a spinal cord lesion. Arm pain or hand weakness typical of brachial plexus dysfunction could signify a lung apex mass. Ipsilateral disorders of extraocular movement in the absence of other brainstem findings suggest a lesion localized to the cavernous sinus. Internal carotid artery dissection must be ruled out in patients presenting with isolated Horner's syndrome and head or neck pain.

Horner's syndrome is a rare complication of thyroid surgery, with less than 30 cases reported in the literature to date [5]. As a result, incidence rates are difficult to establish, although one study estimated the complication rate at 0.2% of thyroidectomies [7]. Based on a review of the reported cases [2–7,12], Horner's symptoms typically first appear between the immediate postoperative period and the second postoperative day and can occur following surgery for both benign and malignant thyroid disease. Approximately 70% of patients are left with a permanent syndrome or incomplete recovery while the remainder recover completely after periods ranging from 3 days to 15 months [7].

Various theories have been proposed to explain how Horner's syndrome develops from thyroidectomy. Anatomical communications between the recurrent laryngeal nerve (RLN) and the cervical sympathetic chain have been reported in 1.5–3.0% of patients [12,13]. Such patients could be at risk for sympathetic nerve trauma during thyroidectomy as a result of isolation or possible manipulation of the RLN [2,7]. Compression of the sympathetic chain with resulting ischaemia could also be caused by postoperative haematoma [2,7]. The inferior thyroid artery may supply branching blood vessels to the cervical sympathetic chain, so ligating this artery during thyroidectomy could inadvertently cut off blood supply

to the nerves [2]. This might occur if ligation were attempted as far laterally as possible in order to avoid RLN damage [3]. De Quervain believed that stretching of the sympathetic chain while retracting the carotid sheath laterally to expose the inferior thyroid artery was the usual cause of sympathetic injury and that the chain itself was occasionally compressed between the tip of the retractor and the vertebral column [3].

Several pharmacologic tests can help confirm the diagnosis of Horner's syndrome. *Cocaine* blocks norepinephrine reuptake at the sympathetic nerve synapse, causing a normal pupil to dilate but having no effect on an eye with impaired sympathetic innervation. After instillation of 10% cocaine eye drops in both eyes, the normal pupil dilates more than the Horner's pupil, exacerbating the anisocoria. Anisocoria of 1 mm or greater 1 h after cocaine administration is diagnostic of Horner's syndrome [9]. *Apraclonidine* is a direct α-adrenergic receptor agonist with weak α1 and strong α2 effects. Pupillary dilation is mediated by α1 receptors while α2 activity is responsible for downregulating norepinephrine release at neuromuscular junctions. Horner's pupils will be supersensitive to α1 effects and will dilate in response to apraclonidine stimulation. Normal pupils, however, will only respond to the α2 activity and will constrict. Consequently, instillation of 0.5% apraclonidine in both eyes of a Horner's syndrome patient will cause a reversal of anisocoria [1].

Once testing with either of the above drugs has confirmed Horner's syndrome, testing with *hydroxyamphetamine* (or its derivative *pholedrine*) is done to help differentiate the site of the sympathetic lesion. Hydroxyamphetamine stimulates the release of stored norepinephrine from postganglionic adrenergic nerve endings, so normal pupils and Horner's pupils affected by central or preganglionic lesions should respond by dilation. A Horner's pupil caused by a third-order neuron lesion will not dilate as well as the normal pupil when 1% hydroxyamphetamine drops are instilled in both eyes. A positive diagnosis for a third-order neuron lesion is made when the anisocoria increases by at least 1 mm. Hydroxyamphetamine testing must be done at least 24 h after the cocaine eye drop test, as the latter may cause a false-negative result [9]. No pharmacologic test differentiates between first- and second-order sympathetic lesions.

Most cases of Horner's syndrome require imaging to identify the causative lesion. Associated neurologic findings and the hydroxyamphetamine test can help guide the clinician in choosing high-yield imaging investigations. Magnetic resonance imaging (MRI) of the brain, upper spinal cord or neck is usually indicated. Computed tomography (CT) scanning of the chest for lung tumours and CT angiography of the carotid arteries for dissection can also be helpful [10].

Horner's syndrome caused by thyroidectomy is typically treated conservatively, as it may resolve spontaneously. While anisocoria is unlikely to be of concern to the patient, ptosis may be corrected surgically with blepharoplasty. Another alternative is the use of topical phenylephrine, an adrenergic agonist which stimulates Müller's muscle. Instillation of phenylephrine eye drops to the affected eye may elevate the upper eyelid as much as 2 mm [1]. There are no treatments available for anhidrosis but few patients find this to be of serious concern.

Complications from surgical positioning

Intraoperative positioning is an essential aspect of surgery that requires effective communication and co-operation between all members of the nursing, anaesthesia and surgical teams. It involves securing the patient's body in place to ensure the best possible surgical exposure while minimizing compromise of their physiologic functions and mechanical stress on their tissues. Safe positioning protects patients from a number of preventable injuries, including pressure ulcers, peripheral nerve injuries and injuries related to neck extension. Reports of such adverse events in thyroidectomy are rare, so incidence rates are difficult to estimate.

Patients are typically positioned supine for thyroidectomy. The patient is placed on their back on the operating table with the spinal column straight and the head extended with a shoulder roll and a head rest. The patient's legs lie extended and uncrossed parallel to the table. Arms are tucked at the sides with palms facing the body or extended less than 90° on padded arm boards with palms facing upward. Some endocrine surgeons prefer a 10–20° reverse Trendelenburg position (supine with head up and feet lowered), which decreases blood loss and postoperative nausea and vomiting in thyroidectomy [14] and may be optimal for ventilating obese patients [15,16].

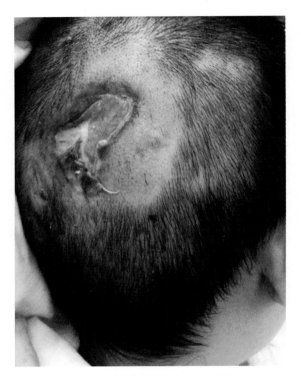

Figure 26.3 Chronic occipital pressure ulcer (stage IV).

Pressure ulcers are lesions caused by unrelieved pressure resulting in localized damage to skin or underlying tissue [17]. These usually occur over bony prominences as soft tissue is compressed against an external surface for a prolonged period of time. Vulnerable body sites in supine position include the occiput, scapula, thoracic vertebrae, elbow, sacrum, coccyx and heel (Figure 26.3) [18]. Pressure ulcers can resemble burns and typically start as a purplish or maroon skin discolouration. They may only become apparent hours to days after surgery and therefore can be missed in the immediate postoperative period. Hospital-acquired pressure ulcers lead to prolonged hospital admission and have been correlated wtih increased mortality and treatment costs [17].

Friction and shear forces often contribute to pressure ulcer formation. Friction injuries can result from skin rubbing against a rough stationary surface such as a positioning device or linen. Shear forces occur when the patient's tissues move but the overlying skin remains immobile, which may result from the patient being lifted without sufficient assistance [19]. In addition, caustic agents such as cleaning solutions or bodily fluids may cause skin breakdown while excessive hydration from pooling of surgical prep solutions or irrigation fluids beneath the patient can lead to maceration and increased permeability to irritants and micro-organisms [18]. External pressure exceeding the normal capillary filling pressure of approximately 32 mmHg occludes local blood flow, causing tissue ischaemia with subsequent skin and subcutaneous tissue necrosis [17]. In supine position, dermal ulcers can result from even 2–3 h of unrelieved pressure on tissues and increase in likelihood with the duration of surgery [18]. Patients with pre-existing vascular compromise have lower thresholds for vascular occlusion and may experience tissue ischaemia at pressures as low as 12 mmHg or after a shorter exposure to occlusive forces [18]. Anaesthesia itself contributes to the formation of pressure ulcers, as muscle relaxation or paralysis prevents the normal function of defence mechanisms against stretching, twisting and compression of tissues [19]. Other risk factors for intraoperative pressure ulcer formation are summarized in Box 26.1.

Positioning aids can prevent tissue injury by redistributing pressure across a larger body surface and limiting excessive stretching. Foam, gel, static air and dynamic air overlays placed directly on the operating room mattress may help reduce the incidence of pressure ulcers [17]. Padding made from these materials should also be used to protect bony prominences and other high-pressure points while pre-existing ulcers should be protected with occlusive dressings. Towels and adhesive drapes can also protect patients from excessive moisture due to pooling of liquids while drawsheets and co-ordinated lifting can reduce shear and friction injuries. Proper positioning includes ensuring that Mayo stands and surgical team members are not pressing against the patient. Importantly, preoperative assessment and documentation of skin integrity and risk factors highlight patients at risk for developing intraoperative pressure ulcers.

Treatment of pressure ulcers depends on their stage (Table 26.1) and is based on several fundamental concepts. Reducing pressure on affected skin surfaces, debriding necrotic tissue, wound cleansing, wound dressing and minimizing bacterial load are the essential components of this process [20]. Just as in the prevention of pressure ulcers, positioning aids are used to reduce mechanical strain on injured tissues. With this aim in mind, patient turning and mobilization are also encouraged in the

---

Box 26.1 Risk factors for development of intraoperative pressure ulcers

- Advanced age
- Medications:
  - Steroids
  - Vasoactive medications
- Co-morbid conditions:
  - Cancer
  - Coronary artery disease
  - Peripheral vascular disease
  - Diabetes mellitus
  - Neurologic disease
  - Respiratory disease
  - Immunodeficiency
- Previous pressure ulcers
- Extracorporeal circulation:
  - Haemodialysis
  - Extracorporeal membrane oxygenation
  - Cardiopulmonary bypass
- Nutritional deficiencies
- Fractures
- Anaemia and low haematocrit levels
- Obesity
- Low serum protein (albumin, globulin)
- Smoking
- Low systemic blood pressure
- Impaired body temperature regulation

Reproduced from Walton-Geer [17] with permission from Elsevier.

---

postoperative period. Ensuring patient comfort with appropriate analgesics is also important throughout the healing period.

Debridement of necrotic tissue reduces bacterial growth to promote wound healing. Various debridement methods are possible but each involves removing eschar to expose granulation tissue. Mechanical debridement usually consists of applying wet-to-dry dressings, which adhere to non-viable tissue. Dead tissue is removed along with the dry dressing during dressing changes. Syringing with normal saline irrigation throughout this process not only cleans the wound but also provides a mechanical force to loosen tissue debris. Sharp debridement entails the use of a scalpel blade to remove thick or extensive eschar, often when the wound becomes infected. Enzymatic debridement with collagenase or fibrinolysin and deoxyribonuclease is useful for treating purulent or fibrinous ulcers when sharp debridement cannot be tolerated

Table 26.1 Pressure ulcer stages and their characteristics [22,55]. Unstageable ulcers should be debrided to determine the appropriate stage.

Ulcer stages	Characteristics
I	Intact skin with non-blanchable redness of a localized area, usually over a bony prominence
II	Partial-thickness loss of dermis presenting as a shallow open ulcer with a red-pink wound bed, without slough. May also present as an intact or open/ruptured serum-filled blister
III	Full-thickness tissue loss. Subcutaneous fat may be visible but bone, tendon or muscle are not exposed. Slough may be present but does not obscure the depth of tissue loss. May include undermining and tunnelling
IV	Full-thickness tissue loss with exposed bone, tendon or muscle. Slough or eschar may be present on some parts of the wound bed. Often includes undermining and tunnelling
Deep tissue injury	Damage to subcutaneous tissue under intact skin. May appear as a localized area of intact bruised skin or as a blood-filled blister

[20,21]. Autolysis refers to the body's natural mechanism of using enzymes and moisture to liquefy and remove hard eschar and slough [20]. This painless process is aided by the use of occlusive dressings which allow moisture to be retained in the wound.

While bacterial colonization of pressure ulcers is inevitable, wound cleansing and debridement are typically sufficient to prevent this from impeding wound healing. Clean ulcers that fail to heal effectively after several weeks of optimal wound care may benefit from the application of topical antibiotics such as silver, mupirocin or bacitracin [20,22].

Systemic antibiotics should only be employed for complicated cases involving advancing cellulitis, osteomyelitis or sepsis.

Advanced wounds (stage III–IV) may benefit from vacuum-assisted closure [23] or surgical intervention, which may involve direct closure, skin grafts or various local or free flaps. Emerging treatment options for pressure ulcers include recombinant growth factors such as platelet-derived growth factor [22]. All pressure ulcer patients benefit from a multidisciplinary approach involving wound care nurses, primary care physicians, physiotherapists and rehabilitation specialists.

Prognosis for pressure ulcers depends on their stage. Over 70% of stage II ulcers heal after 6 months of appropriate treatment, while only approximately 50% of stage III ulcers and 30% of stage IV ulcers heal within this period [20].

Another important complication of incorrect surgical positioning is peripheral nerve injury, which results from ischaemia caused by prolonged stretching or compression of nerve fibres [24]. While few cases of such injuries exist specifically in the thyroid surgery literature, neuropathies commonly reported as a result of prolonged supine intraoperative positioning involve the brachial plexus, ulnar nerve, radial nerve and common peroneal nerve. Each of these may present with pain, muscle weakness or paraesthesia (Table 26.2).

Risk factors for peripheral nerve injury caused by intraoperative positioning are similar to those for pressure ulcers, as both result from similar mechanisms [18,24]. Other patients at risk for nerve injury include those with thin body habitus, pre-existing diabetic or hereditary peripheral neuropathy, deep hypothermia from direct skin cooling and anatomical variants such as cervical ribs [24]. Nerves with increased length are at higher risk of injury and lower extremity nerves are more often injured than those in the upper extremities [24]. Prevention of intraoperative peripheral nerve injuries in supine position should involve awareness of patient risk factors, use of appropriate padding and positioning devices, and avoidance of the positioning errors listed in Table 26.2. Use of somatosensory evoked potentials for intraoperative nerve monitoring can prevent injury but this technology is seldom employed in thyroid surgery. Accurate documentation of any pre- and postoperative nerve injuries and of protective measures taken intraoperatively is important from a medico-legal perspective.

In addition to a detailed neurologic examination, the workup of a peripheral nerve injury requires the use of electromyography (EMG) for more precise localization of the lesion and to document recovery. This helps distinguish positioning injuries from cervical spine pathologies and musculoskeletal issues, as EMG changes in the former should be confined to muscles in the distribution of the injured nerve.

Table 26.2 Causes and clinical features of peripheral nerve injury related to supine intraoperative positioning [18,24].

Nerve	Clinical features	Causes
Brachial plexus	Flaccid paralysis of entire arm with motor dysfunction of wrist and hand. Also presents with lack of sensation in arm and hand	Compression of brachial plexus between clavicle and first rib due to arm hyperabduction (>90°) or arm abduction with lateral flexion of the head to contralateral side
Ulnar	Numbness and tingling in the fourth and fifth digits, pain along medial forearm and hand, weakness of fourth and fifth digit lumbricals and hand intrinsics. May also present with weakness of fourth and fifth digit flexor digitorum profundus	Compression of ulnar nerve in cubital tunnel at elbow due to arm being secured too tightly at patient's side with inadequate elbow padding or due to arm being allowed to slip off edge of mattress or OR bed. May also be due to distal placement of blood pressure cuff
Radial	Weakness of triceps, brachioradialis, wrist extensors, supinator and finger extensors. Sensory deficits of lateral upper arm, posterior arm and forearm, and part of dorsal hand. Deficits vary depending on injury location	Compression of radial nerve due to arm being pushed against rigid structure (i.e. Mayo stand, OR table, vertical bar of anaesthesia screen). May also be due to distal placement of blood pressure cuff
Common peroneal	Foot drop from weakness of foot dorsiflexors and ankle extensors, weakness of ankle eversion, and variable sensory loss on dorsum of foot and lateral leg and ankle	Compression of common peroneal nerve in the popliteal space by knee supports (i.e. hard rolls below knees)

Treatment is conservative and consists primarily of neurogenic pain control with analgesics and agents such as gabapentin. Physiotherapy and mobilization help maintain muscle strength, flexibility and range of motion. Splinting to prevent further injury and assist with activities of daily living can also be useful. Surgery may be beneficial for patients with prolonged injury who fail conservative management. Surgical options include neurolysis, intraoperative evaluation of neuroma incontinuity, resection and grafting of non-conducting nerve lesions, and nerve transposition [24]. Prognosis is variable and depends on the nature, location and severity of nerve injury. Remyelination of injured nerves may take up to several weeks. Nerve fibres affected by Wallerian degeneration require that axons regrow in a distal direction along the length of the degenerated nerve, a process which occurs at a rate of approximately 2–3 mm/day [25]. Depending on the affected nerve, recovery may take anywhere from 20 weeks to 18 months and may be incomplete [24].

A number of complications have also been reported to occur as a result of neck extension during surgery. One such case involved transient bilateral occipital neuropathy after thyroidectomy in a morbidly obese diabetic patient [26]. This effect may have been caused by prolonged direct pressure on the occipital nerves from compression between adipose and muscle tissue. Two reports describe the occurrence of postoperative quadriplegia in

three haemodialysis patients who underwent parathyroidectomy [27,28]. Both reports cite pre-existing cervical stenosis, ischaemic damage due to overstretching of the spinal cord, and occlusion of the vertebral arteries from extreme head rotation as possible aetiologic factors. Patients with Down's syndrome are also at risk for cervical spine injury during head and neck procedures, as 10–20% may have atlantoaxial instability [29]. These cases highlight the impact of co-morbid conditions on positioning-related injuries and show that each member of the healthcare team must be conscious of these issues to provide effective intraoperative patient care.

Post-sternotomy complications

Sternotomy is the surgical division of the sternum for access to the mediastinum and its contents. In the context of thyroid surgery, this procedure is sometimes performed in patients with retrosternal goitre or mediastinal thyroid carcinoma metastases and is done in conjunction with a thoracic surgeon. Major complications from this procedure include sternal malunion, sternal infection and rib fractures.

The term *goiter* is derived from the Latin phrase *tumidum guttur* ('swollen throat') and describes a thyroid gland that is at least twice the normal size, or over 40 g. *Retrosternal* goitres, first described by Albrecht von

Haller in 1749, are defined by some as having more than 50% of their mass lying inferior to the thoracic inlet [30]. Retrosternal goitres are estimated to have a 0.02–0.5% prevalence in the general population and may represent 2–19% of thyroidectomy cases [31]. They commonly present in the fifth decade of life with a female predominance of 3–4:1 [32]. Surgical indications for retrosternal goitre include malignancy, compressive symptoms or acute airway compromise, cosmesis, failure of medical therapy, and diagnosis, as these masses tend not to be amenable to fine needle aspiration [32,33].

Sternotomy is required infrequently for retrosternal goitre, usually as a result of superior vena cava syndrome, recurrent or isolated intrathoracic goitre or low-lying thyroid carcinoma with intrathoracic lymph node involvement [32]. Adequate anatomical exposure of the gland is needed to prevent major bleeding and excessive traction, which may cause damage to the RLNs and other cervical structures. Sternal splitting is estimated to be necessary in only 1–7.5% of retrosternal goitre cases [31,33–35]. Preoperative predictors of the need for sternotomy in such cases include radiologic extension of the mass below the aortic arch [31,34,36], history of previous thyroid surgery [36,37] and CT evidence of adherence to surrounding mediastinal tissues [38]. Median sternotomy in thyroid surgery prolongs hospital stay by 2 days compared with cervical thyroidectomy [34]. Duration of surgery also increases, raising the risk of blood loss and transfusion requirement [31]. CT scanning is essential for surgical planning and should be done for all patients in whom retrosternal goitre is suspected clinically [31].

Overall rates of distant metastasis in thyroid cancer are estimated at 30%, with the majority of lesions arising in the chest [39,40]. Thoracic metastasectomy for various histopathologic subtypes of thyroid cancer is an uncommon but emerging treatment option that has been described in several surgical case series [39–43]. The largest of such studies to date consisted of 48 patients whose pathologies included papillary, follicular, medullary and Hurthle cell thyroid carcinoma [40]. The authors described an overall 5-year postoperative survival rate of 60% and reported no intraoperative mortality.

Most major complications from sternotomy are related to healing. Sternal malunion and incision-related infection are interrelated events occurring in approximately 2–5% of cases and are associated with a mortality rate of 14–47% [44,45]. Malunion of the sternum may be related to sternal closure methods. The basic technique involves sternal reapproximation using a double set of stainless steel wires that pass in and out of the cartilages on each side of the sternum along with appropriate circumferential parasternal wires [46]. In some patients, advanced wiring techniques or rigid support with fixation plates may be required to reinforce the sternum and prevent dehiscence. Risk factors for sternal wound dehiscence include diabetes mellitus, obesity, advanced age, immunosuppression, osteoporosis, renal insufficiency, chronic obstructive pulmonary disease and smoking [44,45,47]. Other risk factors may include transfusions, prolonged critical care admission, steroid use, prolonged postoperative ventilation and surgical chest re-exploration [45,47]. Dehiscence can occur under physiologic loads, especially in high-risk patients.

Clinical signs of sternal separation include local findings of sternal instability, chest wall pain, fluid collection or wound dehiscence. The patient's subjective feelings of throbbing and looseness of the repair can also be indicative of failed closure [45]. Examination of the sternum by x-ray may reveal ruptured wires, wire malposition, sternal dehiscence, fracture and pseudoarthrosis. CT scanning of this region may confirm these findings. Recognition of these features early in the postoperative period may allow for direct sternal reclosure with the use of enhanced techniques for sternal support [45].

Sternal infection involves the layers beneath the skin and subcutaneous tissue while *mediastinitis* refers to further involvement of the organ space. Both are deep space infections directly related to the stability of sternal closure, which is likely technique dependent [45]. Stringent sternotomy closure methods lead to lower infection rates [44]; conversely, subsequent positive wound cultures are indicative of rewiring failure [48]. Atraumatic closure, avoidance of excessive electrocautery, careful attention to aseptic technique and limiting dead space are important principles for avoiding infection. Mediastinal drainage tubes for blood and serous fluid may decrease infection rates and are left in until the second postoperative day. First-generation cephalosporins for antistaphylococcal prophylaxis are given preoperatively and continued until chest drains are removed. Risk factors for sternal wound infection are similar to those for sternal dehiscence [44,45,47]. Presence of a tracheostomy and re-exploration for postoperative haemorrhage may be additional predisposing factors for deep wound infection [45,49].

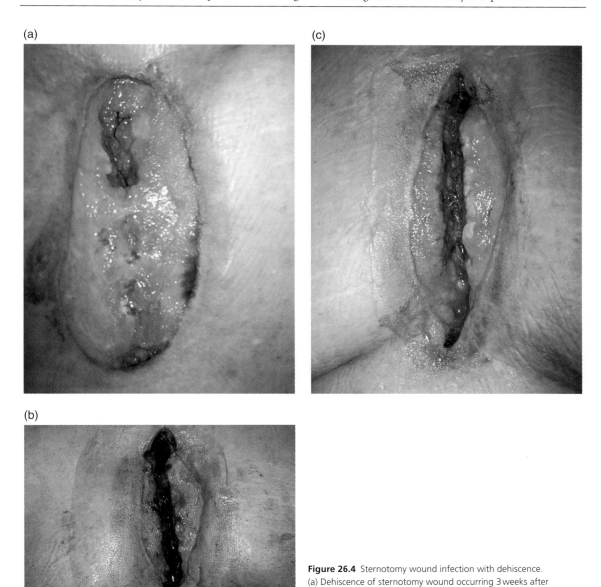

Figure 26.4 Sternotomy wound infection with dehiscence. (a) Dehiscence of sternotomy wound occurring 3 weeks after sternotomy. (b) Sternotomy site immediately after surgical debridement. (c) Granulation and gradual closure of wound after 1 week of healing by secondary intention.

Signs and symptoms of sternal wound infection overlap with those of dehiscence, as these two entities often coincide. In addition, infection usually presents with fever, localized pain or tenderness, erythema, swelling and possibly purulent wound drainage or sepsis (Figure 26.4). Mediastinitis should be considered in patients who exhibit slow postoperative recovery [45]. Chest radiographs can reveal findings of sternal dehiscence while CT scans may highlight fluid collections or other signs of major infection. CT-guided needle aspiration and culture of fluid collections can be diagnostic of infection and help guide further therapy.

Diagnosis of deep sternal wound infection requires prompt operative treatment. Superficial infection may be treated with simple incision and drainage followed by open dressing changes [45]. Mediastinitis requires intraoperative debridement, sternal reclosure and mediastinal antibiotic irrigation. All infected wounds should be cultured intraoperatively. Continuous mediastinal lavage with antibiotics can be achieved using two sets of drainage tubes and allows for primary sternal reclosure [50]. Primary reclosure may also be achieved with the transposition of a vascularized muscle flap, which can fill dead space and help to control infection [51]. Other options include secondary closure with bedside debridement and delayed muscle flap closure [45].

Postoperative management includes culturing the wound site regularly and packing or debriding the wound where necessary. This process may continue after discharge on an outpatient basis. Antibiotic therapy is another mainstay of wound care. Common wound pathogens vary between hospitals, but *Staphylococcus aureus* is the most common, followed by *Staph. epidermidis* [45]. Polymicrobial wound infection has a poor prognosis for wound healing [52]. Initial antibiotic therapy should first be empirical with coverage for gram-negatives, methicillin-resistant gram-positives and anaerobes. Later therapy should be guided by wound cultures. Fungal infection should be considered if the patient fails mediastinal irrigation or long-term antibiotics.

Rib fractures after sternotomy can result from excessively vigorous spreading of or pressure on sternal retractors and from forceful coughing postoperatively [49]. Rib fractures are present in up to 16% of patients [53,54] and usually occur in the first or second rib. Patients typically present with pleuritic chest, subclavicular or shoulder pain and may have point tenderness, deformity or palpable crepitus over the affected ribs. Supine anteroposterior chest x-ray or bone scanning is usually diagnostic. Healing occurs over several weeks but in rare cases recovery may be complicated by brachial plexus injury or Horner's syndrome due to trauma from sharp bony fragments [49]. Prevention includes proper intraoperative arm positioning, controlled retractor spreading and placement of retractors more inferiorly. Patients should also avoid excessive straining or heavy lifting for 2 months after surgery [49].

Acknowledgements

Jeremy Freeman is supported by grants from the Mount Sinai Hospital Foundation of Toronto and from Temmy Latner/Dynacare. The authors would like to thank Dr. Christa Favot for contributing her artistic talents in the creation of Figure 26.2.

References

1 Walton KA, Buono LM. Horner syndrome. Curr Opin Ophthalmol 2003; 14: 357–63.

2 Solomon P, Irish J, Gullane P. Horner's syndrome following a thyroidectomy. J Otolaryngol 1993; 22: 454–6.

3 Smith I, Murley RS. Damage to the cervical sympathetic system during operations on the thyroid gland. Br J Surg 1965; 52: 673–5.

4 Noczynski L, Bielicki F, Dolinski J. [Damage of the cervical part of the sympathetic trunk following surgery on the thyroid gland]. Pol Przegl Chir 1976; 48: 883–7.

5 Italiano D, Cammaroto S, Cedro C, Bramanti P, Ferlazzo E. Horner syndrome following thyroidectomy. Neurol Sci 2011; 32: 531.

6 De Silva WD, de Soysa MS, Perera BL. Iatrogenic Horner's syndrome. a rare complication of thyroid surgery. Ceylon Med J 2010; 55: 136.

7 Cozzaglio L, Coladonato M, Doci R, *et al.* Horner's syndrome as a complication of thyroidectomy. Report of a case. Surg Today 2008; 38: 1114–16.

8 Lyons AJ, Mills CC. Anatomical variants of the cervical sympathetic chain to be considered during neck dissection. Br J Oral Maxillofac Surg 1998; 36: 180–2.

9 Fields CR, Barker FM 2nd. Review of Horner's syndrome and a case report. Optom Vis Sci 1992; 69: 481–5.

10 Harpe KG, Roth RN. Horner's syndrome in the emergency department. J Emerg Med 1990; 8: 629–34.

11 Maloney WF, Younge BR, Moyer NJ. Evaluation of the causes and accuracy of pharmacologic localization in Horner's syndrome. Am J Ophthalmol 1980; 90: 394–402.

12 Reeve TS, Coupland GA, Johnson DC, Buddee FW. The recurrent and external laryngeal nerves in thyroidectomy. Med J Aust 1969; 1: 380–2.

13 Raffaelli M, Iacobone M, Henry JF. The 'false' nonrecurrent inferior laryngeal nerve. Surgery 2000; 128: 1082–7.

14 Tominaga K, Nakahara T. The twenty-degree reverse-Trendelenburg position decreases the incidence and severity of postoperative nausea and vomiting after thyroid surgery. Anesth Analg 2006; 103: 1260–3.

15 Boyce JR, Ness T, Castroman P, Gleysteen JJ. A preliminary study of the optimal anesthesia positioning for the morbidly obese patient. Obes Surg 2003; 13: 4–9.

16 Perilli V, Sollazzi L, Bozza P, *et al.* The effects of the reverse trendelenburg position on respiratory mechanics and blood gases in morbidly obese patients during bariatric surgery. Anesth Analg 2000; 91: 1520–5.

17 Walton-Geer PS. Prevention of pressure ulcers in the surgical patient. AORN J 2009; 89: 538–48; quiz 549–51.

18 McEwen DR. Intraoperative positioning of surgical patients. AORN J 1996; 63: 1059–63, 1066–79; quiz 1080–6.

19 Hoshowsky VM. Surgical positioning. Orthop Nurs 1998; 17: 55–65.

20 Bluestein D, Javaheri A. Pressure ulcers. Prevention, evaluation, and management. Am Fam Physician 2008; 78: 1186–94.

21 Pullen R, Popp R, Volkers P, Fusgen I. Prospective randomized double-blind study of the wound-debriding effects of collagenase and fibrinolysin/deoxyribonuclease in pressure ulcers. Age Ageing 2002; 31: 126–30.

22 Mao CL, Rivet AJ, Sidora T, Pasko MT. Update on pressure ulcer management and deep tissue injury. Ann Pharmacother 2010; 44: 325–32.

23 Argenta LC, Morykwas MJ, Marks MW, DeFranzo AJ, Molnar JA, David LR. Vacuum-assisted closure. State of clinic art. Plast Reconstr Surg 2006; 117: 127 S–142 S.

24 Winfree CJ, Kline DG. Intraoperative positioning nerve injuries. Surg Neurol 2005; 63: 5–18; discussion 18.

25 Stoll G, Muller HW. Nerve injury, axonal degeneration and neural regeneration. Basic insights. Brain Pathol 1999; 9: 313–25.

26 Schulz-Stubner S. Bilateral occipital neuropathy as a rare complication of positioning for thyroid surgery in a morbidly obese patient. Acta Anaesthesiol Scand 2004; 48: 126–7.

27 Wang YC, Huang SY, Lin HT, Hu JS, Chan KH, Tsou MY. Quadriplegia after parathyroidectomy in a hemodialysis patient. Acta Anaesthesiol Taiwan 2011; 49: 32–4.

28 Mercieri M, Paolini S, Mercieri A, *et al.* Tetraplegia following parathyroidectomy in two long-term haemodialysis patients. Anaesthesia 2009; 64: 1010–13.

29 Harley EH, Collins MD. Neurologic sequelae secondary to atlantoaxial instability in Down syndrome. Implications in otolaryngologic surgery. Arch Otolaryngol Head Neck Surg 1994; 120: 159–65.

30 Katlic MR, Wang CA, Grillo HC. Substernal goiter. Ann Thorac Surg 1985; 39: 391–9.

31 Rugiu MG, Piemonte M. Surgical approach to retrosternal goitre. Do we still need sternotomy? Acta Otorhinolaryngol Ital 2009; 29: 331–8.

32 Newman E, Shaha AR. Substernal goiter. J Surg Oncol 1995; 60: 207–12.

33 Singh B, Lucente FE, Shaha AR. Substernal goiter. A clinical review. Am J Otolaryngol 1994; 15: 409–16.

34 Huins CT, Georgalas C, Mehrzad H, Tolley NS. A new classification system for retrosternal goitre based on a systematic review of its complications and management. Int J Surg 2008; 6: 71–6.

35 Rios A, Rodriguez JM, Balsalobre MD, Tebar FJ, Parrilla P. The value of various definitions of intrathoracic goiter for predicting intra-operative and postoperative complications. Surgery 2010; 147: 233–8.

36 Casella C, Pata G, Cappelli C, Salerni B. Preoperative predictors of sternotomy need in mediastinal goiter management. Head Neck 2010; 32: 1131–5.

37 De Perrot M, Fadel E, Mercier O, *et al.* Surgical management of mediastinal goiters: when is a sternotomy required? Thorac Cardiovasc Surg 2007; 55: 39–43.

38 Burns P, Doody J, Timon C. Sternotomy for substernal goitre: an otolaryngologist's perspective. J Laryngol Otol 2008; 122: 495–9.

39 Pak H, Gourgiotis L, Chang WI, *et al.* Role of metastasectomy in the management of thyroid carcinoma: the NIH experience. J Surg Oncol 2003; 82: 10–18.

40 Porterfield JR, Cassivi SD, Wigle DA, *et al.* Thoracic metastasectomy for thyroid malignancies. Eur J Cardiothorac Surg 2009; 36: 155–8.

41 Protopapas AD, Nicholson AG, Vini L, Harmer CL, Goldstraw P. Thoracic metastasectomy in thyroid malignancies. Ann Thorac Surg 2001; 72: 1906–8.

42 Sarrazin R, Brichon PY, Chaffanjon P. [Mediastinal metastasis of differentiated thyroid cancers. Treatment by total mediastinal curettage in 9 cases]. Ann Endocrinol (Paris) 1997; 58: 242–7.

43 Niederle B, Roka R, Schemper M, Fritsch A, Weissel M, Ramach W. Surgical treatment of distant metastases in differentiated thyroid cancer: indication and results. Surgery 1986; 100: 1088–97.

44 Losanoff JE, Jones JW, Richman BW. Primary closure of median sternotomy: techniques and principles. Cardiovasc Surg 2002; 10: 102–10.

45 Losanoff JE, Richman BW, Jones JW. Disruption and infection of median sternotomy: a comprehensive review. Eur J Cardiothorac Surg 2002; 21: 831–9.

46 Robicsek F, Daugherty HK, Cook JW. The prevention and treatment of sternum separation following open-heart surgery. J Thorac Cardiovasc Surg 1977; 73: 267–8.

47 Peivandi AA, Kasper-Konig W, Quinkenstein E, Loos AH, Dahm M. Risk factors influencing the outcome after surgical treatment of complicated deep sternal wound complications. Cardiovasc Surg 2003; 11: 207–12.

48 Murray KD, Pasque MK. Routine sternal closure using six overlapping figure-of-8 wires. Ann Thorac Surg 1997; 64: 1852–4.

49 Weber LD, Peters RW. Delayed chest wall complications of median sternotomy. South Med J 1986; 79: 723–7.

50 Molina JE. Primary closure for infected dehiscence of the sternum. Ann Thorac Surg 1993; 55: 459–63.

51 Jurkiewicz MJ, Bostwick J 3rd, Hester TR, Bishop JB, Craver J. Infected median sternotomy wound. Successful treatment by muscle flaps. Ann Surg 1980; 191: 738–44.

52 Loop FD, Lytle BW, Cosgrove DM, *et al*. J. Maxwell Chamberlain memorial paper. Sternal wound complications after isolated coronary artery bypass grafting. early and late mortality, morbidity, and cost of care. Ann Thorac Surg 1990; 49: 179–86; discussion 186–7.

53 Woodring JH, Royer JM, Todd EP. Upper rib fractures following median sternotomy. Ann Thorac Surg 1985; 39: 355–7.

54 Gumbs RV, Peniston RL, Nabhani HA, Henry LJ. Rib fractures complicating median sternotomy. Ann Thorac Surg 1991; 51: 952–5.

55 National Pressure Ulcer Advisory Panel. Pressure ulcer stages revised by NPUAP. Available at: www.npuap.org/pr2.htm

CHAPTER 27

Late Complications of Thyroid Surgery

Dennis R. Maceri

Department of Otolaryngology – Head and Neck Surgery, Keck School of Medicine, University of Southern California, Los Angeles, CA, USA

Chylous fistula

Leak of chyle (Greek word for 'juice') from the thoracic duct or right lymphatic duct after thyroidectomy is a rare but potentially lethal complication. In the early 1900s, chylous fistula was a well-recognized complication of neck surgery with an associated mortality rate of 12% [1]. This consequence was first reported after neck surgery in 1901 and is estimated to occur in 4.5–8% of patients undergoing thyroidectomy and lateral neck dissection [2]. The rate is increased in reoperation for persistent or recurrent disease [3]. With the addition of a central compartment dissection in thyroidectomy for differentiated thyroid cancer, the risk has been reported by Roh and colleagues to be 1.4% [2].

The leakage develops as a consequence of violation of the main thoracic duct or one of the numerous tributaries and is often missed during the initial operative procedure and recognized only after the resumption of a regular diet. Greenfield and Gottlieb described the various anatomical patterns in a cadaver study of 75 specimens. They found that 45 of 75 thoracic ducts studied terminated on the lateral surface of the internal jugular vein as a single vessel near the junction of the subclavian vein. When the duct did not enter the jugular vein, it entered the subclavian or the innominate. In addition, 10% had multiple terminal duct endings [4]. If recognized intraoperatively, the vessels are ligated or clipped. Having the anesthesiologist ventilate the patient with positive airway pressure (Valsalva manoeuvre) can assist in the recognition of a suspected leak or confirm adequate control of an identified leak.

A delayed chyle leak is heralded by an increase in suction drain output of a milky white liquid after resumption of a diet containing regular fat content. One sees the drain output rapidly increase from an otherwise decreasing rate to 300 cc daily or more. The characteristic colour change from a serosanguinous output to the milky white liquid seen in chylous fistulae is in itself diagnostic. Patients discharged within 24 h and without a drain may present with a fluid collection under the skin in the first week after surgery that shows the characteristic colour upon aspiration. Early recognition and appropriate treatment are essential. In order to confirm the diagnosis, the fluid should be sent for chemical analysis that includes triglycerides, protein level, cell count and chemistries. Rodgers *et al.* reported that if drainage triglyceride levels are higher than 100 mg/dL or higher than the serum triglyceride levels, the diagnosis of chylous fistula is supported [5].

Chyle is a mixture of lymph from the interstitial fluid and emulsified fat absorbed as chylomicrons from the intestinal villa. Chyle contains some protein and an electrolyte composition similar to that of plasma except for a lower calcium content. The leucocyte count ranges from 400 to 6800 cells/mm^3 dominated by T-lymphocytes.

Thyroid Surgery: Preventing and Managing Complications, First Edition. Edited by Paolo Miccoli, David J. Terris, Michele N. Minuto and Melanie W. Seybt.
© 2013 John Wiley & Sons, Ltd. Published 2013 by John Wiley & Sons, Ltd.

Daily drainage can reach 2–4 L/day in high-output leaks [6]. Long chain triglycerides (>10 carbons) make up 70% of the dietary fat and enter the bloodstream through the chylous route whereas medium chain triglycerides (MCT) and short chain triglycerides are absorbed into the portal system directly. It is the fat content that gives chyle the milky colour and greasy texture [7].

Of course, the best treatment for chylous fistula is prevention. Crumley found that the most common site of thoracic duct injury is at the base of the neck lateral to the carotid sheath [8]. The surgeon must be extremely diligent and attentive to detail when dissecting lymph nodes in levels IV, V and VI. When recognized, injury to the duct must be ligated or clipped. Early reports feared that ligation of the thoracic duct was incompatible with life [9]. However, subsequent studies demonstrated that a collateral circulation develops after thoracic duct ligation which allows the return of lymphatic fluid to the venous system and that it is virtually impossible to keep chyle out of the circulation [10]. In an excellent review of the topic and presentation of 15 cases of chylous fistula, Nussenbaum *et al.* advocated that all patients be given a trial of conservative management with dietary restrictions (no-fat diet or MCT diet), pressure dressings and closed suction drainage. They were successful in 80% of their patients. Three patients required reoperation. Their conclusion was that optimal treatment is unclear [11]. Sclerotherapy using tetracycline was described by Metson *et al.* as an adjunct to conservative treatment of chylous fistula. The powdered form of the drug was injected percutaneously in the supraclavicular area and resulted in a rapid decrease in fistula output within hours [12].

Since reoperation for persistent high-output chylous fistula (greater than 500 cc/day) in patients with thyroid cancer is difficult and dangerous due to scar tissue and inflammation, a more conservative approach is desired. Today, the cornerstone of conservative management is reduced dietary intake of long chain triglycerides by implementing a no-fat diet and MCT or keeping the patient nil by mouth and using total parenteral nutrition (TPN) which requires a central line.

The use of somatostatin was first described by Ulibarri in 1990 [13]. Somatostatin or one of its analogues used in conjunction with dietary restriction and suction drainage has revolutionized treatment of this disease. The course of treatment ranges from 3 to 17 days whereas treatment with TPN without somatostatin has a mean time of 35 days to closure [14]. The hormone somatostatin is made in the hypothalamus and travels to the anterior pituitary via the portal system to inhibit the release of growth hormone (GH) as well as thyroid-stimulating hormone (TSH). In the pancreas, the hormone inhibits insulin and glucagon secretion. The effect on the gastrointestinal tract is to reduce chyle production by decreasing intestinal blood flow as well as decreasing gastric, biliary and intestinal secretions. It also decreases the intestinal absorption of fats, reduces the triglyceride concentration in the thoracic duct and reduces lymph flow [15]. Somatostatin can be given by continuous infusion at 6 mg/day or 100–200 µg injected subcutaneously three times a day [16]. The drug octreotide is a long-acting synthetic analogue of somatostatin and is available for clinical use.

Chylous fistulae lead to prolonged hospitalization, potential problems with protein and electrolyte balance and immunological complications. This complication must be recognized immediately and treated appropriately.

Delayed hypocalcaemia following thyroidectomy

Hypoparathyroidism leading to hypocalcaemia is a well-known and feared complication of total thyroidectomy. The resultant hypocalcaemia may be transient or permanent. A postoperative decrease of the serum calcium is frequently observed within 2–5 days after total thyroidectomy, requiring exogenous replacement and potential prolonged hospital stay [17]. Temporary or transient hypocalcaemia is reported to occur in 2–30% of cases. The rate of permanent hypoparathyroidism is reported to be in the range of 0.5–13.8% [18]. The delayed hypoparathyroidism and hypocalcaemia can occur in the first postoperative week and have been reported to occur months and even years following thyroidectomy [19,20]. Of significant concern and consequence is the development of hypocalcaemia after thyroidectomy for Graves' disease [21]. Despite excellent surgical technique and anatomical preservation of the parathyroid glands and their blood supply, theses patients can demonstrate a delayed and rapid drop in serum calcium 2–3 days after total thyroidectomy.

First-line therapy for Graves' disease is traditionally antithyroid drugs (the thionamides) followed by ablation with I^{131} where antithyroid drugs have failed or the patient is intolerant to the medication. As a consequence of perceived higher risks and complications, surgical treatment for Graves' disease is usually reserved for pregnant patients, children and individuals with significant exophthalmos, exceptionally large glands, those who have failed previous radioiodine therapy or because of patient preference. The appropriate operation for Graves' disease is near-total or total thyroidectomy [22]. The advantage of surgical treatment for Graves' disease is that there is immediate relief of symptoms and the recurrence rate of hyperthyroidism is negligible compared to the 22% recurrence rate reported with subtotal thyroidectomy [23]. It is believed that patients undergoing thyroidectomy for Graves' disease are more likely to develop postoperative hypoparathyroidism than those treated with total thyroidectomy for other indications [24]. Symptoms of severe hypocalcaemia include perioral numbness, extremity paraesthesias or myalgias, a positive Chvostek sign (many patients have a positive Chvostek preoperatively) or Trousseau sign.

The mechanism responsible for the increased likelihood of developing postoperative hypocalcaemia in the hyperthyroid patient is not fully understood. Possible explanations include direct surgical trauma to the parathyroid glands or their inadvertent removal. An increase in bleeding in the hypervascular Graves' disease gland as well as adhesions between the thyroid capsule and the parathyroid glands make identification difficult and disruption of blood supply possible. This is especially true when the venous drainage is disrupted which leads to congestion and damage to the parathyroid tissue.

In chronic vitamin D deficiency, there can be an expected secondary hyperparathyroidism with elevated serum parathyroid hormone (PTH) levels. In a study by Erbil et al., the authors demonstrated that their patients with vitamin D-deficient/insufficient states had PTH levels that were normal before surgery [25]. This was felt to be inappropriate since the PTH level should be high in vitamin D deficiency. Chernobilski et al. also reported suppressed PTH and 1,25-dihydroxyvitamin D levels in Graves' patients compared with multinodular goitre cases. They felt that this could be caused by a more severe degree of hyperthyroidism and might be due to an immune-mediated event [26].

It has been shown that when Graves' patients have vitamin D deficiency/insufficiency preoperatively, it is a pre-

dictor for postoperative hypocalcaemia. This was especially true if the serum alkaline phosphatase was also elevated, indicating ongoing bone turnover [25,27]. Thyrotoxic osteodystrophy in Graves' can lead to development of the hungry bone syndrome. This occurs because hyperthyroidism is associated with increased bone resorption and when corrected, calcium returns to the bone which can lower serum calcium levels [28]. The drop in serum calcium due to hungry bone syndrome is transient and should recover if the integrity of the parathyroid glands has been preserved intraoperatively. Furthermore, in the setting of thyrotoxic osteodystrophy associated with hyperthyroidism, the patient is more susceptible to iatrogenic parathyroid gland damage which disrupts the compensatory rise in PTH needed to restore normocalcaemia [29].

The hyperthyroid state has significant impact on bone turnover even after restoration of euthyroid status. Pantazi & Papapetrou found that PTH concentrations remained elevated during the first year of hyperthyroidism treatment, further substantiating the increased bone turnover rate [30]. The theory that manipulation of the gland during thyroidectomy leads to increased release of calcitonin was also considered as a possible explanation for the increased rate of postoperative hypocalcaemia [31]. However, that hypothesis has been shown not to be the case due to the short plasma life of calcitonin [32]. Pesce et al. found that in 68 patients with Graves' disease, those individuals were more likely to require increased dosages of calcium as well as develop tetany after thyroidectomy compared to those undergoing thyroidectomy for other reasons. This trend to develop hypocalcaemia was noted the day after surgery and 1 month later. The authors felt that this was a consequence of alterations in calcium homeostasis [33]. Vescan et al. advocated postoperative PTH levels as a predictor of patients at risk for the development of hypocalcaemia following thyroidectomy. Their data suggest that if the postoperative PTH level 1 h after thyroidectomy is below 1.1 pmol/L, there is a high likelihood of developing hypocalcaemia. This would allow calcium replacement to begin before the serum calcium actually drops [34]. Although the use of immediate postoperative PTH monitoring to predict impending serious hypocalcaemia has potential merits, one has to use this information with caution. Hypocalcaemia, acute and chronic, can exist in the face of normal PTH levels. Therefore, PTH levels must be interpreted with concomitant serum calcium and phosphorus levels. Pattou and colleagues found that when serum calcium remained at 8 mg/dL or less and/or serum phosphorus levels were 4 mg/dL or higher, or both, the risk for postoperative hypocalcaemia was 66% and 69%, respectively [35].

It is recommended that preoperative vitamin D, alkaline phosphatase, calcium and PTH levels be obtained in all Graves' disease patients prior to thyroidectomy. These laboratory parameters assist in the identification of those hyperthyroid patients at risk for postoperative hypocalcaemia. Of course, meticulous dissection of the parathyroid glands with preservation of vascular integrity is essential. Devascularized ischaemic glands should be autotransplanted into the sternocleidomastoid muscle at the end of the procedure.

Thyroid storm

Total thyroidectomy for Graves' disease is reserved for patients who have failed or refused radioiodine therapy or have become intolerant to the antithyroid drugs (the thionamide family) propylthiouracil or methimazole. Preoperative preparation of the hyperthyroid patient is essential to avoid the potentially lethal complication of thyroid storm.

Thyroid storm can be thought of as the end-stage result in the spectrum of hyperthyroidism. Hyperthyroidism is the overproduction of thyroid hormone (T4 and T3) from the thyroid gland. Thyrotoxicosis is excessive thyroid hormone in the circulation and thyroid storm is the extreme manifestation of thyrotoxicosis [36]. The most common cause of thyrotoxicosis is Graves' disease. Graves' disease is mediated by thyroid-stimulating immunoglobulin (TSI) which results in an unregulated excess production of thyroid hormone. In the setting of hyperthyroidism, thyroid storm can be precipitated by any systemic insult such as surgery, trauma, myocardial infarction and pulmonary thromboembolism [37]. In the past, unprepared surgical patients with hyperthyroidism were the most likely to develop thyroid storm. Surgical manipulation of a large gland in the face of hyperthyroidism is associated with a massive release of hormone into the bloodstream.

Although this potentially life-threatening complication most often occurs in the operating room, it can occur up to 36 h into the postoperative period. The high mortality rate associated with thyroid surgery for thyrotoxicosis was due to thyroid storm and in the early 20th century was as high as 20% in less experienced hands [38]. Preparation of the gland prior to surgery with inorganic iodine began in 1923 and antithyroid drug use was started in the 1940s. In the 1960s, β-adrenergic blockade with propranolol was instituted which even further lowered the mortality to less than 1% [39]. Recognition of the early signs and symptoms of the disease is essential for proper treatment. Burch & Wartofsky developed a point system to assess the level of impairment in the various body systems affected in thyroid storm (thermoregulatory, central nervous, gastrointestinal and cardiovascular) [40]. Of course, clinical suspicion of storm in a thyrotoxic patient is most important and should be treated aggressively. Temperature elevations during or after thyroidectomy, in the patient with storm, can range from 100° to as high as 104 °F as the uncontrolled hypermetabolic state progresses. The cardiovascular manifestations of storm include tachycardia and high-output congestive heart failure.

In 1948, Wolff and Chaikoff reported that binding of inorganic iodide in the thyroid was reduced when plasma iodide levels were elevated (acute Wolff–Chaikoff effect). This is an autoregulatory phenomenon of the thyroid gland that inhibits oxidation of iodide (essential in hormone synthesis) in the thyroid when large amounts of iodine are ingested. As a consequence, there is a reduction in thyroid hormone levels in the bloodstream as a result of decreased synthesis and release. The Wolff–Chaikoff effect lasts around 10 days after which the thyroid escapes from the iodine blockade [41]. The escape phenomenon is thought to occur because of decreased iodine transport into the thyroid cell as a consequence of downregulation of the DNA, mRNA and associated proteins that code for the sodium-iodide symporter on the membrane of the thyroid follicular cell [42].

The Wolff–Chaikoff effect allows for adequate preparation of the hyperthyroid patient prior to thyroidectomy and is an adjunct to prevention of thyroid storm. Non-emergency patients are prepared for thyroidectomy; a 10–12-day course of iodine is used in conjunction with continuation of antithyroid drugs and β-adrenergic blockage to achieve a euthyroid state. The iodine is given as a saturated solution of potassium iodide (SSKI) which is prepared from a concentrated solution of 1000 mg/mL. The average dose is 250 mg KI given three times per day for 10 days in adults. For infants, the dose is 2 mg/kg given three times a day. When rapid preoperative preparation of the thyrotoxic patient is necessary, β-adrenergic blockade with propranolol 40–80 mg is given by mouth three or four times a day and continued in the postoperative period. In addition, thionamide drugs, propylthiouracil 200 mg by mouth every 4 h or methimazole 20 mg by mouth every 4 h, are given and continued postoperatively. The β-blockade decreases the conversion of thyroxin (T4) to tri-iodothyronine (T3). Propylthiouracil decreases new hormone synthesis and decreases conversion of T4 to T3. Methimazole inhibits new hormone synthesis [39]. It is extremely important to continue β-adrenergic blockade in the postoperative period because the half-life of T4 is 7–8 days. After thyroidectomy, thionamide treatment can be stopped in 1–3 days if a complete resection has been achieved [38].

Voice and swallowing dysfunction after thyroidectomy

Problems with phonation and swallowing following thyroidectomy are frequently seen and usually due to problems arising from damage to the paired laryngeal nerves. Previously reported studies demonstrate that somewhere between 25% and 90% of patients report abnormal voice within the first few weeks after surgery and that 11–15% have prolonged symptoms lasting 3–6 months [43]. Most commonly, this is due to injury or intentional sacrifice of the recurrent laryngeal nerve (RLN), especially in extensive thyroid cancer [44]. Injury to the external branch of the superior laryngeal nerve (EBSLN) results in a more subtle injury to most patients but can be catastrophic to the patient with a professional voice. The impaired cricothyroid muscle action (the tensor of the larynx) makes it nearly impossible for singers to produce high-pitched sounds [45]. These complications of nerve injury are predictable and measurable in the postoperative period with the use of laryngostroboscopic analysis. The incidence of EBSLN injury has been reported to be anywhere from 0% to 14% and it is frequently overlooked [46]. In order to minimize the potential for EBSLN injury, it is recommended that the superior thyroid pole vessels be identified and individually ligated along the thyroid capsule [47]. Since there is no treatment for this problem, meticulous technique and attention to the anatomical variations of the superior pole vessels are essential.

Swallowing difficulties after thyroidectomy in the absence of laryngeal nerve injury are common complaints

for patients. They complain of dysphagia, tightness of the throat and neck, frequent throat clearing and a globus sensation and must be evaluated for gastro-oesophageal reflux or laryngopharyngeal reflux. A search of the PubMed database does not reveal any studies specifically linking thyroidectomy to the uncovering or precipitation of reflux symptoms and frank disease. It is the author's personal experience, based on numerous post-thyroidectomy videolaryngostroboscopic evaluations, that it is not uncommon to find laryngeal oedema and erythema as well as stringing of secretions at the glottis and supraglottic larynx. These findings are consistent with laryngopharyngeal reflux. Moreover, these patients frequently have a favourable response to protein pump inhibitors.

Many patients suffer short- and long-term voice abnormalities after thyroidectomy but have no evidence of laryngeal nerve injuries [48]. In an excellent study by Lombardi *et al.*, it was demonstrated that thyroidectomy patients frequently complained of voice and swallowing changes even when the surgery was uncomplicated with respect to injury of the RLN or EBSLN [49]. The problem is that the aforementioned complaints do not translate into objective findings. Typical complaints from this cohort of patients after responding to a subjective voice evaluation questionnaire were a hoarse voice, difficulty singing or raising the voice, vocal changes and fatigue during the day and an overall increased effort to speak. The patients were evaluated preoperatively and 3 months post thyroidectomy with videostroboscopy, acoustic voice analysis using a multidimensional voice program and maximum phonation time (MPT) tests. MPT is done by having the patient sustain the vowel 'a' for as long as possible. The authors found that most of these complaints were temporary but without question they were a source of anxiety and frustration[49].

Several explanations have been put forward as to the cause of these problems, including endotracheal intubation [45], modification of the vascular supply and venous drainage of the larynx [50], cricothyroid muscle dysfunction [51], laryngotracheal fixation with impairment of vertical movement of the larynx [45], strap muscle malfunction due to transaction or nerve injury [52], and local pain and oedema as well as a component of psychological reaction to the surgery [50]. Many of the muscular problems, pain, decreased range of motion and lymphoedema are very amenable to treatment by trained physical therapists familiar with the postoperative consequences of thyroidectomy or neck dissection. Henry *et al.* used a Dysphonia Severity

Index (DSI) preoperatively as well as 3 and 6 months after thyroidectomy. The DSI is scored from −5 to +5 where +5 is a normal healthy voice. These measures have been shown to be highly related to clinician-perceived and patient-reported severity of voice handicap [53]. The DSI incorporated measurements of maximum phonation time (MPT in seconds), highest vocal frequency, lowest vocal intensity and jitter. Jitter is an acoustical concept that measures variation of vocal frequencies from the baseline or F^0 frequency. Henry *et al.* recorded patients as having a normal voice versus a negative voice outcome (NVO). The DSI was reduced from baseline in the early post-thyroidectomy period (1–4 weeks) in patients who were found to have long-term NVO [54].

Appropriate preoperative measurements using strobe and a dysphonia index afford the surgeon an opportunity to elucidate pre-existing laryngeal pathology that might be missed with standard mirror or flexible laryngoscopy. Furthermore, the detection of postoperative voice abnormalities facilitates early referral to speech and language professionals for voice therapy. A hard copy of the laryngostroboscopic exam is preserved in the patient record which provides a follow-up reference for the doctor and patient.

The important concept here is that whatever the aetiology of these postoperative complaints, they are significant and potentially life-altering consequences of thyroidectomy. Therefore, the patient needs to be advised of the potential for voice and swallowing dysfunction after surgery. It cannot be stressed enough that preoperative voice evaluation with video laryngostroboscopy and an instrument to measure the degree of dysphonia is critical in the care of these patients.

References

1 Izzard ME, Crowder VL, Southwell KE. The use of Monogen in the conservative management of chylous fistula. Otolaryngol Head Neck Surg 2007; 136: S50–S53.

2 Roh JL, Yoon YH, Park CI. Chyle leakage in patients undergoing thyroidectomy plus central neck dissection for differentiated papillary thyroid carcinoma. Ann Surg Oncol 2008; 15: 2576–80.

3 Noguchi M, Kinami S, Kinoshita K, et al. Risk of bilateral lymph node metastases in papillary thyroid cancer. J Surg Oncol 1993; 52: 155–9.

4 Greenfield J, Gottlieb MI. Variations in the terminal portion of the human thoracic duct. Arch Surg 1956; 73: 955–9.

5 Rogers GK, Johnson JT, Petrzzelli GJ, et al. Lipid and volume analysis of neck drainage in patients undergoing neck dissection. Am J Otolaryngol 1992; 13: 306–9.

6 Tinley NL, Murray JE. Chronic thoracic duct fistula: operative technique and physiologic effects in man. Ann Surg 1968; 167: 1–8.

7 Meyers EN, Dinerman WS. Management of chylous fistulas. Laryngoscope 1975; 85: 835–40.

8 Crumley RL, Smith JD. Postoperative chylous fistula prevention and management. Laryngoscope 1976; 86: 804–13.

9 Loe LH. Injuries to the thoracic duct. Arch Surg 1946; 53: 448–55.

10 Blalock A, Robinson CS, Cunningham RS, et al. Experimental studies on lymphatic blockage. Arch Surg 1937; 34: 1049–71.

11 Nussenbaum B, Liu JH, Sinard RJ. Systematic management of chyle fistula: the Southwestern experience and review of the literature. Otolaryngol Head Neck Surg 2000; 122: 31–8.

12 Metson R, Alessi D, Calcaterra TC. Tetracycline sclerotherapy for chylous fistula following neck dissection. Arch Otolaryngol Head Neck Surg 1986; 112: 651–3.

13 Ulibarri JI, Sanz Y, Fuentes C, et al. Reduction of lymphorrhagia from ruptured thoracic duct by somatostatin. Lancet 1990; 335: 258.

14 Bolger C, Walsh TN, Tanner WA, et al. Chylothorax after esophagectomy. Br J Surg 1991; 78: 587–8.

15 Collard JM, Laterre PF, Boemer F, Reynaert M, Ponlot R. Conservative treatment of postsurgical lymphatic leaks with somatostatin-14. Chest 2000; 117: 902–5.

16 Valentine C, Barresi R, Prinz R. Somatostatin analog treatment of a cervical thoracic duct fistula. Head Neck 2002; 24: 810–13.

17 Pederson WC, Johnson CL, Gaskill HV, et al. Operative management of thyroid disease: technical considerations in a residency training program. Am J Surg 1984; 148: 350–9.

18 Demeester D, Hooghe L, Geertruyden V, et al. Hypocalcemia after thyroidectomy. Arch Surg 1992; 127: 854–7.

19 Bourrel CB, Uzzan B, Tison P, et al. Transient hypocalcemia after thyroidectomy. Ann Otol Rhinol Laryngol 1993; 102: 496–501.

20 Tovi F, Noyek AM, Chapnik JS, Freeman JL. Safety of total thyroidectomy: review of 100 consecutive cases. Laryngoscope 1989; 99: 1233–7.

21 Gann DS, Paone JF. Delayed hypocalcemia after thyroidectomy for Graves' disease is prevented by parathyroid autotransplantation. Ann Surg 1979; 190: 508–11.

22 Wilhelm S, McHenry C. Total thyroidectomy is superior to subtotal thyroidectomy for management of Graves' disease in the United States. World J Surg 2010; 34: 1261–4.

23 Sugino K, Ito K, Nagahama M et al.Surgical management of Graves' disease: 10-year prospective trial at a single institution. Endocr J 2008; 55: 161–8.

24 Welch KC, McHenry CR. Total thyroidectomy: is morbidity higher for Graves' disease than nontoxic goiter? J Surg Res 2011; 170: 96–9.

25 Erbil Y, Ozbey NC, Sari S, et al. Determinants of post-operative hypocalcemia in vitamin D-deficient Graves' patients after thyroidectomy. Am J Surg 2011; 201: 678–84.

26 Chernobilski H, Scharla S, Schmidt-Gayk H, et al. Enhanced suppression of 1,25(OH)2D3 and intact parathyroid hormone in Graves' disease as compared to toxic multinodular goiter. Calcif Tissue Int 1988; 42: 5–12.

27 Yamashita H, Noguchi S, Murakami I, et al. Predictive risk factors for postoperative tetany in female patients with Graves' disease. J Am Coll Surg 2001; 192: 465–8.

28 Michie W, Stowers JM, Duncan T, et al. Mechanism of hypocalcemia after thyroidectomy for thyrotoxicosis. Lancet 1971; 1: 508–9.

29 Biet A, Zaatar R, Strunski V, et al. Postoperative complications in total thyroidectomy for Graves' disease: comparison with multinodular benign goiter surgery. Ann Otolaryngol Chir Cervicofac 2009; 126: 190–5.

30 Pantazi H, Papapetrou PD. Changes in parameters of bone and mineral metabolism during therapy for hyperthyroidism. J Clin Endocrinol Metab 2000; 85: 1099–106.

31 Wilkin TJ, Paterson CR, Isles TE, et al. Post thyroidectomy hypocalcemia: a feature of the operation or the thyroid disorder. Lancet 1977; 1: 621–2.

32 McHenry CR, Speroff T, Wentworth D, et al. Risk factors for post-thyroidectomy hypocalcemia. Surgery 1994; 116: 641–5.

33 Pesce CE, Shiue Z, Tsai HL, et al. Postoperative hypocalcemia after thyroidectomy for Graves' disease. Thyroid 2010; 20: 1279–83.

34 Vescan A, Witterick I, Freeman J. Parathyroid hormone as a predictor of hypocalcemia after thyroidectomy. Laryngoscope 2005; 115: 2105–8.

35 Pattou F, Combemale F, Fabre S, et al. Hypocalcemia following thyroid surgery: incidence and prediction of outcome. World J Surg 1998; 22: 718–24.

36 Larsen PR, Davies TF. Thyrotoxicosis. In: Larsen PR, Rosenberg HM (eds) Williams Textbook of Endocrinology, 10th edn . Philadelphia: WB Saunders, 2002: 374–421.

37 Goldberg PA, Inzucchi SE. Critical issues in endocrinology. Clin Chest Med 2003; 24: 583–606.

38 Nayak BN, Burman K. Thyrotoxicosis and thyroid storm. Endocrinol Metab Clin North Am 2006; 35: 663–8.

39 Langley RW, Burch HB. Perioperative management of the thyrotoxic patient. Endocrinol Metab Clin North Am 2003; 32: 519–34.

40 Burch HB, Wartofsky L. Life-threatening thyrotoxicosis. Thyroid storm. Endocrinol Metab Clin North Am 1993; 22: 263–77.

41 Wolff J, Chaikoff IL. Plasma inorganic iodide as a homeostatic regulator of thyroid function. J Biol Chem 1948; 174: 555–64.

42 Eng PHK, Cardona GR, Fang SL, et al. Escape from the acute Wolff–Chaikoff effect is associated with a decrease in thyroid sodium/iodide symporter messenger ribonucleic acid and protein. Endocrinology 1999; 140: 3404–10.

43 De Pedro NI, Fae A, Vartanian JG, et al. Voice and vocal self-assessment after thyroidectomy. Head Neck 2006; 28: 1106–14.

44 Rosato L, Carlevato MT, de Toma G, Avenia N. Recurrent laryngeal nerve damage and phonetic modifications after total thyroidectomy: surgical malpractice only or predictable sequence? World J Surg 2005; 29: 780–3.

45 Stojadinovic A, Shaha AR, Orlikoff RF, et al. Prospective functional voice assessment in patients undergoing thyroid surgery. Ann Surg 2002; 236: 823–32.

46 Dursun G, Sataloff R, Spiegal J, et al. Superior laryngeal nerve paresis and paralysis. J Voice 1996; 10: 206–11.

47 Bellantone R, Boscherini M, Lombardi CP, et al. Is the identification of the external branch of the superior laryngeal nerve mandatory in thyroid operations? Results of a randomized prospective study. Surgery 2001; 130: 1055–9.

48 Pereria JA, Girvent M, Sancho JJ,Parada C, Sitges-Serra A. Prevalence of long-term upper aero-digestive symptoms after uncomplicated bilateral thyroidectomy. Surgery 2003; 133: 18–22.

49 Lombardi CP, Raffaelli M, d'Alatri L, et al. Voice and swallowing changes after thyroidectomy in patients without inferior laryngeal nerve injuries. Surgery 2006; 140: 1026–34.

50 Debruyne F, Ostyn F, Delaere P, Wellens W. Acoustic analysis of the speaking voice after thyroidectomy. J Voice 1997; 11: 479–82.

51 Siagra DL, Montesinos MR, Tacchi VA, et al. Voice changes after thyroidectomy: recurrent nerve injury. J Am Coll Surg 2004; 199: 556–60.

52 Hong KH, Kim YK, Phonatory characteristics of patients undergoing thyroidectomy without laryngeal nerve injury. Otolaryngol Head Neck Surg 1997; 117: 399–404.

53 Wuyts FL, Bodt MS, Molenbergs G, et al. The Dysphonia Severity Index: an objective measure of voice quality based on a multiparameter approach. J Speech Lang Hearing Res 2000; 43: 796–809.

54 Henry LR, Helou LB, Solomon NP, et al. Functional voice outcomes after thyroidectomy: an assessment of the Dysphonia Severity Index (DSI) after thyroidectomy. Surgery 2010; 147: 861–70.

CHAPTER 28

Post-thyroidectomy Distress: Voice and Swallowing Impairment Following Thyroidectomy

Mira Milas[1] *and Zvonimir Milas*[2]

[1] Department of Endocrine Surgery, Endocrinology and Metabolism Institute, Cleveland Clinic, Cleveland, OH, USA

[2] Department of Head and Neck Surgery, University of Texas M.D. Anderson Cancer Center, Orlando, FL, USA

Introduction

There is a spectrum of symptoms that affect the upper aerodigestive system and that are commonly experienced after thyroid surgery. These range from minor and temporary disturbances of voice, speech and swallowing to serious dysfunction of the speaking or singing voice that impairs quality of life. Surgeons have traditionally been aware of and emphasize the need to achieve optimum voice preservation in individuals who require thyroid surgery. On this topic, for example, literature widely covers the recognition and prevention of potential complications related to the laryngeal nerves, availability of diagnostic modalities to evaluate the voice, and treatment options to rehabilitate the voice [1–5]. There are more subtle changes that can occur in the absence of laryngeal nerve injury. These include the subjective perception by patients that their voice is gravelly or weak, that the process of swallowing is more difficult or that something 'pulls', 'hurts' or 'feels stuck' in the neck. Many of these symptoms promptly resolve or are interpreted in the wider context of postoperative healing, making deeper inquiry by physicians and patients less likely. Only more recently have these postoperative symptoms garnered interest and become the subject of case-based analysis

[6–10]. Much progress is still required to raise awareness about such impairments.

This chapter focuses on contemporary issues in 'post-thyroidectomy distress', defined as problems affecting the functions of voice and swallowing that affect a patient's daily life or professional activities, whether they experience spontaneous resolution or cause permanent disability. Understanding the causes of voice and swallowing impairment can lead to improved patient education preoperatively, attention to technique intraoperatively, and ability to provide reassurance or direct therapy postoperatively.

Issues of voice impairment

General principles, prevalence and anatomy

The voice is a complex product, resulting from the actions of many anatomical components that cover the head and neck, respiratory and upper abdominal regions. Most important, and also most relevant to thyroid surgery, are the laryngeal nerves that lie in proximity to the planes of dissection during thyroidectomy: the recurrent laryngeal nerves (RLN) and the external branches of the superior

Thyroid Surgery: Preventing and Managing Complications, First Edition. Edited by Paolo Miccoli, David J. Terris, Michele N. Minuto and Melanie W. Seybt.

laryngeal nerves (EBSLN). They are at risk from operative manoeuvres and from underlying thyroid disease, most notably extrathyroidal or lymphatic extranodal invasion by thyroid cancers. The anatomy of these structures was described in detail in a preceding chapter. Additionally, reviews by several groups have emphasized and described the postoperative changes that can make reoperative exploration challenging and pose higher risks of laryngeal nerve injury [2,5,11–13].

The reported prevalence of RLN injuries after thyroid surgery varies widely. Randolph compiled the following statistics current for 2010 [1]. Transient RLN paresis rates appear to average around 10%, based on a meta-analysis of 27 published articles with over 25,000 patients undergoing thyroidectomy. Permanent RLN paralysis rates are reported to be as low as 0% to as high as 18.6%, depending on the method of laryngeal evaluation. A Scandinavian quality registry of thyroid and parathyroid procedures described a 4.3% rate of immediate vocal cord paralysis in 2008. This report, and a British registry which identified a 2.5% rate, relied on surgeon-reported data from settings which do not routinely use postoperative laryngoscopy. The RLN paralysis rate doubled in the Scandinavian registry, when directed at data from patients who had routine postoperative laryngoscopy. In contrast to these fortunately modest numbers, the incidence of voice impairments directly after thyroid surgery, and as a general perioperative symptom, has been reported in as many as 41–84% of patients [9].

Recurrent laryngeal nerve paralysis can exist in a patient with a normal voice. Conversely, there can be significant voice change when RLN and EBSLN functions are confirmed by laryngoscopy or other examinations to be normal. Therefore, the reassurance a surgeon may gain about the status of laryngeal nerves by simply listening to the sound of their patient's voice is limited. It is not possible to conclude reliably that a normal preoperative voice equates to normal or unaffected laryngeal nerves. Similarly, it is impossible to feel relieved that a normal voice upon extubation or immediately postoperatively indicates that the laryngeal nerves were uninjured during surgery. Conversely, significant voice changes or hoarseness in the immediate perioperative period does not necessarily reflect permanent RLN paralysis. A functional assessment of laryngeal nerve function is ultimately necessary preoperatively and on subsequent evaluations to define the character of the voice deficit and expectations for recovery. Attentiveness to details about the voice during longitudinal follow-up is likewise valuable, even though it may not be the primary focus of care, such as in thyroid cancer patients.

A number of experts advocate routine pre- and postoperative laryngeal examination of patients undergoing thyroid surgery [1,2,14]. Preoperative assessment of the larynx can objectively define the status of the voice in reference to vocal cord function and identify unsuspected intrinsic and extrinsic laryngeal abnormalities. Some thyroid conditions are more likely to affect the voice preoperatively. These include Graves' disease or severe thyroiditis, large compressive goitres and invasive thyroid malignancies [5,15]. The prevalence of invasive thyroid disease, reflected by vocal cord dysfunction or invasiveness into adjacent anatomical structures (trachea, oesophagus, strap muscles), was 6% in several recent series [2,15]. In a group of 365 patients undergoing surgery at a large tertiary thyroid referral centre, laryngoscopy detected preoperative vocal cord paralysis in 4% of patients [2]. Notably, however, this rate was 71% for a subset of 21 patients whose final pathology confirmed invasive thyroid cancer and whose presentation was a self-discovered neck mass, although the majority of these patients (67%) did not exhibit or notice voice change at presentation. In the remaining 344 patients whose operations were performed for benign disease, preoperative vocal cord paralysis was found in only one (0.3%) who had a massive substernal goitre. This study further went on to describe that vocal cord paralysis, if seen on preoperative laryngoscopy and viewed as a screening test for invasive thyroid cancer, had sensitivity of 76% and specificity of 100%. Thus, the surgeon's knowledge of the patient's vocal cord function translates into more informed patient counselling and facilitates appropriate operative planning.

The considerable prevalence of identifiable deficits preoperatively emphasizes how insufficient symptomatic voice assessment and radiographic evaluation can be. However, not all surgeons incorporate the practice of routine preoperative laryngoscopy and, indeed, several authors have argued that vocal fold examination before thyroid surgery is unnecessary (summarized in Farrag et al. [14]). Many factors contribute to differing viewpoints, including philosophical and operative preferences acquired during surgical training, referral bias and patient population differences that affect the type of thyroid disease treated by a surgeon or institution. There are also differences in study design and findings that may support selective use of laryngoscopy.

Nature of the impairment

Changes in the speaking or singing voice range from barely noticeable to severe. They can also be categorized according to the presence or absence of injuries to the RLN and EBSLN, and according to the subjective or objective determination of changes. The voice is a very personal attribute and subtle alterations not audible to a listener may be instantly apparent to the individual having thyroid surgery [1]. Subjective assessments include descriptions of fatigue, difficulty with changing the pitch of the voice, perception that the voice has a lower frequency, and changes in the singing voice [16]. The complexity of the voice also means that deficits are rarely simply classified with the presence or absence of 'hoarseness'. The patient may explain the change in very vivid or practical terms ('my voice sounds deeper', 'I cannot hum quite as high', 'my voice rumbles like gravel', 'it's just not the same'). Postoperative voice disorders without laryngeal nerve palsy are considered permanent when the changes persist beyond 6–12 months after thyroid surgery [17].

Unilateral vocal cord palsy or paresis may be completely asymptomatic in 50% of patients [8,18]. In others, the changes can be subtle. Attentiveness to listen to the strained sound of a cough is important. Also, more can be learned by asking the patient about voice changes than by waiting for them to volunteer information. Of course, the profound dysphonia seen with RLN palsy or paresis manifests as a raspy, hoarse and weak voice whose sound trails away with prolonged conversation. The ability to shout is impaired. The patient can experience fatigue from the sheer effort of producing speech and dyspnoea from a more restricted airway. Choking upon swallowing liquids is a concerning sign of RLN palsy long before this is confirmed by laryngoscopy.

Pereira *et al.* describe the non-specific alterations of the voice after surgery including tiredness, weakness and change in voice pitch higher or lower [10]. To others who listen to them, patients will have ostensibly clear, strong and normal voices. To their own hearing or perception, however, patients will judge their voice to be abnormal or different from their normal phonation. Patients with excellent preoperative vocal performance – actors, sing-

ers, teachers – are more prone to notice such subtle and non-specific changes. These types of patients are also more likely to experience usually transient reductions in their vocal performance [9]. Men and women do not differ dramatically in the pattern of voice alterations after thyroidectomy [9].

Lombardi *et al.* provide a timeline of resolution of non-specific voice changes in patients with known intact laryngeal nerve function [19]. Data were analysed based on patient self-reporting of symptoms utilizing a questionnaire. The prevalence of patients with preoperative voice symptoms of any kind was 38%. At 1 week and 1 month after surgery, this figure was 80% but improved to 64% by 3 months after surgery. These statistics are worthy of attention. They imply that over 50% of patients will still notice voice impairments long after their initial postoperative care has ended, particularly for benign thyroid disease. In a follow-up study using the same questionnaire and extending prospective monitoring to 1 year after surgery, 34% of patients still reported some kind of voice symptom [6]. Lombardi and colleagues also demonstrated that techniques involving less dissection (minimally invasive videoscopic thyroidectomy or MIVAT) had fewer subjective and objective voice deficits at all timepoints [7]. Musholt *et al.* corroborate this observation with data that the singing voice is undisturbed after limited cervical interventions – thyroid nodulectomy, MIVAT and minimally invasive parathyroid operations [9].

It is interesting to consider each type of voice symptom and to what degree it resolved after surgery. For example, 80% of patients exhibited hoarseness at 1 week postoperatively, 54% at 1 month, and 41% at 3 months. For the remaining symptoms analysed, the prevalence at these same timepoints is indicated in parentheses: weak and breathy voice (46%, 26%, 31%), difficulty singing and yelling (64%, 79%, 64%), lower-pitched voice (41%, 31%, 26%), monotonous voice (36%, 26%, 20%), reduced air intake capacity during speech (46%, 64%, 54%), voice fatigue (41%, 31%, 31%), unpredictable clarity of voice (26%, 36%, 31%), and great difficulty speaking (36%, 46%, 41%). These changes were noticeable throughout the day in 54% of patients during the first week after surgery, and then in 46% and 31% by 1 and 3 months after surgery, respectively. Knowledge of these details can help a surgeon counsel patients appropriately and manage their expectations of surgery.

Aetiology

Box 28.1 provides a comprehensive list of causes of voice impairment following thyroid surgery. The clearest mechanisms arise from iatrogenic physical injury to the laryngeal nerves. These can take the form of partial or complete transection, or injury by cautery, ligating devices/sutures or sharp dissection. They can also, significantly, be the result of traction or stretch manoeuvres that are necessary for the normal mobilization of the thyroid during surgery. Although sometimes required by the disease process (laryngeal nerve resection with invasive malignancy), many of these injuries are inadvertent, may go unrecognized during surgery, and may indeed be unavoidable. Reoperative thyroid surgery or central neck dissections can be particularly challenging because of distorted anatomical planes and scarring from prior operation [13].

Intubation is a known cause of RLN injury and dysphonia [17,20]. Although viewed by many to be rare as a solitary explanation of RLN paralysis, endotracheal intubation accounted for up to 11% of such injuries in some large series summarized by Myssiorek [5].

Intubation can lead to inflammation or oedema of the vocal folds. In other cases, the anterior branch of the RLN can be compressed between the lateralized arytenoid cartilage, thyroid cartilage and inflated cuff from the endotracheal tube. If RLN injury is suspected after intubation, nerve compression must be distinguished from arytenoid dislocation [5]. Viral infections, such as herpes zoster triggered after local trauma from the intubation, have been suggested as an unusual cause of vocal cord dysfunction [21].

The perivisceral nerve plexus integrates motor, sensory and autonomic functions of the pharynx and larynx (Figure 28.1). It is postulated to play a role in the dysphonia and voice changes that occur despite intact laryngeal nerve function, and recent physiological investigations have provided data to support this theory [22].

Box 28.1 Aetiology of voice and swallowing impairments following thyroidectomy

Causes beyond surgeon control
Endotracheal intubation (vocal cord oedema, arytenoid dislocation)
Preoperative/pre-existing changes in patient health

Laryngeal nerve injury or dysfunction
Recurrent laryngeal nerve (RLN) paralysis
RLN paresis
External branches of the superior laryngeal nerves (EBSLN) paralysis
External branches of the recurrent laryngeal nerves (EBRLN) paresis

Normal laryngeal nerve function
Normal healing changes (inflammation)
Seroma/mild haematoma/oedema
Local pain in neck
Psychological reaction to stress of operation
Alterations in vascular supply or venous drainage of larynx
Cricothyroid muscle injury/oedema/dysfunction
Strap muscle dysfunction caused by denervation or transaction
Laryngotracheal fixation with impaired vertical movement
Cervical perivisceral nerve plexus disturbance
Greater extent of dissection/more invasive surgical techniques

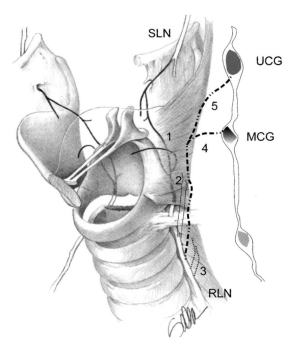

Figure 28.1 Perivisceral neural plexus. The complex anatomical arrangements of the perivisceral cervical neural plexus connect the autonomic system (UCG, upper cervical ganglion and MCG, middle cervical ganglion) to the major laryngeal nerves (RLN, recurrent laryngeal nerve and SLN, superior laryngeal nerve). Shown are the branches from the RLN to the SLN (1, Galen's nerve), from the RLN to oesophagus (2) and pharynx (3), and between the RLN, UCG and MCG (4,5). Adapted from the work of Randolph [1,2], Pereira [10] and Henderson [36].

The strap muscles, particularly the sternothyroid muscles, are thought to influence the extreme ranges of vocal pitch [23]. The degree of voice deficit produced because of division of the sternohyoid and sternothyroid muscles is unknown [8]. However, studies suggest that division of these muscles to enhance exposure of the superior thyroid pole and its vascular pedicle does not aggravate dysphonia or other acoustic voice parameters [23]. Manoeuvres to divide the strap muscles can be applied if needed at the discretion of the surgeon. Familiarity with vascular and neural anatomy investing the sternothyroid and sternohyoid muscles is useful [13,24,25]. Transection should be directed towards a superior aspect of the muscles with preservation of the ansa cervicalis innervation (Figure 28.2). When appropriate, such as in a reoperative field with anatomical distortion or with the strap muscles densely adherent to the midline, a retrograde approach to the thyroid bed can be used. This exposes the thyroid bed via the lateral border of the strap muscles, opening the plane along the medial edge of the sternocleidomastoid muscle [13].

Conceptually, it is logical to expect that normal postoperative inflammation and oedema may affect the voice. Little more than inferential data exist to support this, such as the study by Wang et al. showing that intraoperative corticosteroid administration improved the course of transient postoperative RLN palsy [26]. Musholt et al. demonstrated that smoking does not worsen postoperative voice changes [9].

Evaluation and management

Laryngeal exam is a fundamental component of evaluating postoperative hoarseness. While excellent at defining deficits related to the RLN, laryngoscopy by itself is relatively weaker at detecting EBSLN deficits. Phonation characteristics at rest and with speech can be examined using continuous cold light. Stroboscopy can additionally be performed to describe the mucosal wave of the vocal folds during phonation of the prolonged vowel 'i'. Thus, videolaryngostroboscopy (VLS) is often preferred and more advantageous in diagnosing the specific deficit of the laryngeal nerve and predicting functional outcomes [4]. VLS can even serve as a non-invasive means to identify subtle alterations in cricothyroid muscle function.

Complete paralysis of tje RLN will result in the ipsilateral vocal cord being fixed in the paramedian position, with no muscle tone or mobility. The glottis cannot close completely and the movements of the bilateral folds are asymmetrical. The paralysed vocal fold has a greatly reduced or completely absent mucosal wave. RLN paresis or incomplete paralysis means that the vocal fold is slightly mobile and has some muscle tone. Also, the

(a)

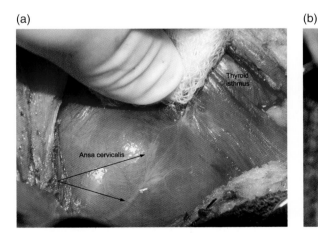

(b)

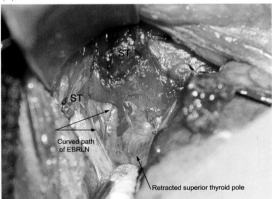

Figure 28.2 Surgical views of the ansa cervicalis and external branch of the superior laryngeal nerve. Branches of the ansa cervicalis are shown as fine white filaments towards the superior end of the sternothyroid muscle, distended over the bulge of the underlying right thyroid lobe. (a) Division of this muscle was necessary to expose the enlarged superior thyroid pole in this patient with a huge goitre from Graves' disease. This is preferably done in a region between the ansa fibres and the insertion of the sternothyroid muscle into the thyroid cartilage (where the surgeon's fingertip is in the photo). (b) Once performed, this illustration shows how the exposure allows identification of the external branch of the recurrent laryngeal nerve (EBRLN). The transected ends of the sternothyroid (ST) are also seen.

glottis closure is better, and the mucosal wave is reduced, but present. There is still asymmetry in movement of the bilateral folds, in direct proportion to the number of affected neurons [4]. Musholt *et al.* nicely demonstrate the range of possible deficits as seen on VLS [9].

Even though laryngeal electromyography (EMG) assessment may be the likely 'gold standard' to diagnose EBSLN impairment, few specialists elect to perform this study routinely. Instead, they may seek to observe features on VLS that can imply EBSLN neuropathy. Detailed extensively in other publications [3,4], these features are listed here for general awareness: (1) thin, short and bowed unilateral vocal fold; (2) oblique glottis deviating to the paretic side posteriorly because of the tonus of the unaffected cricothyroid muscle; (3) vocal fold lag ('sluggish' motion) or absence of brisk adduction/abduction; (4) lack of tension in one vocal fold only; (5) irregular vibratory motions during phonation; and (6) lower vertical plane ('scissoring' action during phonation) of the paretic vocal fold. The mucosal wave is asymmetrical because the wave is late on the affected fold.

Other specialized methods exist to conduct acoustic, aerodynamic and glottographic tests. These report very specific metrics of pitch, range, intensity, singing quality, and acoustic parameters. The Dysphonia Severity Index (DSI), for example, was first applied to study thyroidectomy patients by Henry *et al.* only as recently as 2010 [27]. The DSI represents an objective multivariate model of acoustic measures that are scored and weighted to provide a report of vocal function. These include maximum phonation time, highest vocal frequency, lowest vocal intensity and percent jitter. Elaborating on the details of these tools is beyond the scope of this chapter, but the reader is directed to the excellent publications of Soylu [4], Meek [3], Stojadinovic [8,27], Randolph [1,2], Van Lierde [28] and Akyildiz [29].

Between these objective and somewhat invasive techniques of assessing voice function and the subjective, entirely patient-reported scales discussed below exist other methods of voice evaluation. These can be described as clinician-determined voice assessments. One is the GRBAS perceptual rating of voice quality. A digital audio tape recording is made of a patient reading a specific passage and presented to an expert speech and language therapist blinded to the clinical history. The voice is rated on overall quality and also five specific parameters (grade, roughness, breathiness, asthenia and strain – GRBAS).

These ratings can be performed by different experts or reanalysed by the same expert after a specified time interval. Another example is the Vocal Performance Questionnaire (VPQ) that provides a numerical rating of the patient's vocal performance and impact on quality of life. Originally composed of 12 questions, a modified VPQ version has 10 questions rated on a five-point scale (1 – no adverse effect to 5 – severe effect). Thus, a total severity score has the range of 10 minimum (normal voice performance) to 50 maximum (severely dysphonic voice performance).

There are subjective measures of voice changes that rely on patient self-assessment. Two that were employed in recent studies are detailed in Box 28.2. The Voice Handicap Index (VHI-10) is a self-administered, 10-item assessment of voice alterations. The scores across the categories are added and range from 0 (no voice impairment) to 40 (highest impairment) [30]. The Lombardi Subjective Voice Evaluation Questionnaire was specifically developed for thyroidectomy patients [6,7,19]. It was the tool used to define short-term and long-term voice changes prospectively for patients undergoing conventional open and video-assisted minimally invasive thyroidectomy. It also contains 10 questions that can accrue a maximum total impairment score of 40.

Although there are many informative modalities of voice evaluation, the reality is that most patients will not be eager to undergo extensive evaluations when they perceive their voice to be normal. Likewise, many surgeons may also feel that deeper investigation and objectively recording the status of the larynx become less mandatory when voice outcomes appear satisfactory.

The management of voice impairment after thyroidectomy depends on the nature of the underlying problem. In the absence of RLN injury, management may consist of providing clear information to the patient about the expected course of improvement, providing reassurance and support, and directing re-evaluation and referral to a speech therapist as needed.

After RLN injury, the prognosis for recovery of function is often unpredictable [12]. Although reinnervation may occur, this may not restore movement of the larynx for normal or improved voice functionality. As presented by Ludlow, the mechanisms behind this discrepant effect are many and include misdirection of reinnervating exons from motor neurons to the wrong muscle and preferential innervation of some but not all opposing muscles [12].

Box 28.2 Subjective assessment measures of voice impairment

Voice Handicap Index (VHI-10)
Patient indicates how often, in the past month, the itemized symptoms occurred: 0 (never), 1 (almost never), 2 (sometimes), 3 (almost always) and 4 (always). The total score is added for a range of 0 (no impairment) to 40 (maximum impairment).
1 My voice makes it difficult for people to hear me
2 People have difficulty understanding me in a noisy room
3 My voice difficulties restrict my personal and social life
4 I feel left out of conversations because of my voice
5 My voice problem causes me to lose income
6 I feel as though I have to strain to vocalize
7 The clarity of my voice is unpredictable
8 My voice problem upsets me
9 My voice makes me feel handicapped
10 People ask, 'What's wrong with your voice?'

Lombardi Subjective Voice Evaluation Questionnaire
Patient rates each change as occurring 0 (never), 1 (nearly never), 2 (sometimes), 3 (often) or 4 (always).The total score is the sum of all responses with possible score ranging from 0 to 40 (maximum deficits).
1 My voice is hoarse
2 My voice is breathy and weak
3 I have difficulty in singing and yelling
4 The pitch of my voice is lowered
5 My voice is monotonous
6 I run out of air when I talk
7 My voice changes during the day
8 I use a great effort to speak
9 The clarity of my voice is unpredictable
10 I feel vocal fatigue

Speech and voice therapy is valuable and recommended for all patients who experience voice impairment with laryngeal nerve injury after thyroidectomy. In addition, options of surgical interventions can be considered for voice rehabilitation and include endoscopic injection medialization, transcervical implant medialization, arytenoid repositioning, and RLN reinnervation with ansa cervicalis, vagus or free nerve grafts [31–35].

The absence of effective treatment of EBSLN palsy and the poor prospects for recovery make prevention a more crucial management strategy than anything else [8]. The technical approaches used to maximize EBSLN integrity include excellent exposure of the superior thyroid pole, isolation and ligation of individual superior pole vascular branches at the level of the thyroid capsule rather than higher, deliberate identification of the EBSLN when possible, and neuromonitoring for the EBSLN [4,13]. For the EBSLN, and especially the RLN, there is no substitute for knowledge of regional anatomy and delicate conduct of the operation [1,2,5,11,13].

Issues of swallowing impairment

General principles, prevalence and anatomy

A variety of subjective and ill-defined aerodigestive symptoms exist after thyroidectomy. It is not uncommon for patients to notice and inquire about altered sensations related to swallowing at their initial postoperative visit. Most experienced surgeons recognize that they often field such questions and provide reassurance that the sensations are temporary and not detrimental. Rarely do they affect quality of life to a degree that demands urgent or focused attention. Patients may not be eager to participate in studies. The pertinence of this factor for obtaining meaningful data is demonstrated in one recent questionnaire-based study: of 127 eligible patients who signed informed consent to participate, only 39 (31%) completed post-thyroidectomy questionnaires [19]. Sometimes swallowing symptoms are attributed to irritation from endotracheal intubation or can be entirely dismissed from consideration by physicians. Few have therefore investigated swallowing impairment after thyroid surgery with well-designed and controlled studies to really quantify the meaning of 'often' and the duration of 'temporary'.

In 2003, Pereira *et al.* led efforts to define the prevalence of upper aerodigestive symptoms (UADS) after uncomplicated bilateral thyroidectomy [10]. Patients with known RLN injury, vocal cord dysfunction before surgery, cancer recurrence, associated laryngeal or pharyngeal disorders and chronic pulmonary disease were excluded. The study reported that minor UADS were equally as common preoperatively in patients undergoing thyroidectomy (15%) as in those undergoing cholecystectomy (13%), with the exception of a sensation of 'neck strangling' that could be viewed as a specific symptom of thyroid enlargement (5% versus none, respectively). Compared to cholecystectomy patients, the prevalence of UADS definitely worsened among thyroidectomy patients, where slightly over half (52% versus 25%, p = 0.002) reported one or more of the following symptoms: voice changes (28% versus 3% for cholecystectomy, p = 0.0002), dysphagia (15% versus 3%, p=0.02), strangling sensation (22% versus none, p=0.0001), cough (7% versus 11%, p=ns), sore throat (20% versus 15%, p=ns), and incidence of common cold-type symptoms per year (about 1/yr each, p=ns). The worsening of UADS after thyroidectomy occurred both in terms of more or worse symptoms in those patients who reported preoperative changes and of *de novo* UADS in those who were asymptomatic preoperatively. The authors also observed that, despite the high incidence of these symptoms, no patient specifically requested medical care to evaluate or alleviate the symptoms.

More elaborate studies with the same goal were carried out by Lombardi *et al.* between 2006 and 2009 [6,7,19]. Again, these were conducted in patients without laryngeal nerve injuries. In their early series, the authors identified that at least one-third of patients and as many as two-thirds experienced some type of swallowing change at 1 week after surgery. These changes gradually improved by 1 month and 3 months after surgery. Yet even at the 3-month time period, they were five times more prevalent than what was reported preoperatively. The follow-up study in 2009 corroborated many of these findings and also suggested that minimally invasive techniques of thyroidectomy reduce early postoperative swallowing deficits [6,7]. Nevertheless, some degree of swallowing impairment after thyroid surgery persisted beyond 3 months in 30% of patients. In some circumstances, the swallowing symptoms were reported more frequently and persisted longer than voice changes. Finally, in the first prospectively designed study of long-term swallowing outcomes after thyroidectomy, Lombardi *et al.* were able to show that, by 1 year after surgery and in the absence of laryngeal nerve injury, swallowing symptoms were the same as or better than preoperatively [6].

There are complex sensory, motor and autonomic innervations to the pharynx that can be damaged during thyroidectomy even when RLNs are intact [10]. The anatomical observation highlighted in all the above studies is the presence of a perivisceral nerve plexus that contributes to hyoid-epiglottic dynamics. This anatomy was appreciated even in earlier literature describing side-effects of thoracic surgeries in the 1970s [36]. The perivisceral nerve plexus may be more important to the functions of the larynx and pharynx than previously appreciated (see Figure 28.1). In 2004, Ludlow presented innovations in the status of knowledge about sensory function in laryngeal control and pharyngeal

dysphagia [12]. At that time, as now, it was unclear whether motor deficits follow sensory deficits or whether both coincide to produce significant pharyngeal dysphagia. Unfortunately, the fine calibre branches of this plexus may be less visible or recognizable, vary from patient to patient and according to underlying thyroid pathology, and are less amenable to be consciously protected or preserved. Preserving their integrity nevertheless seems to be important in minimizing the postoperative changes seen after thyroid surgery.

Nature of the impairment

The type, duration and prevalence of swallowing distress are difficult to know for certain, given the infrequent literature on the subject. The emerging concept is that distinct swallowing changes are more common after thyroid surgery than has previously been appreciated. Adding to the complexity is the lack of consistent terminology to use in describing symptoms, the variability of symptoms experienced by individual patients, and also the tendency by patients and physicians to cluster everything into 'swallowing problems'. At the severe end of the spectrum, laryngeal nerve injury can lead to profound dysphagia (difficulty in the passage of solids and liquids from mouth to stomach) and aspiration. Odynophagia, or pain with swallowing, is a term rarely used in publications related to thyroid surgery. It is not entirely the same as a 'sore throat' which occurs commonly after surgery. At the less severe end of the spectrum, for example, patients may describe a 'strangling sensation', akin to that of a foreign body in the pharynx or having a 'too tightly buttoned shirt collar'. It is unclear whether Pereira *et al.* interpreted these descriptions to mean globus pharyngeus [10]. Often called simply globus, this refers to a sensation of a ball (literal translation from Latin) or 'lump in the throat' generally unaccompanied by dysphagia. It is more noticeable during an 'empty swallow'. The precise mechanism is unclear. Considered a sign of laryngopharyngeal irritation, globus can be seen with gastro-oesophageal reflux, postnasal drip, excessive throat clearing, thyroid enlargement, stress and other psychological influences [37].

Globus may be associated with as many as one-third of patients with a thyroid mass. It can also be expected to improve after thyroid surgery in 80% of patients, especially those with histological evidence of thyroiditis or extremely large goitres [37–41]. In a study that used a questionnaire aimed at globus-type symptoms (Glasgow-

Edinburgh Throat Scale or GETS), thyroidectomy was not found to exacerbate globus symptoms in a randomly selected group of patients at 3 and 12 months postoperatively [41]. It is difficult to compare the scope of conclusions in this study to those of Lombardi and Pereira [6,7,10,19]. The latter do not specifically use the term globus, although their swallowing impairment evaluations seem to ask similar questions as the GETS.

In some of the most detailed insights about post-thyroidectomy swallowing problems available from the work of Lombardi and colleagues, we learn of the following expected deficits [19]. The percentage of patients who experience using great effort to swallow was 54% at 1 week, 25% at 1 month, and 15% at 3 months postoperatively. At the same intervals, patients also reported feeling a throat obstacle during swallowing (31%, 25%, 10%), irritation during bolus transit (64%, 41%, 5%), coughing during bolus transit (41%, 25%, 31%) and sensation of a foreign body in the throat (41%, 41%, 36%). When patients undergoing conventional open thyroidectomy were compared to those having MIVAT, they experienced more swallowing impairment in these categories at the 1-week timepoint, but not by 1 and 3 months after surgery. From a series of robotic thyroidectomy patients, Lee *et al.* likewise observed that open thyroidectomy results in significantly worse swallowing symptoms at 1 week and 3 months after surgery, compared to the robotic approach [30].

Aetiology

In contrast to thyroidectomy-related voice changes, the basis of swallowing symptoms is rarely studied with radiological or other interventional methods. Alterations in swallowing dynamics or physiology have not been precisely defined after thyroid surgery. The list of causes of swallowing impairment in Box 28.1 overlaps with causes of voice change. RLN injury is one example – there are direct, small branches to the oesophagus from the RLN that, when the main trunk of the RLN sustains injury, impair swallowing function (see Figure 28.1). Conceptually here also, it is logical to expect that normal postoperative inflammation and oedema, or strap muscle division, may affect swallowing function, though few data are published to support this.

Preoperative oesophageal disorders may exist but yet be undiagnosed. Following thyroid surgery, these can mimic swallowing impairment or symptoms due to surgery [42]. One study contemplated whether dysfunc-tion of oesophageal transit (seen in 55% of patients) was due to the hypothyroidism associated with ^{131}I administration for thyroid cancer, but found a similarly high rate in patients operated on for follicular adenoma [43]. Dysphagia from hypocalcaemia due to post-thyroidectomy hypoparathyroidism has also been reported [44].

Evaluation and management

Awareness that problems with swallowing can occur after thyroid surgery is the beginning of any effective evaluation and therapy. To that end, preoperative assessment for symptoms of swallowing impairment should be part of a comprehensive medical history at initial consultation. Laryngoscopy may be valuable in this context, just as it has been advocated for the preoperative voice assessment, to discern the integrity of RLN function or detect pharyngeal irritation and inflammation.

It is important to consider the possibility that underlying gastro-oesophageal reflux (GORD) leads to laryngitis or pharyngitis exacerbating post-thyroidectomy symptoms. GORD may even be present (undiagnosed) preoperatively. In one study, evaluation with fibreoptic VLS and videofluoroscopic swallowing study (VFSS) was perfomed preoperatively in patients with goitre who complained of voice and swallowing changes. GORD was evident in 68% by VLS and 50% by VFSS. The symptoms persisted in 75% of patients 3 months after thyroidectomy, with throat discomfort in 91%. Although there was not an internal control group in this study, these rates are higher than reported at the same postoperative time period in other series. The authors advocate screening for underlying GORD in patients with swallowing and voice symptoms prior to thyroid surgery and recommend starting appropriate antireflux therapy (proton pump inhibitors) after surgery [42].

A number of patient self-assessment tools and questionnaires have been applied to the study of post-thyroidectomy swallowing deficits. These are provided as a practical reference with all questions itemized in Box 28.3. Except for voice specialists and those with academic interest in the topic, few surgeons are acquainted with these swallowing evaluation tools, much less use them routinely. The *Swallowing Impairment Index (SIS-6)* is a self-administered, six-item assessment of symptoms related to dysphagia and validated for diagnosis of impairment. It can also be used to evaluate non-voice throat symptoms such as cough, choking and throat

Box 28.3 Examples of index measures of swallowing impairment

Swallowing Impairment Index (SIS-6)

Patient indicates how often, in the past month, the itemized symptoms occurred: 0 (never), 1 (almost never), 2 (sometimes), 3 (almost always) and 4 (always). The total score is added for a range of 0 (no impairment) to 24 (maximum impairment).

1. It requires great effort to swallow
2. I feel a throat obstacle during swallowing
3. I feel pharyngeal annoyance during bolus transit
4. I cough during bolus transit
5. I feel a sensation of a foreign body in my pharynx
6. I have some difficulties swallowing fluids

Lombardi Subjective Swallowing Evaluation Questionnaire

Patient rates each change as occurring 0 (never), 1 (nearly never), 2 (sometimes), 3 (often) or 4 (always).The total score is the sum of all responses with possible score ranging from 0 to 20 (maximum deficits).

1. I use a great effort to swallow
2. I feel a throat obstacle during swallowing
3. I feel pharyngeal annoyance during bolus transit
4. I cough during bolus transit
5. I feel sensation of foreign body in pharynx

Glasgow-Edinburgh Throat Scale

Patient rates each change from 0 (unaffected) to 7 (unbearably affected).

1. Feeling of something stuck in the throat
2. Pain in the throat
3. Discomfort/irritation in the throat
4. Difficulty in swallowing food
5. Throat closes off
6. Swelling in the throat
7. Catarrh in the throat
8. Can't empty throat when swallowing
9. Wanting to swallow all the time
10. Food sticking when swallowing
11. How much time do you spend thinking about your throat?
12. At present, how annoying do you find your throat sensation?

clearing. The score assigned to the patient's impairment ranges from 0 (no swallowing impairment) to a maximum of 24 (highest impairment) [30]. The *Lombardi Subjective Swallowing Evaluation Questionnaire* was specifically developed for thyroidectomy patients and used to define short-term and long-term changes prospectively for patients undergoing conventional open and video-assisted minimally invasive thyroidectomy

[6,7,19]. There are five questions that can accrue a maximum total impairment score of 20. The *Glasgow-Edinburgh Throat Scale* is more applicable to the general evaluation of globus pharyngeus from a variety of causes. This index contains the largest number of questions (12) asking for deficits to be graded along the broadest spectrum of changes (seven gradations) [41,45].

On the topic of swallowing impairment after thyroid surgery, discerning specific management recommendations from the published literature is very difficult. Prevention by means of minimizing dissection as much as possible seems prudent and has support from objective data [7,30,46]. Awareness of the prevalence, nature and time course of these changes is useful to educate both surgeons and patients. Providing such information can perhaps lessen anxiety and distress about the changes. Other than the cautious reminder to consider treatment of GORD, there is no pharmacotherapy. Referral to a speech and swallowing specialist is appropriate, especially when the swallowing deficits arise from laryngeal injury. These experts can provide directions in handling solid and liquid components of meals to lessen chances of aspiration and to optimize the effort of swallowing. For the non-specific spectrum of swallowing problems that occur with normal laryngeal function, no rehabilitation programme is clearly described in literature. Eventually with time, these symptoms may resolve on their own.

Conclusion

Surgeons should inform patients that temporary voice and swallowing symptoms are common after thyroidectomy, with mild symptoms affecting the majority of patients for several months and even up to a year after surgery. Fortunately, most of these consequences have a self-limited time course and will improve without specific treatment. Serious and permanent injury to laryngeal nerves, resulting in impaired voice and swallowing functions, is fortunately rare when performed by experienced thyroid surgeons [1,2,47].

When significant impairments exist or there is suspected laryngeal nerve injury, thoughtful evaluation is necessary to define the aetiology of the problem. Laryngoscopy is a key component of this process, and provides the most useful information when performed both pre- and postoperatively. More elaborate assessment using stroboscopy and other highly specialized voice analysis tools can be determined on an individualized basis. Referral to voice and speech therapists is essential. Surgical options are available to rehabilitate vocal function with a paralysed RLN. Fewer management options exist to identify and improve deficits in swallowing seen after thyroid surgery.

The best management of both voice and swallowing distress after surgery remains preventive. This consists of knowledgeable and meticulous surgical technique and understanding of the relevant anatomy and disease processes requiring thyroid operations [48]. The RLN should be routinely identified and every care taken to preserve it. Similarly, operative methods to preserve the EBSLN should be followed whenever possible. Care should be taken to limit dissection. Although this has been shown to minimize postoperative symptoms following MIVAT and robotic approaches, reducing unnecessary dissection as a principle can be stressed for conventional open techniques as well [7,30,46,49].

Further academic study of the topics of voice and swallowing distress after thyroidectomy would be welcome. There is extensive literature addressing laryngeal nerve injury but the topic of voice change with intact laryngeal nerves has received much less attention, and swallowing deficits the least. Multidimensional voice outcomes measures already exist. Perhaps innovative options to evaluate swallowing function could be developed. Even a vocabulary to better match the described changes in swallowing would be an improvement.

Voice preservation has been a hallmark goal of excellent thyroid surgery. A newer addition to this goal can be for surgeons to gain understanding of the more subtle impairments that affect speech and swallowing. These are not insignificant. Greater awareness of these consequences of thyroid surgery can aid the surgeon in the key goals of patient care when addressing complications – information, counsel, reassurance and restoration of function.

References

1 Randolph GW. The importance of pre- and postoperative laryngeal examination for thyroid surgery. Thyroid 2010; 20(5): 453–8.

2 Randolph GW, Kamani D. The importance of preoperative laryngoscopy in patients undergoing thyroidectomy: voice, vocal cord function, and the preoperative detection of invasive thyroid malignancy. Surgery 2006; 139(3): 357–62.

3 Meek P, Carding PN, Howard DH, Lennard TW. Voice change following thyroid and parathyroid surgery. J Voice 2008; 22(6): 765–72.

4 Soylu L, Ozbas S, Uslu HY, Kocak S. The evaluation of the causes of subjective voice disturbances after thyroid surgery. Am J Surg 2007; 194(3): 317–22.

5 Myssiorek D. Recurrent laryngeal nerve paralysis: anatomy and etiology. Otolaryngol Clin North Am 2004; 37(1): 25–44.

6 Lombardi CP, Raffaelli M, De Crea C, et al. Long-term outcome of functional post-thyroidectomy voice and swallowing symptoms. Surgery 2009; 146(6): 1174–81.

7 Lombardi CP, Raffaelli M, d'Alatri L, et al. Video-assisted thyroidectomy significantly reduces the risk of early post-thyroidectomy voice and swallowing symptoms. World J Surg 2008; 32(5): 693–700.

8 Stojadinovic A, Shaha AR, Orlikoff RF, et al. Prospective functional voice assessment in patients undergoing thyroid surgery. Ann Surg 2002; 236(6): 823–32.

9 Musholt TJ, Musholt PB, Garm J, et al. Changes of the speaking and singing voice after thyroid or parathyroid surgery. Surgery 2006; 140(6): 978–88; discussion 988–9.

10 Pereira JA, Girvent M, Sancho JJ, et al. Prevalence of long-term upper aerodigestive symptoms after uncomplicated bilateral thyroidectomy. Surgery 2003; 133(3): 318–22.

11 Morton RP, Whitfield P, Al-Ali S. Anatomical and surgical considerations of the external branch of the superior laryngeal nerve: a systematic review. Clin Otolaryngol 2006; 31(5): 368–74.

12 Ludlow CL. Recent advances in laryngeal sensorimotor control for voice, speech and swallowing. Curr Opin Otolaryngol Head Neck Surg 2004; 12(3): 160–5.

13 Richer SL, Wenig BL. Changes in surgical anatomy following thyroidectomy. Otolaryngol Clin North Am 2008; (4): 1069–78.

14 Farrag TY, Samlan RA, Lin FR, Tufano RP. The utility of evaluating true vocal fold motion before thyroid surgery. Laryngoscope 2006; 116(2): 235–8.

15 Brauckhoff M, Machens A, Thanh PN, et al. Impact of extent of resection for thyroid cancer invading the aerodigestive tract on surgical morbidity, local recurrence, and cancer-specific survival. Surgery 2010; 148(6): 1257–66.

16 Page C, Zaatar R, Biet A, Strunski V. Subjective voice assessment after thyroid surgery: a prospective study of 395 patients. Indian J Med Sci 2007; 61(8): 448–54.

17 De Pedro Netto I, Fae A, Vartanian JG, et al. Voice and vocal self-assessment after thyroidectomy. Head Neck 2006; 28(12): 1106–14.

18 Rueger R. Benign disease of the thyroid gland and vocal cord paralysis. Laryngoscope 1974; 84: 897–907.

19 Lombardi CP, Raffaelli M, d'Alatri L, *et al*. Voice and swallowing changes after thyroidectomy in patients without inferior laryngeal nerve injuries. Surgery 2006; 140; 1026–34.

20 Dralle H, Kruse E, Hamelmann WH, et al. Not all vocal cord failure following thyroid surgery is recurrent paresis due to damage during operation. Statement of the German Interdisciplinary Study Group on Intraoperative Neuromonitoring of Thyroid Surgery concerning recurring paresis due to intubation. Chirurgie 2004; 75(8): 810–22.

21 Marie JP, Keghian J, Mendel I, *et al*. Post-intubation vocal cord paralysis: the viral hypothesis. Eur Arch Otorhinolaryngol 2001; 258: 285–6.

22 Timon CI, Hirani SP, Epstein R, Rafferty MA. Investigation of the impact of thyroid surgery on vocal tract steadiness. J Voice 2010; 24(5): 610–13.

23 Henry LR, Solomon NP, Howard R, *et al*. The functional impact on voice of sternothyroid muscle division during thyroidectomy. Ann Surg Oncol 2008; 15(7): 2027–33.

24 Meguid EA, Agawany AE. An anatomical study of the arterial and nerve supply of the infrahyoid muscles. Folia Morphol (Warsz) 2009; 68(4): 233–43.

25 Wang RC, Puig CM, Brown DJ. Strap muscle neurovascular supply. Laryngoscope 1998; 108(7): 973–6.

26 Wang LF, Lee KW, Kuo WR, *et al*. The efficacy of intraoperative corticosteroids in recurrent laryngeal nerve palsy after thyroid surgery. World J Surg 2006; 30(3): 299–303.

27 Henry LR, Helou LB, Solomon NP, *et al*. Functional voice outcomes after thyroidectomy: an assessment of the Dsyphonia Severity Index (DSI) after thyroidectomy. Surgery 2010; 147(6): 861–70.

28 Van Lierde K, d'Haeseleer E, Wuyts FL, *et al*. Impact of thyroidectomy without laryngeal nerve injury on vocal quality characteristics: an objective multiparameter approach. Laryngoscope 2010; 120(2): 338–45.

29 Akyildiz S, Ogut F, Akyildiz M, Engin EZ. A multivariate analysis of objective voice changes after thyroidectomy without laryngeal nerve injury. Arch Otolaryngol Head Neck Surg 2008; 134(6): 596–602.

30 Lee J, Nah KY, Kim RM, *et al*. Differences in postoperative outcomes, function, and cosmesis: open versus robotic thyroidectomy. Surg Endosc 2010; 24(12): 3186–94.

31 Crumley RL. Update: ansa cervicalis to recurrent laryngeal nerve anastomosis for unilateral laryngeal paralysis. Laryngoscope 1991; 101(4 Pt 1): 384–7; discussion 388.

32 Lee WT. Ansa cervicalis-to-recurrent laryngeal nerve anastomosis for unilateral vocal fold paralysis: experience of a single institution. Ann Otol Rhinol Laryngol 2008; 117(1): 40–5.

33 Wang W, Chen D, Chen S, *et al*. Laryngeal reinnervation using ansa cervicalis for thyroid surgery-related unilateral vocal fold paralysis: a long-term outcome analysis of 237 cases. PloS One 2011; 6(4): e19128.

34 Lorenz RR, Esclamado RM, Teker AM, *et al*. Ansa cervicalis-to-recurrent laryngeal nerve anastomosis for unilateral vocal fold paralysis: experience of a single institution. Ann Otol Rhinol Laryngol 2008; 117(1): 40–5.

35 Miyauchi A, Inoue H, Tomoda C, *et al*. Improvement in phonation after reconstruction of the recurrent laryngeal nerve in patients with thyroid cancer invading the nerve. Surgery 2009; 146(6): 1056–62.

36 Henderson RD, Boszko A, van Nostrand AW, Pearson FG. Pharyngoesophageal dysphagia and recurrent laryngeal nerve palsy. J Thorac Cardiovasc Surg 1974; 68(4): 507–12.

37 Remacle M. The diagnosis and management of globus: a perspective from Belgium. Curr Opin Otolaryngol Head Neck Surg 2008; 16(6): 511–15.

38 Burns P, Timon C. Thyroid pathology and the globus symptom: are they related? A two year prospective trial. J Laryngol Otol 2007; 121(3): 242–5.

39 Adler JT, Sippel RS, Schaefer S, Chen H. Preserving function and quality of life after thyroid and parathyroid surgery. Lancet Oncol 2008; 9(11): 1069–75.

40 Greenblatt DY, Sippel R, Leverson G, *et al*. Thyroid resection improves perception of swallowing function in patients with thyroid disease. World J Surg 2009; 33(2): 255–60.

41 Maung KH, Hayworth D, Nix PA, *et al*. Thyroidectomy does not cause globus pattern symptoms. J Laryngol Otol 2005; 119(12): 973–5.

42 Fiorentino E, Cipolla C, Graceffa G, *et al*. Local neck symptoms before and after thyroidectomy: a possible correlation with reflux laryngopharyngitis. Eur Arch Otorhinolaryngol 2011; 268(5): 715–20.

43 Purizhanskii II, Lyzhina VD, Ogneva TV, *et al*. The esophageal transport function in patients with nodular goiter and in patients operated on for thyroid cancer. Med Radiol 1989; 34: 25–8.

44 Ratanaanekchai T, Art-smart T, Vatanasapt P. Dysphagia after total laryngectomy resulting from hypocalcemia: case report. J Med Assoc Thai 2004; 87(6): 722–4.

45 Deary IJ, Wislon JA, Harris MB, *et al*. Globus pharyngeus: development of a symptom assessment scale. J Psych Res 1995; 39: 203–13.

46 Terris DJ. Effect of video-assisted thyroidectomy on the risk of early postthyroidectomy voice and swallowing symptoms. World J Surg 2008; 32(5): 701.

47 Mitchell J, Milas M, Barbosa G, *et al*. Avoidable reoperations for thyroid and parathyroid surgery: effect of hospital volume. Surgery 2008; 144(6): 899–906; discussion 906–7.

48 Bliss R, Gauger PG, Delbridge LW. Surgeon's approach to the thyroid gland: surgical anatomy and the importance of technique. World J Surg 2000; 24: 891–7.

49 Ikeda Y, Takami H, Sasaki Y, Takayama J, Niimi M, Kan S. Clinical benefits in endoscopic thyroidectomy by the axillary approach. J Am Coll Surg 2003; 196(2): 189–95.

PART VII

New Issues: Complications
Following Minimally Invasive
and Robotic Techniques

CHAPTER 29

Minimally Invasive Techniques Performed Through the Neck Access

Paolo Miccoli,[1] *Michele N. Minuto*[2] *and Valeria Matteucci*[1]

[1] Department of Surgery, University of Pisa, Pisa, Italy
[2] Department of Surgical Sciences (DISC), University of Genoa, Genoa, Italy

Introduction

Among endoscopic or video-assisted procedures, the two most widely performed operations currently are minimally invasive video-assisted thyroidectomy (MIVAT) and transaxillary robot-assisted thyroidectomy. The former is widely diffused in western countries, as affirmed by Terris' statement: 'the technique most widely practiced in the United States' [1], whereas the latter is more popular in eastern countries [2]. Both techniques can be responsible for different and unique complications that are described in two separate chapters of this book.

The more specific complications of the MIVAT technique will be discussed here. We will focus in particular on the unique aspects and management of well-known complications (e.g. postoperative bleeding) during and after this minimally invasive procedure, and on how to avoid them.

It is obvious that complications specific to conventional thyroidectomy can also occur after an endoscopic and/or video-assisted procedure. Additionally, no report has demonstrated that video-assisted or endoscopic thyroidectomy has any significant benefit in terms of inferior laryngeal nerve injury or postoperative hypoparathyroidism. Since these typical complications are extensively discussed in other parts of this book, in this chapter we will focus only on the adverse events that are unique to the MIVAT technique, and that can occur

more frequently (although still very rarely) when carrying out these operations.

It is also necessary to point out that the complication rate of the MIVAT procedure should be theoretically lower than that of conventional thyroidectomy, due to the restrictive indications for this approach. In fact, most, if not all, cases selected to undergo MIVAT are represented by smaller masses, with no macroscopic extrathyroidal extension and no grossly metastatic lymph nodes. This means that generally the 'easiest' cases are the ideal candidates for this surgery. As a consequence, when considering the published series, particular attention should be paid when examining complications. An excessive rate, surpassing that of conventional surgery, should not be tolerated unless produced inside a learning curve or in a population with a well-demonstrated higher incidence (e.g. those affected with thyroid cancer; see also Chapter 1) or unless the populations compared (MIVAT versus standard thyroidectomy) are identical in terms of size of the thyroids treated and preoperative diagnosis.

It is evident from literature, then, that the complication rate is very similar when comparing MIVAT with standard open thyroidectomy. In the most recent review article on this topic [3], among all the examined papers, no group reported any difference between these techniques in terms of hypoparathyroidism or recurrent nerve palsy. It should be added, however, that this result may also be related to the low numbers of patients analysed in the

Thyroid Surgery: Preventing and Managing Complications, First Edition. Edited by Paolo Miccoli, David J. Terris,
Michele N. Minuto and Melanie W. Seybt.
© 2013 John Wiley & Sons, Ltd. Published 2013 by John Wiley & Sons, Ltd.

various series reported throughout the literature. This would have made it impossible to achieve statistical significance considering both the limited number of patients examined and the extremely low incidence rate of the complications themselves.

Postoperative haematoma

This is an extremely rare complication after MIVAT, especially when compared to the traditional surgery, and there are two main reasons for this. First, the thyroids treated with this surgery are essentially small (thus have a limited blood supply) when compared to other bulky thyroid diseases requiring conventional thyroidectomy. Second, Harmonic® technology (which is the only haemostatic device used in MIVAT) is characterized by early haemostasis. This means that any failure of the instrument results in immediate bleeding, thus reducing the postoperative (or delayed) bleeding to almost zero (see Chapter 12).

Intraoperative management

During the operation we strongly recommend dedicating a few seconds to careful inspection of the edges of the large vessels dissected with the instrument immediately after they have been ligated (particularly those of the upper pedicle), in search of any minimal bleeding that might predict failure of the instrument. Even a small amount of oozing from a cut vessel should not be ignored, since it is a sure sign of an imperfect sealing, and should be treated with a second passage of the instrument. If in doubt, a small vascular clip can be applied rather than relying too greatly on ultrasonic coagulation (Video 29.1). This simple precaution allows the surgeon to prevent significant bleeding that might lead to conversion to conventional thyroidectomy and jeopardize an otherwise straightforward MIVAT.

Postoperative management

Since generally no drain is used in MIVAT, even minimal oozing might result in a swelling in the central neck that is easily recognized in the first hours after surgery. When the swelling is stable in the first few postoperative hours, and does not cause any respiratory distress, conservative treatment is generally indicated. Some surgeons prefer a compressive dressing to be applied on the neck. These limited bleedings generally come from the strap muscles and teguments and they tend to stop quite easily.

In cases of haematomas seriously impairing the respiration, an urgent surgical exploration is mandatory, with the patient under general anaesthesia with tracheal intubation, to guarantee the correct ventilation. We mainly favour an endoscopic evaluation first, reopening the incision, cleaning up the surgical field and exploring the operative space carefully, searching for the source of the bleeding. If the bleeding comes from the upper pedicle and the vessel is not easy to reach and to control, a quick conversion is strongly advised. This can be obtained by simply enlarging the former incision by no more than 2 cm on both sides.

In our personal series consisting now of more than 2000 cases, postoperative bleeding leading to impairment of respiratory function requiring a surgical reoperation occurred in only 0.2% of cases. This result is confirmed in a recent review of the literature [3]. In five of the most recent papers (out of a total of 21 examined) where this complication was noted and compared with conventional thyroidectomy, a postoperative haematoma requiring surgical reoperation has never been described, confirming the extreme rarity of this event.

Skin damage/cosmetic issues

Generally after the first few MIVAT cases performed, the surgeon realizes that the edges of the skin are not perfectly vital and may demonstrate superficial areas of demarcation. These burns are generally very limited and would not be considered a serious complication unless they result in an unfavourable cosmetic outcome, as one main advantage of MIVAT is the excellent aesthetic outcome.

The trauma may occur during the first phase of the procedure, when preparing the access with monopolar electrocautery through the skin and strap muscles. With the narrow incision, the blade of the cautery can inadvertently injure the skin, leading to skin necrosis. Therefore, it is mandatory to isolate the blade of the electrocautery all along its length with a rubber or silicone sheath, leaving only the very tip of the instrument free (Figure 29.1). This will prevent burns to the skin edges when the cautery device touches the edge of the wound, which is almost impossible to avoid in this limited space.

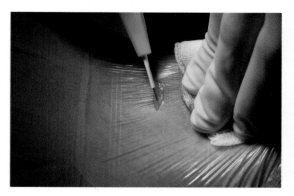

Figure 29.1 To help prevent skin burns during a MIVAT procedure, the blade of the electrocautery is inactivated by a rubber cover. The only working part of the instrument is the tip.

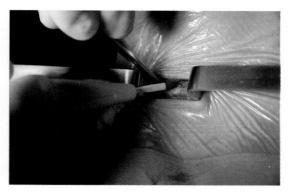

Figure 29.2 The rubber cover prevents burning especially during opening of the linea alba. Notice also the Tegaderm® sheath covering the operative area of the neck, which can prevent superficial burns.

A second phase when skin damage can occur is during the last dissection of the thyroid lobe, which is performed under direct vision and follows the conventional rules of open thyroidectomy. The Harmonic® instrument, that has an active sheath of around 3 cm in length, may accidentally come into contact with the skin, creating burns that are superficial and not necrotic (the temperatures are much lower than those of conventional electrocautery), but that can affect the cosmetic outcome. To avoid this sort of damage, we recommend covering the operative area with an isolating dressing (Figures 29.1, 29. 2) such as Tegaderm®, and to always be aware of the angle of the Harmonic® during the dissection (an assistant can pay better attention to the skin edges and their contact with the instrument). The surgeon should additionally note that the blade of the instrument that is considered 'inactive' (see Chapter 12) can nonetheless transmit a temperature that can cause damage to the skin. For this reason, one should also avoid contact of this blade with the skin.

If at the end of the intervention the surgeon realizes that minimum damage has occurred at the skin margins, this portion of skin can usually be excised, leaving the margins vital and intact. This will ensure the cosmetic result will not be affected and the incision size would remain exactly the same (see Chapter 16).

Apart from the individual propensity of every patient, which is highly unpredictable, a possible reason for the occurrence of a keloid is excessive traction on the skin margins. Gentle retraction is highly advisable for this reason. The retractors must be applied on the strap muscles (see Chapter 6, Figure 6.2b) and never on the skin to avoid wound edge ischaemia, which is the main factor responsible for an unfavourable cosmetic outcome. Additionally, the surgeon should not hesitate to enlarge an incision when the extraction of the lobe is difficult. Frequently, simply cutting the strap muscles a few millimetres transversely without enlarging the skin incision will allow a big nodule to be delivered without stretching the margins of the wound. Also, the skin can be remodelled, as already described, with the scalpel at the end of the operation if the margins appear damaged.

Injuries to the trachea and the carotid artery

Tracheal injury

The narrow operative space that is typical of the MIVAT procedure has contributed to some rare complications that might appear more frequently than expected, especially when considering the already cited relative 'ease' of this approach. A tracheal injury that is superficial (in most cases) or deeper is an occurrence that is never reported in the literature, maybe because of its irrelevant influence on the global postoperative outcome (when the lesion is superficial it is generally not treated at all). Nevertheless, a surgeon with significant experience in MIVAT operations who has never experienced this problem is rarely found. This lesion may be due to the nature of the operation itself, together with the use of the Harmonic® instrument in such a limited space. The active sheath of the instrument is relatively large and creates temperatures that, even if relatively low, can still damage the surrounding structures. Tracheal damage can generally occur when dissection of the isthmus is performed, and is generally caused by the tip of the instrument (when the damage is deeper and very limited) or by the relatively 'inactive' sheath of the instrument (see Chapter 12), that can conduct a temperature high enough to produce a superficial lesion of the trachea. It is strongly suggested to always have complete visual control of the tip of the instrument during all phases of the surgery, and to pay particular attention to the 'inactive' sheath of the Harmonic® so as to avoid contact with the extremely delicate structures.

The proper management of a tracheal lesion is discussed in Chapter 17.

Carotid artery injury

This is an extremely rare complication that has never been described in the literature but occurred in one case out of more than 2000 in our series. Generally, optimal visualization of this artery is obtained utilizing the endoscope. Once isolated, the carotid should be retracted laterally to expose the thyroid space before dividing the upper pedicle. If the artery is not constantly in view, it might be injured with the tip of the Harmonic® (see Chapter 12). Since this part of the instrument has the highest temperature and is the most distal, it is sometimes difficult to visualize clearly in the endoscopic view. We recommend always having the tip of the Harmonic® in perfect view, and always obtaining proper dissection of the whole carotid sheath during the access to the operative space (similar to traditional open surgery) before the dissection of the upper pedicle, and to always have the carotid artery completely loaded (and therefore protected) under the retractor of the assistant.

An event that can facilitate injury of the carotid is kinking of the carotid artery, not uncommon in elderly patients where, moreover, the carotid sheath is particularly vulnerable because of atherosclerosis. It is also worth noticing that older patients may be less demanding in terms of cosmetic outcome, and less likely to undergo a MIVAT procedure, due to the nature of the thyroid diseases that are the most indicated for this minimally invasive operation.

Undoubtedly, this complication is an indication for immediate conversion to open surgery to dissect the carotid artery and immediately repair the injury. This is extensively discussed in Chapter 18.

Conclusion

A MIVAT procedure demonstrates exactly the same mortality and morbidity as traditional thyroidectomy, in terms of the complications that are unusual in this surgery. Inferior laryngeal nerve damage and hypoparathyroidism have been shown to be identical in all the series reported in the literature [1,4]. Reviewing the literature and our series as well, there seems to be no specific morbidity from this technique although some extremely rare events have been recorded in our own experience and seem to be related to the peculiarity of the instruments used rather than to the technique itself. In particular, all the rare injuries described (tracheal and carotid artery injury in particular) are due to the nature of the Harmonic® device, which produces moderate-to-high temperatures in a very narrow space. This led us to confirm, once again, that a proper learning curve in the use of such an instrument is mandatory when starting a MIVAT series.

References

1 Terris D, Angelos P, Steward D, Simental A. Minimally invasive video assisted thyroidectomy: a multi institutional North American experience. Arch Otolaryngol Head Neck Surg 2008; 134: 81–4.

2 Lee J, Yun JH, Nam KH, Soh EY, Chung WY. The learning curve for robotic thyroidectomy: a multicenter study. Ann Surg Oncol 2011; 18: 226–32.

3 Miccoli P, Materazzi G, Baggiani A, Miccoli M. Mini-invasive video assisted surgery of the thyroid and parathyroid glands: a 2011 update. J Endocrinol Invest 2011; 34: 473–80.

4 Miccoli P, Bellantone R, Mourad M, Walz M, Raffaelli M, Berti P. Minimally invasive video-assisted thyroidectomy: multiinstitutional experience. World J Surg 2002; 26(8): 972–5.

Videoclip

This chapter contains the following videoclip. They can be accessed at: www.wiley.com/go/miccoli/thyroid

Video 29.1 Intraoperative management of bleeding from a right upper pedicle during a MIVAT procedure. Even a small amount of oozing from a cut vessel should not be ignored; a vascular clip can be applied rather than relying on further ultrasonic coagulation.

CHAPTER 30

Minimally Invasive Techniques Performed Through Other Accesses

Kee-Hyun Nam[1] and William B. Inabnet III[2]

[1] Department of Surgery, Yonsei University College of Medicine, Seoul, Korea
[2] Division of Metabolic, Endocrine and Minimally Invasive Surgery, Mount Sinai Medical Center, New York, NY, USA

Introduction

The technique of thyroidectomy was standardized by Theodor Kocher (1841–1917), who introduced ligation of the four principal arteries, leading to reduction of mortality from 12.8% in 1883 to less than 0.5% 15 years later [1]. Conventional open thyroidectomy still remains the most widely used approach for thyroid excision. Conventional thyroidectomy usually has a long incision line in the anterior neck that can lead to keloid formation or hypertrophic scar. Thyroid disease is more common in women and the incidence of thyroid disease in young women is increasing [2]; women tend to be more conscious of the cosmetic outcome that results from conventional open thyroidectomy.

In the evolution from traditional thyroid surgery, Michel Gagner [3] performed the first endoscopic parathyroidectomy in 1996 and Hüscher [4] performed the first video-assisted thyroid lobectomy in 1997, followed by Gagner and Inabnet in 1998. Miccoli *et al.* [5] developed a minimally invasive video-assisted thyroidectomy (MIVAT) which was performed under direct and endoscopic vision using conventional instruments. Its advantages over conventional thyroidecotmy include improved magnification of cervical anatomy, improved cosmesis, less postoperative pain and decreased tissue trauma. However, indications for MIVAT are confined to

small tumours because the working space is too small to handle a large tumour [6]. Shimizu *et al.* modified the transcervical approach for application to large tumours, but operative scars measuring up to about 4 cm, just below the clavicle, tended to be hypertrophic [7].

During the same period, minimally invasive endoscopic thyroidectomy was performed through a cervical approach by Inabnet [8]. Compared to MIVAT, which requires a centrally located incision, endoscopic thyroidectomy by a cervical approach allows for a smaller incision size and superior ergonomics when an angled endoscope is used. However, the main disadvantages of the cervical approach were difficulty in maintaining the working space and visible scars on the neck (albeit much smaller). These disadvantages led to the evolution of remote-access endoscopic thyroidectomy, a novel surgical technique to resect the thyroid gland remote from the neck, thus resulting in no scar in the neck and transferring the scar to an area that is covered by natural position or clothing. With the remote approach, other investigators developed scarless (in the neck) endoscopic thyroidectomy using the axillary approach [9] and the breast approach [10]. In these approaches, there has been no reported mortality. However, new complications have been encountered that are not routinely or previously associated with conventional open thyroidectomy.

Thyroid Surgery: Preventing and Managing Complications, First Edition. Edited by Paolo Miccoli, David J. Terris, Michele N. Minuto and Melanie W. Seybt.
© 2013 John Wiley & Sons, Ltd. Published 2013 by John Wiley & Sons, Ltd.

According to methods for the creation of working space, remote-access endoscopic thyroidectomy can be divided into CO_2 gas insufflation methods and gasless methods using an external retractor. Carbon dioxide-related complications may develop when endoscopic thyroidectomy is performing using CO_2 insufflation. And endoscopic thyroidectomy using an external retractor tends to be more invasive than conventional thyroidectomy and may develop its own related complications because it requires a wide skin flap for creation of the working space. To further contribute to the risk of complication, the learning curve of remote-access endoscopic thyroidectomy is steep. There is a need for familiarization with 'new anatomy'. Most surgeons are comfortable with conventional open thyroidectomy but in the remote approach to the gland, the vector of surgery is inferiorly or laterally, which is not what most are accustomed to. For this reason, the perioperative complication rate in remote approaches may increase during the initial period of the learning curve.

In this chapter, a brief summary of each surgical technique of remote-access thyroid surgery and its advantages and disadvantages will be described, to allow better understanding of the technique-related complications. Then, the complications and their management will be described in detail.

Axillary endoscopic thyroidectomy using CO_2 insufflation

The axillary approach reported by Ikeda *et al.* utilizes three ports located in the axillary region [9]. In this technique, the cosmetic results seemed excellent because there were no operative scars in either the neck or anterior chest. However, the three ports were located in such a narrow area that interference of the surgical instruments occurred frequently.

The patient is placed in the supine position, with the neck slightly extended, under general anaesthesia. The arm on the tumour side is lifted up, exposing the axilla, along the clavicular line. A 30 mm skin incision is made in the axilla and the lower layer of the platysma is separated through the upper layer of the pectoralis major muscle, manually at first and then with a vein harvesting system. A 12 mm trocar is inserted through this incision and a purse-string suture is placed to prevent both gas leakage and trocar slippage out of the wound. Carbon dioxide is then insufflated up to 4 mmHg and a flexible laparoscope is inserted through the trocar. Then, two additional 5 mm trocars are inserted inferior to the 30 mm skin incision under endoscopic guidance. Endoscopic scissors are used for additional blunt and sharp dissection to enlarge the space in the anterior chest and the subplatysmal space. The anterior border of the sternocleidomastoid muscle is separated from the sternohyoid muscle. The thyroid gland is exposed by splitting the sternothyroid muscle. The sternothyroid muscle is severed at the upper pole of the thyroid gland, which is then completely explored from the lateral side.

Next, with the thyroid tissue retracted upward, the lateral wall of the trachea is identified. The upper pole of the thyroid is resected with laparoscopic coagulating shears slim (LCSs) (Johnson & Johnson Medical). In the second part of the procedure, the lower pole of the thyroid is grasped, retracted upward, and divided from the fat and inferior thyroid vein with LCSs. The lateral portion of the thyroid gland is retracted medially to remove tissue around it using endoscopic scissors or LCSs. After this manoeuvre, the recurrent laryngeal nerve can usually be seen crossing the inferior thyroid artery, and the perithyroid fascia is cut carefully to avoid injuring it and the parathyroid glands. The parathyroid glands are identified during dissection and are left intact. The thyroid is dissected from the trachea. Finally, the isthmus is cut with LCSs and a hemithyroidectomy is performed. The specimen is placed in a plastic bag and extracted through the 30 mm skin incision. Before completing the operation, a 3 mm closed suction drain is placed under the platysma through the site of the most inferior 5 mm trocar in the axillary wound, to prevent development of a cervical haematoma. To achieve wound closure, the adipose tissue is sutured with 3-0 absorbable thread and the subcutaneous layers are tightly sutured with 4-0 absorbable monofilament thread with an atraumatic needle, followed by fixing of the skin with tape only.

Breast endoscopic thyroidectomy using CO_2 insufflation

The breast approach (BA) reported by Ohgami *et al.* utilized three ports passing through two circumareolar incisions and one parasternal incision [10]. The BA method improved narrow-angled instrumentation, but was problematic due to the resulting hypertrophic scars on the anterior chest.

Axillo-bilateral breast approach with CO$_2$ insufflation

Shimazu *et al.* [11] modified the BA method to develop the axillo-bilateral breast approach (ABBA). They reported that ABBA is feasible for removing large goitres sized 5–6 cm and described excellent cosmetic results. Furthermore, due to the multiangular nature of this approach, it seemed easy to perform compared with the axillary approach. However, this method is limited by difficulty visualizing both lobes of the thyroid.

Bilateral axillo-breast approach with CO$_2$ insufflation

Choe *et al.* [12] modified the ABBA method and developed a new endoscopic thyroid procedure by using the bilateral axillo-breast approach (BABA) after performing 25 ABBA operations. The BABA method was able to obtain optimal visualization of major structures including recurrent laryngeal nerves, superior and inferior thyroid arteries and parathyroid glands, as well as both lobes of the thyroid, utilizing two ports passing through two circumareolar incisions and two axillary incisions (Figure 30.1).

Under general anaesthesia, patients were placed in the supine position with neck extension using a shoulder pillow. Both arms are mildly abducted to provide for insertion of 5 mm ports. Diluted (1:200,000) epinephrine solution is injected into the subcutaneous space in both breasts and the subplatysmal space in the neck to reduce bleeding during dissection. After making two incisions on both axillae (12 mm, 5 mm), subcutaneous and subplatysmal dissection is performed bluntly with the use of a Rochester clamp and vascular tunneller.

After establishing the required working space of the anterior chest, two 5 mm incisions are made on both upper circumareolar areas. (Figure 30.2) The working space is extended to the level of the thyroid cartilage superiorly and to the medial border of each sternocleidomastoid muscle laterally. The working space is established with CO$_2$ insufflation at a pressure up to 6 mmHg.

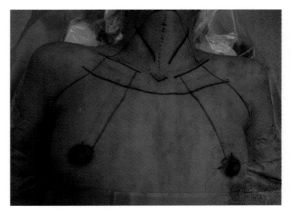

Figure 30.1 Two circumareolar incisions and two axillary incisions in the BABA approach. The lines shown on the anterior chest wall and neck represent the anatomical landmarks and extent of dissection. Courtesy of Prof. Y. K. Youn, Seoul National University, Seoul, Korea.

Division in the midline is done with electrocautery or Harmonic® (Ethicon, Cincinnati, OH).

The isthmic portion of the thyroid gland are resected and thyroid lobectomy is performed. The specimen is retrieved through the 12 mm port with a plastic bag.

The advantages of BABA endoscopic thyroidectomy are as follows;
1) the procedures are same as conventional open thyroidectomy,
2) BABA gives symmetric view of bilateral thyroid lobes and gives an optimal visualization of major structures during the operation,
3) no interference between each instruments due to the ports are remote from each other, and as mentioned above,
4) good cosmetic results with no visible scar.

Gasless transaxillary endoscopic thyroidectomy

To maintain the working space constantly during the operation, a gasless transaxillary approach was developed by Chung and colleagues in Korea [13]. Working with bioengineers, these surgeons developed a unique external retractor which can be connected with a continuous suction line by a canal in the midline of the retractor blade. In this method, the surgeon approaches the thyroid compartment between the sternocleidomastoid (SCM) bellies

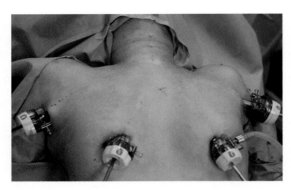

Figure 30.2 Two 5 mm ports inserted via the circumareolar incisions and one 12mm and one 5 mm ports via the bilateral axillary incisions in the BABA approach. Courtesy of Prof. Y. K. Youn, Seoul National University, Seoul, Korea.

and dissects along the anterior surface of the carotid sheath and drops the carotid sheath just below the strap muscle. This approach enables the surgeon to conduct a complete ipsilateral central compartment node dissection (CCND) from the carotid artery to the substernal notch and the prelaryngeal area including the para-oesophageal lymph nodes. Another benefit of this approach is that the anterior surface of the SCM (sternal head) and strap muscle is not dissected. This enables the surgeon to preserve the sensory nerve around the anterior neck area and postoperative hypaesthesia in this region can be avoided.

However, the transaxillary gasless endoscopic thyroidectomy also has some pitfalls. This method is more invasive and needs more operation time than conventional open thyroidectomy due to the wide dissection from the axilla to the anterior neck area. The approach to the contralateral superior pole of thyroid using this method is difficult. However, Chung and co-workers [13] solved this problem by conducting a subcapsular dissection of the anterior thyroid surface to create a working space until the contralateral lobe is exposed. They usually use a 45° scope which enables downward vision to more easily identify the contralateral superior pole of thyroid.

The patient was positioned in a supine position on a small shoulder roll. The ipsilateral arm was placed on an arm board and extended cephalad to expose the axilla. A vertical line was marked from the sternal notch to the hyoid in the midline. A 5–6 cm skin incision was made along the line marked in the axilla at the posterior aspect of the pectoralis (Figure 30.3). The arm was placed in its natural position to confirm that the marked incision

would be hidden in the axilla postoperatively. A second skin incision (0.5 cm in length) was made on the medial side of the anterior chest wall for insertion of endoscopic instruments on an imaginary horizontal line starting from the lower end of the axillary incision and extending 5–6 cm (Figure 30.4).

Dissection was performed using electrocautery above the pectoralis major muscle to create a space using serially longer retractors to elevate the skin, subcutaneous tissue and platysma. The space was opened superiorly, the omohyoid was retracted superficially and posterolaterally or divided, and the sternohyoid and sternothyroid muscles were elevated from the thyroid gland. To main-

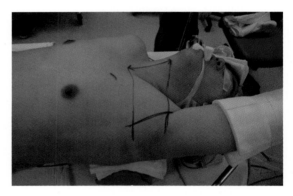

Figure 30.3 Patient position and skin markings for the gasless transaxillary approach, showing the primary incision within the anterior axillary fold and the small incision on the anterior chest wall. Courtesy of Prof. W. Y. Chung, Yonsei University, Seoul, Korea.

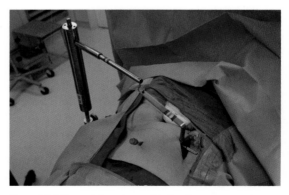

Figure 30.4 External view after positioning the retractor and inserting trocars in the gasless transaxillary approach. Courtesy of Prof. W. Y. Chung, Yonsei University, Seoul, Korea.

tain a working space, a spatula-shaped external retractor (Chung's thyroid retractor) with table mount lift was placed under the strap muscles and secured to the table mount lift. For endoscopic thyroidectomy, under the endoscopic guidance of an assistant, dissection and resection were performed using a fine endoscopic dissector and Harmonic™ Scalpel. The operation proceeded in the same manner as conventional open thyroidectomy.

Complications

Recurrent laryngeal nerve injury

Recurrent laryngeal nerve (RLN) injury is one of the most serious complications in endocrine surgery. It is related to significant morbidity and frequent malpractice claims [14]. The current policy of visual identification of the RLN tracing along the whole cervical course is the gold standard to reduce the risk of permanent RLN injury. Therefore, endocrine surgeons should be aware of the anatomical variability of the RLN. In instances of embryological malformation of the aortic arch in terms of retro-oesophageal right subclavian artery, the nerve passes with a more median course directly to the larynx (non-recurrent laryngeal nerve). Although the reported incidence of non-recurrent laryngeal nerve is less than 1%, the surgeon performing thyroidectomy especially on the right lobe should always bear in mind the possible existence of a non-recurrent laryngeal nerve.

During endoscopic cervical exploration, the recurrent laryngeal nerve can be exposed at different levels: caudally, at the crossing with the common carotid artery, in the neighbourhood of the inferior thyroid artery, and cranially, at Berry's ligament, a dense tissue of the posterior thyroid capsule near the cricoid cartilage and upper tracheal rings.

Permanent RLN injury is very rare in the procedure of remote-access endoscopic thyroidectomy if performed by an experienced surgeon, because visualization of these vital structures might actually be easier with the excellent magnification obtained with the endoscope through intense focused lighting within the closed operative space, although the nerve cannot be palpated directly as in conventional open thyroidectomy. Intraoperative electrical nerve stimulation of the surgical field in addition to visualization of the RLN can be used to delineate the presence, function and possibly the course of the RLN by observing contractions of the cricopharyngeus muscle [15–17].

Damage to the recurrent laryngeal nerve may be caused by different mechanisms: cutting, clamping or stretching of the nerve, nerve skeletonization, local compression of the nerve due to oedema or haematoma, or thermal injury by electrocoagulation or Harmonic™ Scalpel. Studies of remote-access endoscopic thyroidectomy have demonstrated that rates of temporary recurrent laryngeal nerve damage are 2.1%, 3.6% and 2.8% in the axillary, breast and axillo-breast approaches, respectively [18]. These incidences are within an acceptable range compared with the 2% rate of transient palsy in conventional thyroidectomy [19].

Transient cord palsy, which is often caused by oedema or axon damage by excessive nerve stretching, seldom lasts more than 4–6 weeks. It is necessary to be cautious when using the Harmonic™ Scalpel when the nerve is in close proximity because there is a potential collateral transfer of energy that may result in its injury. It is recommended that the RLN should not be touched directly with the blade just after it has been used, and that it is possible to use an ultrasonic surgical device at a distance of 3 mm from the RLN for less than 20 sec at level 3 [20]. To maintain these distances, the RLN must be endoscopically visualized during surgery of the neck.

When function of the RLN is not recovered within 6–12 months postoperatively, permanent damage to the RLN should be considered. If inadvertent cutting or clamping of the RLN is encountered intraoperatively, primary repair of the nerve using microsurgical techniques and epineural sutures or a reinnervation from the ansa cervicalis nerve can be attempted [21]. Even if the nerve is reanastomosed, the dysfunctioning vocal cord will probably never completely recover [22,23]. Recently, injection laryngoplasty has been described as a good treatment option for unilateral permanent RNL palsy suffered by patients during remote-access endoscopic thyroidectomy, because it does not require an external skin incision on the neck [24].

When creating a working space for gasless endoscopic thyroidectomy via the axillary approach, which presents novice surgeons with unfamiliar new anatomy, incorrect dissection of the carotid sheath and strap muscles to exposure the thyroid gland may lead to accidental injury to the vagus or RLN [25]. Therefore, surgeons should be well acquainted with the anatomical relationships between the SCM, strap muscles and thyroid gland.

Bilateral RLN injury is the most serious complication of thyroid surgery and results in a near midline position of the vocal cords and airway obstruction. As its rate was reported to be 0.4% in conventional total thyroidectomy [19], it may occur in endoscopic total thyroidectomy through remote access. Importantly, because gasless axillary endoscopic total thyroidectomy is conducted by only one side approach and does not routinely include identification of the contralateral RLN nerve due to the operative technique that resects the contralateral lobe through a subcapsular dissection, it may carry the risk of bilateral RLN palsy. To prevent it, it would be better to perform a bilateral procedure after the surgeon gradually extends the extent of thyroidectomy to overcome the learning curve. The use of nerve monitoring may also decrease the incidence of bilateral RLN palsy, because if the signal is lost in an ipsilateral nerve, the contralateral dissection can be staged.

If bilateral RLN injury is not observed intraoperatively, it may be diagnosed directly after extubation or during the early postoperative phase. The patient should be reintubated without delay and treated systemically with corticosteroids. In the presence of reversible nerve injury, extubation under controlled conditions may be possible in most cases after 24–72 h and no further treatment may be necessary. In cases of persisting respiratory obstruction, reintubation and tracheostomy may need to be carried out immediately. If the vocal cords fail to recover after a waiting period of 9–12 months, permanent tracheostomy or transverse laser cordotomy can be considered [26].

Injury to the external branch of the superior laryngeal nerve

Because injury to the external branch of the superior laryngeal nerve (EBSLN) shows less severe symptoms than injury of the RLN, this complication is less easily recognized and it may be difficult to assess its manifestation [27].

Because evaluation by laryngoscopy can be quite difficult, the most accurate test for postoperative assessment of superior laryngeal nerve palsy is laryngeal electromyography. The superior laryngeal nerve, like the RLN, originates from the main trunk of the vagus nerve outside the jugular foramen. It passes anteromedially on the thyrohyoid membrane where it is joined by the

superior thyroid artery and vein. At about the level of the hyoid bone, it divides into two branches. The external laryngeal nerve innervates the cricothyroid muscle and the internal branch provides sensory innervation of the supraglottic larynx. The internal laryngeal nerve separates into three branches that communicate with the recurrent laryngeal nerve posterior to the cricoid cartilage. Injuries to the internal branch are rare during thyroid or parathyroid surgery.

According to Cernea's widely accepted classification for the course of the EBSLN [28,29], Cernea type 1 is where the nerve crosses medially into the cricothyroid muscle more than 1 cm cranial to the upper pole of the thyroid lobe; it occurs in about two-thirds of cases. Cernea type 2a is where the EBSLN remains cranial to the upper pole of the thyroid gland. Cernea type 2b is where the most caudal position of the EBSLN lies below the upper pole of the thyroid gland; it occurs in 20%. This location has definite surgical importance because of an increased risk of injury during the dissection and ligation of the superior thyroid pedicle.

In order to avoid damage during ligation of the superior thyroid pedicle, the vessels of the upper pole should be dissected individually and ligated as caudally as possible on the surface of the thyroid. In addition, the tip of the Harmonic™ Scalpel or electrocautery should not be touched directly on the cricothyroid muscle just after activation.

Since the cricothyroid muscle is a tensor of the vocal cord, injury to the EBSLN often results in voice weakness, loss of voice range and inability to perform high-pitch phonation. Especially in singers, injury to this nerve is a serious problem.

Hypoparathyroidism

Although the pathogenesis of post-thyroidectomy hypocalcaemia is multifactorial, damage to the parathyroid glands in the form of direct injury, unrecognized inadvertent removal or indirect injury by devascularization of the gland are the most common causes. For these reasons, it is essential for preventing hypoparathyroidism that the surgeon should understand the anatomical variations of the parathyroid glands and identify the glands during surgery.

The superior parathyroid glands are usually located lateral and posterior to the RLN at the level of Berry's ligament and are the parathyroid glands that are usually the easiest to preserve during endoscopic thyroidectomy. The inferior parathyroid glands are almost always located anterior to the RLN and caudal to where the RLN crosses the inferior thyroid artery. The criteria that can differentiate the parathyroid glands are (1) the position, (2) mobility independent of the thyroid gland, (3) brownish colour, (4) smooth, finely granular surface, (5) presence of vascular pedicle, (6) easy bleeding on manipulation, (7) the presence of a small fatty hood.

In conventional thyroidectomy, permanent hypoparathyroidism resulting in lifetime disability occurs in less than 1% of patients [30,31], whereas transient postoperative hypocalcaemia which recovers within 6 months after surgery is much more common, with a range of 4–42% [32–34]. However, its incidence in remote-access endoscopic thyroidectomy has not been well investigated because there are only a few published reports. Transient and permanent hypoparathyroidism in gasless transaxillary endoscopic thyroidectomy occurred in 3.2% and 0%, respectively [13]. The BABA approach also showed a similar pattern in that transient and permanent hypoparathyroidism occurred in 3.0% and 0% [12]. Based on these results, there is no evidence that endoscopic thyroidectomy is associated with an increased incidence of hypoparathyroidism. Magnification by endoscopy is rather helpful to identify the parathyroid glands. With a cumulative experience of endoscopic thyroidectomy, surgical identification of the parathyroid gland will likely become easier. In addition, it should be pointed out that hypoparathyroidism is associated with thermal injury by the Harmonic™ Scalpel in endoscopic thyroidectomy [35]. Therefore, it is recommended that the inactive blade be the nearest to the parathyroid gland during cutting and coagulation.

If safe dissection of a parathyroid gland is technically not feasible or its viability has been compromised, the gland should be removed, cut into small fragments, and implanted into a muscle pocket in the sternocleidomastoid muscle or pectoralis major muscle (especially in axillary endoscopic thyroidectomy). The site of autotransplantation should be marked in case the tissue transplanted subsequently becomes pathological. With advances in knowledge of the specific anatomical features of the parathyroid gland and meticulous surgical technique, permanent hypoparathyroidism in remote-access endoscopic thyroidectomy should be low.

Bleeding

Surgeons have always been concerned with bleeding and haemostasis since these may sometimes have devastating consequences. Like all areas of surgery, thorough haemostasis is critical in thyroid surgery because a small amount of bleeding can often obscure the operative field, making surgery more hazardous. Intraoperative bleeding can increase the possibility of injury to the RLN and the parathyroid glands because of tissue staining, making identification more difficult. Furthermore, haematoma formation after thyroid surgery is of particular concern as it may lead to life-threatening airway obstruction. This is due to the rapid rise in pressure within a closed space, with subsequent laryngeal oedema and airway obstruction.

Because remote-access endoscopic thyroidectomy uses only energy devices such as the Harmonic™ Scalpel and the electrocautery for all haemostatic manoeuvres, surgeons should be very familiar with use of these devices before attempting endoscopic thyroidectomy.

Postoperative bleeding is characterized by respiratory distress, pain or cervical pressure, dysphagia and increased drain output. Perioperative bleeding may be decreased by having the patient in a reverse Trendelenburg position, with the head elevated 20°. If the surgeon is uncertain about the dryness of the operative field, a Valsalva manoeuvre, which elevates the intrapulmonary pressure to 40 cmH$_2$0 and facilitates recognition of bleeding vessels, can be performed by the anaesthetist prior to wound closure. Postoperatively, patients should be placed in a low Fowler position with the head and shoulders elevated 10–20° to keep a negative pressure in the veins.

In the majority of patients, symptomatic haemorrhage with airway oedema and obstruction occur between 4 and 6h after the initial operation [36]. Since in approximately 20% of cases the onset of haematoma symptoms is reported beyond 24h postoperatively, the surgeon should warn patients who undergo ambulatory surgery about the risk of delayed bleeding [37].

Although the incidence of symptomatic haemorrhage requiring reoperation amounts to 0.1–1.5% in conventional thyroidectomy [19,32,36–38], its incidence following remote-access endoscopic thyroidectomy is not well known because of the paucity of reports. In a large study of gasless transaxillary endoscopic thyroidectomy, chest wall haematoma which originated from a tiny bleeder in the anterior surface of the strap muscle and pectoralis major muscle occurred in 0.6% of the patients [13]. The haematomas were easily controlled and evacuated at the bedside without difficulty. Because gasless transaxillary endoscopic thyroidectomy has a wide operative space, through which intraoperative and postoperative bleeding can be drained well, major haematoma formation with airway compression rarely occurs in this approach.

In contrast, axillary and BABA approaches with gas insufflation have required conversion to open surgery due to intraoperative bleeding [12,39]. This implies that a small amount of bleeding may not only obscure the operative field but make the operation more difficult in an insufflation approach. Moreover, a small haematoma may lead to life-threatening airway obstruction due to a small operative space. Although no postoperative major haematoma in an insufflation approach has yet been reported, if it is recognized, making a new incision on the anterior neck should be considered to evacuate the haematoma and relieve airway pressure. In case of significant respiratory distress, emergency bedside haematoma evacuation is required, if necessary in combination with endotracheal intubation. The requirement for tracheotomy either in the emergency setting or due to persisting airway obstruction after haematoma removal is generally a rare event.

Complications induced by CO_2 gas insufflation

Complications induced by insufflation have been encountered during the initial trials of endoscopic neck surgery using CO_2 gas. Massive subcutaneous emphysema, severe hypercarbia and severe tachycardia were observed during surgery in patients who underwent endoscopic transcervical parathyroidectomy using CO_2 insufflation [3,40]. Relatively high pressures of CO_2 were applied for insufflation (15–20 mmHg). Although one reported patient resumed spontaneous respiration, patients in whom massive subcutaneous emphysema develops may need ventilatory support to normalize haemodynamics.

After this experience, in trials of the axillary approach described by Ikeda et al. [9], the breast approach reported by Ohgami et al. [10], the ABBA approach [11] and the BABA approach [12], low-pressure CO_2 insufflation (4–6 mm Hg) was applied. The surgeons were still able to obtain a satisfactory operative view and stable haemodynamics in which the end-tidal CO_2 pressure and the

PCO_2 in arterial blood were maintained under 40 mmHg in all patients during surgery, without requiring hyperventilation. They have experienced no complications induced by CO_2 gas insufflation.

It is recommended by Ohgami et al. that a loose rubber bandage be applied to the face around the mandible during surgery to prevent extension of subcutaneous emphysema to the face [10]. Therefore, it is a current opinion that CO_2 insufflation for endoscopic thyroid or parathyroid surgery is safe if insufflation is maintained at low pressures.

In the BABA approach, one case of pneumothorax developed not via mechanical injury of the chest wall but by high-pressure ventilation during general anaesthesia [12]. This pneumothorax was easily resolved by chest tube insertion.

Brachial plexus injury

In the gasless transaxillary approach, some patients experienced mild shoulder pain due to postoperative neuropathy of the brachial plexus [35]. This spontaneously resolved within a few months without disability. This postoperative neuropathy of the brachial plexus remains a relatively frequent and poorly understood complication. Previously, brachial plexus injury has occurred after abdominal operation with the patient positioned on the operative table with the arm restrained on a board in abduction, external rotation and extension [41–43]. Lesions of the brachial plexus are often regarded as stretch-induced neuropathies [44] due to malposition. Several positions of the upper quadrant (arm and neck) that elongate the length of the nerve bedding of the brachial plexus and median nerve and have been associated with perioperative neuropathies include shoulder girdle depression, abduction greater than 90°, lateral rotation of the arm, lateral flexion of the patient's head to the opposite side, full elbow extension and forearm supination [45,46].

Onset of symptoms is characterized by paraesthesias and weakness, yet pain is not a prominent sign. The recovery starts 2–3 weeks later, with gradual sensory recovery, followed by lower and upper plexus strength recovery after conservative treatment [41]. The differential diagnosis between brachial plexus neuropathy and ulnar nerve neuropathy is important, as the prognosis of brachial plexus neuropathy is generally better [47].

In the axillary approach, the neck is extended and the lesion-side arm is raised and fixed to shorten the distance from axilla to anterior neck. For this reason, inadvertent hyperextension of the arm may injure the brachial nerve plexus. Therefore, it is recommended that the arm should be best positioned in the natural extension position because this does not load the nervous system. Surgeons should be aware of the brachial plexus injury in order to make an early diagnosis and begin treatment. Also, the anaesthesiologist should know the risks of malpositioning in order to help prevent nerve injuries.

With awareness of risk factors and positioning which are likely to cause injury to the brachial plexus, careful positioning of the upper extremity can prevent injury and potential disability to the patient.

Seroma

Among the remote approach methods, the approach in which seroma has most commonly developed is gasless transaxillary endoscopic thyroidectomy. This method is more invasive and needs more operation time than open surgery due to the wide dissection from the axilla to the anterior neck area. For this reason, chest wall seroma has occurred in 1.5% of patients [13]. In general, seromas resolve easily with repeated needle aspiration and compression dressings on the chest wall.

Oesophageal injury

In a report about BABA [12], one case of oesophageal perforation near the site of the superior thyroid artery ligation was observed 9 days after surgery. Therefore, re-exploration was performed and then gauze packing was maintained for 25 days and eventually the patient recovered. It was suspected that there was a possibility of thermal injury to the oesophagus at the moment of superior thyroid artery ligation with the Harmonic™ Scalpel. If thermal oesophageal injury is recognized intraoperatively, it is generally recommended that direct suturing and total parenteral nutrition for 2–3 days be pursued.

Conclusion

Remote-access thyroid surgery can be performed safely and offers numerous advantages over conventional open thyroid surgery and neck-based video-endoscopic approaches. A good understanding of possible complications and how to prevent them will help maximize patient safety.

References

1 Kocher T. Uber kropfextirpation und ihre Folgen. Arc Klin Chirurg 1883; 29: 254–337.

2 Park JG. Korea Central Cancer Registry cancer incidence in Korea 1999–2001. Seoul: Ministry of Health and Welfare, 2005.

3 Gagner M. Endoscopic subtotal parathyroidectomy in patients with primary hyperparathyroidism. Br J Surg 1996; 83: 875.

4 Hüscher CS, Chiodini S, Napolitano C, Recher A. Endoscopic right thyroid lobectomy. Surg Endosc 1997; 11: 877.

5 Miccoli P, Berti P, Bendinelli C, Conte M, Fasolini F, Martino E. Minimally invasive video-assisted surgery of the thyroid: a preliminary report. Langenbecks Arch Surg 2000; 385: 261–4.

6 Bellantone R, Lombardi CP, Bossola M, et al. Video-assisted vs conventional thyroid lobectomy: a randomized trial. Arch Surg 2002; 137: 301–4; discussion 305.

7 Shimizu K, Akira S, Jasmi AY, et al. Video-assisted neck surgery: endoscopic resection of thyroid tumors with a very minimal neck wound. J Am Coll Surg 1999; 188: 697–703.

8 Gagner M, Inabnet WB 3rd. Endoscopic thyroidectomy for solitary thyroid nodules. Thyroid 2001; 11: 161–3.

9 Ikeda Y, Takami H, Sasaki Y, Kan S, Niimi M. Endoscopic neck surgery by the axillary approach. J Am Coll Surg 2000; 191: 336–40.

10 Ohgami M, Ishii S, Arisawa Y, et al. Scarless endoscopic thyroidectomy: breast approach for better cosmesis. Surg Laparosc Endosc Percutan Tech 2000; 10: 1–4.

11 Shimazu K, Shiba E, Tamaki Y, et al. Endoscopic thyroid surgery through the axillo-bilateral-breast approach. Surg Laparosc Endosc Percutan Tech 2003; 13: 196–201.

12 Choe JH, Kim SW, Chung KW, et al. Endoscopic thyroidectomy using a new bilateral axillo-breast approach. World J Surg 2007; 31: 601–6.

13 Kang SW, Jeong JJ, Yun JS, et al. Gasless endoscopic thyroidectomy using trans-axillary approach: surgical outcome of 581 patients. Endocr J 2009; 56: 361–9.

14 Kern KA. Medicolegal analysis of errors in diagnosis and treatment of surgical endocrine disease. Surgery 1993; 114: 1167–73; discussion 1173–64.

15 Marcus B, Edwards B, Yoo S, et al. Recurrent laryngeal nerve monitoring in thyroid and parathyroid surgery: the University of Michigan experience. Laryngoscope 2003; 113: 356–61.

16 Scheuller MC, Ellison D. Laryngeal mask anesthesia with intraoperative laryngoscopy for identification of the recurrent laryngeal nerve during thyroidectomy. Laryngoscope 2002; 112: 1594–7.

17 Eltzschig HK, Posner M, Moore FD Jr. The use of readily available equipment in a simple method for intraoperative

monitoring of recurrent laryngeal nerve function during thyroid surgery: initial experience with more than 300 cases. Arch Surg 2002; 137: 452–6; discussion 456–7.

18 Tan CT, Cheah WK, Delbridge L. 'Scarless' (in the neck) endoscopic thyroidectomy (SET): an evidence-based review of published techniques. World J Surg 2008; 32: 1349–57.

19 Rosato L, Avenia N, Bernante P, et al. Complications of thyroid surgery: analysis of a multicentric study on 14,934 patients operated on in Italy over 5 years. World J Surg 2004; 28: 271–6.

20 Owaki T, Nakano S, Arimura K, Aikou T. The ultrasonic coagulating and cutting system injures nerve function. Endoscopy 2002; 34: 575–9.

21 Aynehchi BB, McCoul ED, Sundaram K. Systematic review of laryngeal reinnervation techniques. Otolaryngol Head Neck Surg 2010; 143: 749–59.

22 Chou FF, Su CY, Jeng SF, Hsu KL, Lu KY. Neurorrhaphy of the recurrent laryngeal nerve. J Am Coll Surg 2003; 197: 52–7.

23 Damrose EJ, Huang RY, Ye M, Berke GS, Sercarz JA. Surgical anatomy of the recurrent laryngeal nerve: implications for laryngeal reinnervation. Ann Otol Rhinol Laryngol 2003; 112: 434–8.

24 Lee SW, Kim JW, Chung CH, et al. Utility of injection laryngoplasty in the management of post-thyroidectomy vocal cord paralysis. Thyroid 2010; 20: 513–17.

25 Kang SW, Lee SC, Lee SH, et al. Robotic thyroid surgery using a gasless, transaxillary approach and the da Vinci S system: the operative outcomes of 338 consecutive patients. Surgery 2009; 146: 1048–55.

26 Fewins J, Simpson CB, Miller FR. Complications of thyroid and parathyroid surgery. Otolaryngol Clin North Am 2003; 36: 189–206, x.

27 Friedman M, LoSavio P, Ibrahim H. Superior laryngeal nerve identification and preservation in thyroidectomy. Arch Otolaryngol Head Neck Surg 2002; 128: 296–303.

28 Cernea CR, Ferraz AR, Furlani J, et al. Identification of the external branch of the superior laryngeal nerve during thyroidectomy. Am J Surg 1992; 164: 634–9.

29 Cernea CR, Ferraz AR, Nishio S, Dutra A Jr, Hojaij FC, dos Santos LR. Surgical anatomy of the external branch of the superior laryngeal nerve. Head Neck 1992; 14: 380–3.

30 Shaha AR, Burnett C, Jaffe BM. Parathyroid autotransplantation during thyroid surgery. J Surg Oncol 1991; 46: 21–4.

31 Olson JA Jr, DeBenedetti MK, Baumann DS, Wells SA Jr. Parathyroid autotransplantation during thyroidectomy. Results of long-term follow-up. Ann Surg 1996; 223: 472–8; discussion 478–80.

32 Bergamaschi R, Becouarn G, Ronceray J, Arnaud JP. Morbidity of thyroid surgery. Am J Surg 1998; 176: 71–5.

33 Herranz-Gonzalez J, Gavilan J, Matinez-Vidal J, Gavilan C. Complications following thyroid surgery. Arch Otolaryngol Head Neck Surg 1991; 117: 516–18.

34 Flynn MB, Lyons KJ, Tarter JW, Ragsdale TL. Local complications after surgical resection for thyroid carcinoma. Am J Surg 1994; 168: 404–7.

35 Jeong JJ, Kang SW, Yun JS, et al. Comparative study of endoscopic thyroidectomy versus conventional open thyroidectomy in papillary thyroid microcarcinoma (PTMC) patients. J Surg Oncol 2009; 100: 477–80.

36 Shaha AR, Jaffe BM. Practical management of post-thyroidectomy hematoma. J Surg Oncol 1994; 57: 235–8.

37 Burkey SH, van Heerden JA, Thompson GB, Grant CS, Schleck CD, Farley DR. Reexploration for symptomatic hematomas after cervical exploration. Surgery 2001; 130: 914–20.

38 Lacoste L, Gineste D, Karayan J, et al. Airway complications in thyroid surgery. Ann Otol Rhinol Laryngol 1993; 102: 441–6.

39 Ikeda Y, Takami H, Niimi M, Kan S, Sasaki Y, Takayama J. Endoscopic thyroidectomy and parathyroidectomy by the axillary approach. A preliminary report. Surg Endosc 2002; 16: 92–5.

40 Gottlieb A, Sprung J, Zheng XM, Gagner M. Massive subcutaneous emphysema and severe hypercarbia in a patient during endoscopic transcervical parathyroidectomy using carbon dioxide insufflation. Anesth Analg 1997; 84: 1154–6.

41 Brill S, Walfisch S. Brachial plexus injury as a complication after colorectal surgery. Tech Coloproctol 2005; 9: 139–41.

42 Brieger GM, Korda AR, Houghton CR. Abdomino perineal repair of pulsion enterocele. J Obstet Gynaecol Res 1996; 22: 151–6.

43 Milsom JW, Ludwig KA, Church JM, Garcia-Ruiz A. Laparoscopic total abdominal colectomy with ileorectal anastomosis for familial adenomatous polyposis. Dis Colon Rectum 1997; 40: 675–8.

44 Warner MA. Perioperative neuropathies. Mayo Clin Proc 1998; 73: 567–74.

45 Gagnon J, Poulin EC. Beware of the Trendelenburg position during prolonged laparoscopic procedures. Can J Surg 1993; 36: 505–6.

46 Romanowski L, Reich H, McGlynn F, Adelson MD, Taylor PJ. Brachial plexus neuropathies after advanced laparoscopic surgery. Fertil Steril 1993; 60: 729–32.

47 Britt BA, Gordon RA. Peripheral nerve injuries associated with anaesthesia. Can Anaesth Soc J 1964; 11: 514–36.

CHAPTER 31

Complications of Robotic Thyroidectomy

David J. Terris and Michael C. Singer

Department of Otolaryngology – Head and Neck Surgery, Georgia Health Sciences University, Augusta, GA, USA

Introduction

The field of thyroid surgery has evolved considerably over the past 8–10 years. After more than a century of performing thyroidectomy essentially the way it was described by Theodor Kocher, there are a number of minimally invasive and remote-access options now available to surgeons and patients.

Innovative thyroid surgery has progressed in one of two essential directions. On one hand, a number of investigators have pioneered techniques to reduce the extent of dissection and minimize the length of incision required [1–3]. The second avenue of innovation has focused on achieving the complete absence of neck scars. This second approach actually requires considerably more extensive dissection, with the sole benefit of no visible scar [4–6]. Remote-access and robotic thyroidectomy are discussed in greater detail in other chapters. The two principal options that have emerged in the past 18–36 months include the robotic axillary thyroidectomy (RAT) [7] and the robotic facelift thyroidectomy (RFT) [8].

Complications that may be associated with robotic thyroidectomy comprise many of the same complications that can occur with a thyroidectomy of any type. As these are covered in comprehensive detail in prior chapters, the focus of this chapter will be those complications that are unique to (or more likely to occur during) remote-access robotic thyroidectomy. Since RAT and

RFT approaches are substantially different, they will be covered separately below.

Complications of robotic axillary thyroidectomy

This approach, which was pioneered, refined and popularized by Chung and his colleagues in Seoul, South Korea [7], places the access portal in the axilla, with or without an additional presternal port. Because this method requires crossing of the clavicle, somewhat awkward positioning of the arm is needed in order to optimize the access. This arm positioning, as well as the vector of approach, is responsible for most of the potential complications that are unique to this procedure.

The Chung group has reported a very robust and successful experience that now exceeds 2000 patients [9] and has been performed with a low complication profile. Many of the complications described below occurred with the exportation of the procedure to a North American population.

Brachial plexopathy

The original description of the positioning required for this procedure has the arm extended above the head (Figure 31.1). This positioning has the potential to put

Thyroid Surgery: Preventing and Managing Complications, First Edition. Edited by Paolo Miccoli, David J. Terris, Michele N. Minuto and Melanie W. Seybt.
© 2013 John Wiley & Sons, Ltd. Published 2013 by John Wiley & Sons, Ltd.

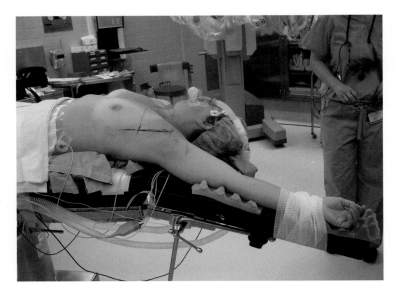

Figure 31.1 The robotic axillary thyroidectomy procedure requires crossing the clavicle to reach the thyroid gland. The arm is positioned above the head in order to rotate the clavicle downward and optimize the exposure.

the brachial plexus on stretch, and during the prolonged operative intervention has resulted in numerous episodes of temporary arm paralysis [10–12]. While these have all resolved (some requiring up to several months), this is a very unwelcome outcome following routine thyroid surgery. Some investigators have reverted back to the positioning described by Ikeda [4], wherein the arm is crossed over the top of the face (Figure 31.2), and still others have advocated for routine bilateral brachial plexus monitoring during the thyroidectomy to mitigate this complication [13].

Visceral injury: oesophageal perforation

Because of the vector of approach, the oesophagus is placed at considerably higher risk than with the typical conventional (ventral) approach. A number of unpublished incidents of perforation (and even one case of oesophageal transection) have occurred during thyroidectomy (Figure 31.3). Cautious and meticulous technique should allow the surgeon to minimize this risk despite the direction of surgical approach. Management is predicated upon prompt recognition, with subsequent steps dictated by the severity of injury. These may include intravenous antibiotics, incision and drainage, oesophagostomy and occasionally oesophageal reconstruction.

Visceral injury: tracheal perforation

While tracheal perforation may occur during any type of thyroidectomy approach, it has recently been described during the course of robotic axillary thyroidectomy [14]. Once again, the vector of approach may be a contributing factor, along with the substantially reduced haptic feedback associated with robotic surgery. When these occur, there is usually no doubt about the diagnosis. The options include primary repair or a tracheostomy followed by stepwise removal of the tracheostomy.

Retained thyroid tissue

Perhaps because of the unfamiliar anatomical planes and direction of approach, the inadvertent retention of substantial thyroid remnant tissue has been described [12]. Particularly in an era where endocrinology consultants demand ever more thorough thyroidectomies, this substantial oversight should be avoided. In a related complication, the inability to adequately access the thyroid gland has resulted in known retention of an unacceptably large remnant of thyroid tissue. Patients should be advised of the potential need to open the neck and if necessary, conversion should be considered.

Carotid sheath violation

In verbal communications, cases of excessive blood loss exceeding 1 L of blood have been reported. This has

Figure 31.2 An alternative method for positioning the arm during axillary thyroid surgery was proposed by Ikeda and colleagues [4]. It is likely that this technique promotes less stretching of the brachial plexus, thereby reducing the likelihood of arm paralysis.

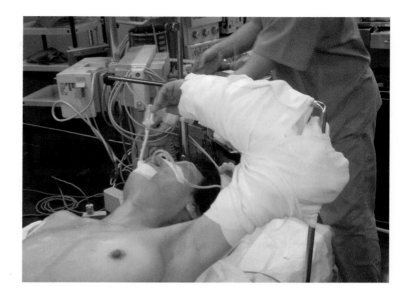

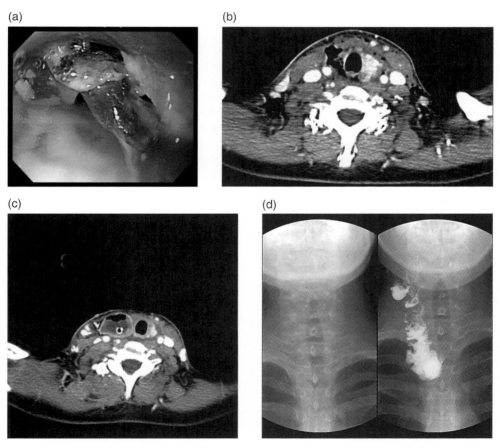

Figure 31.3 A major complication that has been associated with axillary thyroidectomy is oesophageal perforation (and even one case of transection). In the case illustrated here, an endoscopic examination of the oesophagus (a) reveals granulation tissue associated with the violation of the oesophageal wall. A computed tomographic (CT) scan (b) demonstrates air in the region of the perforation. After failed incision and drainage and even temporary oesophagostomy, a jejunal free flap repair was necessary to reconstruct the oesophagus, as seen in the CT scan (c) and the barium swallow (d).

occurred from poor control of a superior thyroid artery, and during the initial dissection as a result of inadvertent transection of the external jugular vein. In at least one additional case, an injury to the internal jugular vein has been suffered and required repair. While the vessel was controlled robotically, strong consideration should be given to opening the neck in the event of major vessel injury, or when blood loss exceeds 500 cc.

Chest wall hypaesthesia

Because of the significant undermining of the cutaneous flap, extensive and prolonged hypaesthesia in the chest wall region has been described with axillary approaches [15]. While it may be anticipated that this will resolve, this should be included as part of the informed consent process. No specific treatment is necessary nor is effective.

Complications of robotic facelift thyroidectomy

Because of some of the substantial complications that have occurred in the United States with the attempt to import the robotic axillary thyroidectomy technique, a novel robotic thyroid surgical approach has been described by Singer *et al.* [16]. This incorporates a number of previously described principles in a hybrid approach. It uses as its access port a facelift type of incision (Figure 31.4) and dissection planes which are inherently more familiar to head and neck surgeons. No special positioning is required since the clavicle is not crossed in order to access the thyroid compartment. There are potential complications that are unique to this approach. Only a modest number of robotic facelift thyroidectomies have been performed (especially relative to the robotic axillary thyroidectomy) and it is possible that additional complications will emerge over time.

Greater auricular nerve hypaesthesia

As the musculocutaneous flap is developed on top of the sternocleidomastoid muscle, the dissection plane should remain dorsal to the greater auricular nerve and the external jugular vein. Even when the greater auricular nerve is completely preserved, the patient will experience a temporary hypaesthesia in the distribution of this

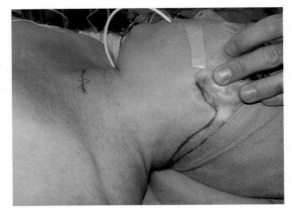

Figure 31.4 The novel robotic facelift thyroidectomy is performed through a facelift incision located in the postauricular crease, and extending across to the occipital hairline. This results in a completely hidden scar. Reproduced from Terris *et al.* [17], with permission from Lippincott Williams and Wilkins.

nerve. This sensation returns typically over a period of several weeks to several months. The nerve may also be inadvertently transected. However, as has been true with parotid surgery, even when the nerve is transected the patient can anticipate complete or nearly complete return of sensory function. No specific management is required. The importance of laying the foundation of patient expectations cannot be overemphasized.

Neck pain

While all patients who undergo thyroid surgery will experience some degree of cervical incisional pain or anterior neck pain from the thyroid dissection, we have observed qualitatively that patients who undergo robotic facelift thyroidectomy seem to have above average neck discomfort. This likely relates to the disruption of the plane along the sternocleidomastoid muscle and between this muscle and the strap muscles. While this discomfort resolves promptly, we believe it is worth mentioning to our patients in order to help calibrate their expectations.

Seroma

The area of dissection required to reach and remove the thyroid gland with remote-access surgery is considerably greater than that needed with conventional and minimally invasive techniques. The potential space created may occasionally result in seroma formation.

Prevention of this complication consists of absolute haemostasis at the time of surgery and limitation of postoperative activities for 7–10 days. The use of drains is ineffective. In most cases that occur, no specific management is needed. Incision and drainage with application of a pressure dressing should be necessary only in the event of skin ischaemia or excessive pain.

Remote-access surgery: general

An adverse characteristic of virtually all remote-access surgery (while not necessarily representing a complication) is the necessarily prolonged surgical time associated with these procedures. Because of the resulting lengthier anaesthesia time, these techniques should be reserved primarily for healthy patients. Appropriate precautions must be taken to guard against complications that may be associated with prolonged anaesthesia, including deep venous thrombosis, urinary retention and atelectasis.

Finally, the extensive dissection required in order to reach the thyroid compartment from any remote-access location should logically be associated with a lengthier healing process and increased healing time. While this has not proven to be problematic for our patients, its likelihood should be acknowledged.

Conclusion

Remote-access and robotic thyroidectomy techniques represent an important new avenue of options for patients undergoing thyroidectomy who are particularly reluctant to suffer a visible neck scar. Novel and non-standard complications may be associated with these techniques, and strategies for their avoidance should be pursued. The informed consent process should include acknowledgement of these complications in addition to those associated with conventional thyroidectomy.

References

1 Miccoli P, Berti P, Materazzi G, Minuto M, Barellini L. Minimally invasive video-assisted thyroidectomy: five years of experience. J Am Coll Surg 2004; 199(2): 243–8.

2 Lombardi CP, Raffaelli M, Princi P, de Crea C, Bellantone R. Video-assisted thyroidectomy: report on the experience of a single center in more than four hundred cases. World J Surg 2006; 30(5): 794–800.

3 Terris DJ, Angelos P, Steward D, Simental A. Minimally invasive video-assisted thyroidectomy: a multi-institutional North American experience. Arch Otolaryngol Head Neck Surg 2008; 134(1): 81–4.

4 Ikeda Y, Takami H, Sasaki Y, Takayama J, Niimi M, Kan S. Clinical benefits in endoscopic thyroidectomy by the axillary approach. J Am Coll Surg 2003; 196(2): 189–95.

5 Jeryong K, Jinsun L, Hyegyong K, et al. Total endoscopic thyroidectomy with bilateral breast areola and ipsilateral axillary (BBIA) approach. World J Surg 2008; 32(11): 2488–93.

6 Lee KE, Koo do H, Kim SJ, et al. Outcomes of 109 patients with papillary thyroid carcinoma who underwent robotic total thyroidectomy with central node dissection via the bilateral axillo-breast approach. Surgery 2010; 148(6): 1207–13.

7 Kang SW, Jeong JJ, Yun JS, et al. Robot-assisted endoscopic surgery for thyroid cancer: experience with the first 100 patients. Surg Endosc 2009; 23(11): 2399–406.

8 Terris DJ, Singer MC, Seybt MW. Robotic facelift thyroidectomy: II. Clinical feasibility and safety. Laryngoscope 2011; 121(8): 1636–41.

9 Lee J, Kang SW, Jung JJ, et al. Multicenter study of robotic thyroidectomy: short-term postoperative outcomes and surgeon ergonomic considerations. Ann Surg Oncol 2011; 18(9): 2538–47.

10 Kang SW, Lee SC, Lee SH, et al. Robotic thyroid surgery using a gasless, transaxillary approach and the da Vinci S system: the operative outcomes of 338 consecutive patients. Surgery 2009; 146(6): 1048–55.

11 Landry CS, Grubbs EG, Morris GS, et al. Robot assisted transaxillary surgery (RATS) for the removal of thyroid and parathyroid glands. Surgery 2011; 149(4): 549–55.

12 Kuppersmith RB, Holsinger FC. Robotic thyroid surgery: an initial experience with North American patients. Laryngoscope 2011; 121(3): 521–6.

13 Kandil E, Winters R, Aslam R, Friedlander P, Bellows C. Transaxillary gasless robotic thyroid surgery with nerve monitoring: initial experience in a North American center. Minim Invasive Ther Allied Technol 2012; 21(2): 90–5.

14 Lee S, Ryu HR, Park JH, et al. Excellence in robotic thyroid surgery: a comparative study of robot-assisted versus conventional endoscopic thyroidectomy in papillary thyroid microcarcinoma patients. Ann Surg 2011; 253(6): 1060–6.

15 Yoon JH, Park CH, Chung WY. Gasless endoscopic thyroid-ectomy via an axillary approach: experience of 30 cases. Surg Laparosc Endosc Percutan Tech 2006; 16(4): 226–31.

16 Singer MC, Seybt MW, Terris DJ. Robotic facelift thyroidectomy: I. Preclinical simulation and morphometric assessment. Laryngoscope 2011; 121(8): 1631–5.

17 Terris DJ, Singer MC, Seybt MW. Robotic facelift thyroidectomy: patient selection and technical considerations. Surg Laparosc Endosc Percutan Tech 2011; 21(4); 237–42.

PART VIII

Iatrogenic Hypothyroidism, Metabolic Effects of Post-thyroidectomy Thyroid Hormone Replacement, and Quality of Life after Thyroid Surgery

CHAPTER 32

Iatrogenic Hypothyroidism and Its Sequelae

Paolo Vitti and Francesco Latrofa
Department of Endocrinology and Metabolism, University Hospital of Pisa, Pisa, Italy

Introduction

Hypothyroidism is defined as the lack of action of thyroid hormones on target tissues. It can be due to transient or permanent thyroid failure (primary hypothyroidism), lack of thyroid stimulation by thyroid-stimulating hormone (TSH) (secondary or central hypothyroidism) and resistance to thyroid hormone. Primary hypothyroidism is induced by iatrogenic factors, autoimmune thyroid disease, subacute thyroiditis, severe iodine deficiency, natural goitrogens, infiltrative diseases (amyloidosis, scleroderma) and congenital abnormalities.

Iatrogenic hypothyroidism can be permanent, when induced by treatment leading to permanent thyroid damage, or reversible, when caused by drugs interfering with thyroid function (Box 32.1). Thyroidectomy and radioiodine (^{131}I) therapy, which are employed for treatment of multinodular goitre, Graves' disease and thyroid carcinoma, and external radiotherapy, used for malignant neck or head tumours, cause permanent hypothyroidism. Conversely, treatment with antithyroid drugs and other agents induce hypothyroidism which is reversible in most circumstances.

In primary hypothyroidism, clinical hypothyroidism is characterized by low concentrations of thyroid hormones and high levels of serum TSH, subclinical hypothyroidism by an isolated rise of TSH levels.

Aetiology

Surgical hypothyroidism

The incidence of surgical hypothyroidism varies from 10% to 70% [1]. The broad differences in reported incidence are mainly caused by the extent of surgery (subtotal thyroidectomy, total or near-total thyroidectomy, lobectomy or hemithyroidectomy), which influences the amount of residual thyroid tissue, and the type (subclinical or clinical) of hypothyroidism investigated. Other factors influencing the incidence of hypothyroidism are the underlying thyroid disease (autoimmune or non-autoimmune thyroid disease) and the damage to thyroid vessels during the surgical procedure. Hypothyroidism is transient when the thyroid remnant is sufficient to undergo hyperplasia under the stimulus of elevated levels of TSH and to produce an adequate amount of thyroid hormones. Additional factors that can restore euthyroidism after partial thyroidectomy are rising levels of TSH receptor-stimulating autoantibodies (TSAb) in patients with Graves' disease and development of autonomy in the thyroid remnant in patients with nodular goitre. On the other hand, co-existent Hashimoto's thyroiditis, which influences the function of the thyroid remnant, can contribute to the development of hypothyroidism in patients who are euthyroid after partial thyroidectomy. These mechanisms may require a long

Thyroid Surgery: Preventing and Managing Complications, First Edition. Edited by Paolo Miccoli, David J. Terris, Michele N. Minuto and Melanie W. Seybt.

Box 32.1 Causes of iatrogenic hypothyroidism

Surgery:

- subtotal thyroidectomy
- total and near-total thyroidectomy
- lobectomy-hemithyroidectomy

External and internal radiation:

- ^{131}I therapy
- external radiotherapy

Drugs interfering with:

- TSH secretion
- thyroid hormone synthesis and secretion
- absorption of levothyroxine
- metabolism of tetra-iodothyronine and tri-iodothyronine

Other drugs

---

period to develop and therefore transient hypothyroidism can last for many months or years after partial thyroidectomy before evolving into euthyroidism. One series reported that 20% of patients who were hypothyroid shortly after subtotal thyroidectomy were euthyroid at 6 months [2] and another series reported that 37% of patients were euthyroid at 1 year [3].

Subtotal thyroidectomy

In the past, in order to avoid postsurgical hypothyroidism, patients with Graves' disease were treated with subtotal thyroidectomy. However, the attempt to obtain euthyroidism by leaving a sufficient amount of thyroid remnant was frequently unsuccessful and this practice increased the risk of recurrent hyperthyroidism but did not avoid the occurrence of hypothyroidism. The rate of hypothyroidism after subtotal thyroidectomy ranged from 3% to 75% [4,5]. Postsurgical hypothyroidism developed mostly within 1 year after surgery. Subclinical hypothyroidism was common and frequently transient. In addition, 79% of patients changed their clinical status during a follow-up of 12 years and about half of those who were hypothyroid 6 years after surgery became euthyroid by 12 years [6]. Therefore, Graves' patients treated with subtotal thyroidectomy need to be followed for decades because of the possible late occurrence of hypothyroidism or hyperthyroidism.

Subtotal thyroidectomy for toxic or non-toxic multinodular goitre is correlated with a risk of developing

hypothyroidism of less than 15% but is associated with a recurrence rate of 10–20% at 10 years and 40% at 30 years after surgery [4].

Total and near-total thyroidectomy

Postsurgical hypothyroidism is the expected outcome of total and near-total thyroidectomy performed for Graves' disease, toxic and non-toxic multinodular goitre and thyroid carcinoma. The long-term changes reported after subtotal thyroidectomy are not observed when Graves' hyperthyroidism is treated with total thyroidectomy.

Lobectomy-hemithyroidectomy

Patients who undergo lobectomy for an autonomously functioning nodule or a toxic solitary nodule may develop transient subclinical hypothyroidism postoperatively [7] but are usually euthyroid 10 years after thyroidectomy, with an incidence of hypothyroidism of 14–22% [8,9].

External and internal radiation

The thyroid can be exposed to internal and external radiation. Internal radiation can be the consequence of indirect exposure after environmental disasters (fallout) or therapeutic irradiation with ^{131}I. External radiation is the consequence of direct exposure after environmental disasters or therapeutic irradiation for diseases of the head and neck.

Radioiodine therapy

Radioiodine is used for the treatment of hyperthyroidism due to Graves' disease or toxic multinodular goitre and to reduce the volume of large non-toxic multinodular goitre.

The majority of Graves' patients treated with high doses ($\geq$370 MBq or $\geq$5.6 MBq per gram of thyroid tissues) of ^{131}I develop hypothyroidism: 70% at 10 years [4]. Lower doses of ^{131}I induce hypothyroidism in about 10% of patients after 1 year but in more than 50% after 11–15 years [4] and are associated with a higher rate of persistent hyperthyroidism [10]. The recommendation is therefore to administer a dose of ^{131}I sufficient to induce hypothyroidism because attempts to attain euthyroidism are often followed by recurrence of hyperthyroidism or late onset of hypothyroidism.

Hypothyroidism is less frequent after treatment with ^{131}I of toxic multinodular goitre (6–7% 1–5 years after 555 MBq) [11] or autonomously functioning thyroid adenoma (6–13% 1–10 years after 555–740 MBq) [12] because of the presence of some thyroid tissue that is suppressed and therefore not vulnerable to ^{131}I damage. Indeed, hypothyroidism is reported to be more common when ^{131}I uptake is present in extranodular thyroid tissue.

Post ^{131}I hypothyroidism is more common after treatment of non-toxic multinodular goitre: in 22% of patients 5 years after 3.7 MBq per gram of thyroid tissue [13] and in 100% of patients 8 years after 740–1850 MBq [14].

External radiotherapy

Subclinical or clinical hypothyroidism develops in 20–50% of patients treated with external radiotherapy (25 Gy or more) to the neck for Hodgkin's or non-Hodgkin's lymphomas [15]. Higher doses of radiation are associated with a higher frequency of hypothyroidism, whereas shielding of the thyroid may reduce the risk of hypothyroidism. Hypothyroidism usually occurs within 2–5 years after radiotherapy but has been reported also within 1 year, as well as many years later.

Hypothyroidism develops in 10–50% of patients after external radiotherapy for neck or head tumours [16]. It normally develops within 1 year and is usually subclinical. Patients treated with total bone irradiation for anaplastic anaemia or acute leukaemia develop hypothyroidism in 25% of cases, mostly within 1 year; hypothyroidism is usually subclinical and transient [17].

Drugs

Some drugs can affect thyroid function, in either the presence or absence of pre-existing thyroid dysfunctions, whereas others can interfere with assays measuring thyroid hormones. Hypothyroidism can also be the effect of overtreatment with antithyroid drugs.

Drugs interfering with thyroid-stimulating hormone secretion

Dopamine, the glucocorticoids and the somatostatin analogues (octreotide and others) inhibit TSH secretion and cause central hypothyroidism (normal or low TSH and low T4). However, prolonged treatment with glucocorticoids or somatostatin analogues rarely induces a persistent reduction of TSH levels and therefore permanent hypothyroidism is rare. Glucocorticoids can also modify thyroid function by reducing the levels of circulating thyroxine-binding globulin (TBG), inhibiting T4 deiodination and increasing renal clearance of iodine.

Dopamine antagonists (metoclopramide and domperidone) can cause a transient increase of TSH levels in patients with pre-existing hypothyroidism. β-Carotene, used for the treatment of T-cell cutaneous lymphoma, can cause central hypothyroidism.

In all cases the drug effect on TSH production is transient and after drug withdrawal, TSH secretion is restored. When prolonged treatment is required, levothyroxine (LT4) can be administered.

Drugs interfering with thyroid hormone synthesis and secretion

Chronic treatment with lithium carbonate induces sublinical hypothyroidism in 20% and clinical hypothyroidism in an additional 20% of patients. In the presence of thyroid autoimmunity, treatment with lithium may increase thyroid autoantibody concentration and may induce subclinical or overt hypothyroidism.

The administration of a large amount of iodine can induce hypothyroidism, particularly in patients with chronic autoimmune thyroiditis or other thyroid diseases. The daily administration of 1–2 mg of iodine suppresses thyroid hormone synthesis (Wolff–Chaikoff effect). In the normal thyroid, this suppression is followed by the restoration of thyroid hormone production (escape from Wolff–Chaikoff effect). In patients with chronic autoimmune thyroiditis, the thyroid gland is unable to escape from the acute Wolff–Chaikoff effect after the iodine load and therefore cannot resume normal hormone synthesis [18]. Many substances containing iodine usually employed in clinical practice (particularly for computed tomography scan and coronarography) release variable amounts of iodine.

Amiodarone-induced hypothyroidism is more common than amiodarone-induced thyrotoxicosis in iodine-sufficient areas and can affect both subjects with normal thyroid function and those with chronic autoimmune thyroiditis. Female sex and positive thyroid peroxidase autoantibodies (TPOAb) represented a relative risk of 7.9 and 7.3, respectively, for amiodarone-induced hypothyroidism and when both were present the risk was 13.5 [18]. In addition, amiodarone-induced hypothyroidism is more frequently persistent in TPOAb-positive and more commonly transient in TPOAb-negative patients. The concomitance of hypothyroidism does not contraindicate the use of amiodarone and requires careful treatment with LT4.

Aminoglutethimide, sulphonamides and sulphonylureas can occasionally cause a slight reduction of the levels of thyroid hormones and an increase of TSH, but hypothyroidism is uncommon.

Some monovalent cations (thiocyanates, perchlorate and nitrate) reduce iodine uptake of thyroid follicular cells. Perchlorate is occasionally used for treatment of thyrotoxicosis.

Drugs interfering with the absorption of levothyroxine

Eighty percent of LT4 administered orally is absorbed through the jejunum and the upper tract of the ileum. Cholestyramine, colestipol, aluminium hydroxide, ferrous sulphate and sucralfate reduce the absorption of the hormone in patients treated with LT4, inducing hypothyroidism. This consequence can be avoided by administering LT4 and the drug a few hours apart.

Drugs interfering with the metabolism of tetra-iodothyronine and tri-iodothyronine

Phenobarbital, rifampicin, phenytoin and carbamazepine can increase the catabolism of T4 and T3 by interfering with the enzymes involved. This effect does not influence the concentration of thyroid hormones in normal subjects while it can cause hypothyroidism in patients being treated with LT4.

Other drugs

The development of thyroid autoantibodies, transient thyrotoxicosis, hypothyroidism or thyrotoxicosis followed by hypothyroidism has been reported after treatment with cytokines such as interferon (IFN)-α, IFN-β, interleukin (IL)-2 and granulocyte macrophage colony-stimulating factor (GM-CSF). Seven to 40% of patients treated with IFN-α develop hypothyroidism. Female sex and pre-existing circulating antibodies are risk factors for thyroid dysfunction [19]. However, in 15% of patients with no evidence of thyroid autoimmunity, treatment with IFN-α will induce high serum TPO autoantibody or thyroid dysfunction [20].

The tyrosine kinase inhibitor sunitinib can induce permanent primary hypothyroidism or transient hypothyroidism, probably by inducing a destructive thyroiditis [21].

Clinical presentation

When thyroid damage is severe, a mild to severe clinical hypothyroidism ensues. In other cases the first finding is a slightly elevated TSH concentration without symptoms and signs of hypothyroidism (subclinical hypothyroidism). Clinical expression of hypothyroidism is mainly influenced by its pace of development and the patient's age. When progression of hypothyroidism is rapid, as after total thyroidectomy or withdrawal of replacement therapy, symptoms are well recognized whereas when it is slow, as in chronic autoimmune thyroiditis, its appearance may be insidious and its severity variable. In the elderly, hypothyroidism may be particularly insidious and severe and may eventually lead to myxoedema coma.

Symptoms of overt hypothyroidism in adulthood

Overt hypothyroidism of adulthood induces changes in almost every organ system.

Cutaneous changes are frequent and include cold intolerance, nail abnormality, thickening and dryness of hair and skin, oedema of hands, face and eyelids, change in shape of face, malar flush, non-pitting oedema, alopecia and pallor. Unusual coldness of the arms and legs is common.

Multiple alterations of the cardiovascular system are present. Bradycardia parallels the decrease in body metabolic rate. Loss of the inotropic and chronotropic actions of the thyroid hormones reduces myocardial contractility, and thus both stroke volume and heart rate and consequently cardiac output at rest. Narrowing of pulse pressure, prolongation of circulation time and decreased blood flow to the tissues are due to the increase of peripheral vascular resistance at rest and reduction of blood volume. Because myocardial oxygen consumption is decreased more than blood supply to the myocardium, angina is uncommon. The haemodynamic alterations at rest resemble those of congestive heart failure but in response to exercise, cardiac output increases and peripheral vascular resistance decreases normally, unless the hypothyroid state is severe. As a consequence of the increase of peripheral resistance, blood pressure rises mildly. All these cardiovascular alterations induce few symptoms. The occurrence of angina before or after the beginning of substitutive treatment indicates the presence of coronary artery disease.

Respiratory troubles are rarely a serious complaint in hypothyroid patients. However, fatigue and particularly dyspnoea on exertion are reported commonly by hypothyroid patients. The severity of hypothyroidism parallels the incidence of impaired ventilatory drive. Carbon dioxide narcosis may be a cause of myxoedema coma. Sleep apnoea syndrome and upper airway obstruction can be present.

Poor appetite can be a leading symptom in hypothyroid patients. Weight gain is reported by most patients but is of modest amount and due largely to retention of fluid. True obesity is uncommon. Constipation is frequent and is due to lowered food intake and decreased peristaltic activity. Gaseous distension may be a troublesome symptom. As a result of decreased energy metabolism and heat production, the basal metabolic rate is low, the appetite decreases and patients experience cold intolerance and slightly low basal body temperature.

In adults, severe hypothyroidism induces neurological symptoms such as somnolence, slow speech, impaired cognitive functions, loss of initiative, memory defects, headache, paraesthesia, deafness and vertigo. An unusual complacency, fatigue and pronounced somnolence or even lethargy should suggest the possibility of severe hypothyroidism. Cerebellar ataxia is present in rare cases of long-standing hypothyroidism. Sensory phenomena are common. Numbness and tingling of the extremities are frequent, as well as carpal tunnel syndrome and other mononeuropathies which cause nocturnal paraesthesia and pain. Deafness is a characteristic symptom of hypothyroidism and is due to both conduction and nerve impairment. Serous otitis media is common. Vestibular abnormalities and night blindness can be present. Psychiatric symptoms are common and include depression, bipolar disorders and affective psychosis. Reasoning power is preserved, except in the terminal stage. The emotional level seems low and irritability is decreased. Hypothyroidism should be suspected in any patient presenting with depression.

Muscle symptoms including myalgia, stiffness, cramps, slowness of movement and easy fatigability are often the predominating features and sometimes the sole manifestations of hypothyroidism. Hoffman's syndrome identifies the hypothyroid adult with increased muscle mass due to pseudohypertrophy, which mainly involves gastrocnemius, deltoid and trapezius muscles.

Articular and muscular pain and stiffness of the extremity may mistakenly suggest the diagnosis of rheumatoid arthritis or polymyalgia rheumatica. Bleeding symptoms are uncommon.

Hypothyroid women of fertile age have changes in cycle length and amount of bleeding. Oligomenorrhoea is the most common symptom; amenorrhoea, polymenorrhoea and menorrhagia are also reported. Severe hypothyroidism in women is associated with diminished libido and failure of ovulation. Hypothyroidism is associated with more fetal wastage and abortion in the first trimester. In adult men hypothyroidism may cause diminished libido and impotence.

Ocular manifestations typical of Graves' ophthalmopathy are uncommon in autoimmune hypothyroidism.

Physical findings

The main physical findings of overt hypothyroidism include changes of skin, face, hands, voice, thyroid and reflexes.

The epidermis is dry, rough, cool and covered with fine superficial scales, as a consequence of decreased cutaneous metabolism, reduced secretion of sweat and sebaceous glands, vasoconstriction and hyperkeratosis of the stratum corneum. Subcutaneous fat may be increased, particularly above the clavicles. The hands and feet show a broad appearance, due to thickening of subcutaneous tissue. The diffuse pallor and waxy surface are due to vasoconstriction, excess fluid and mucopolysaccharide accumulation in the dermis and to eventual co-existent anaemia. Yellowish discoloration of the skin is caused by elevation of carotene concentrations. The face is puffy, pale and expressionless at rest; sometimes it appears round or moon-like. The palpebral fissure may be narrowed. The tongue is usually large. The voice is husky, low-pitched and coarse, and speech is slow. The hair is sparse, dry, dull and coarse, grows slowly and falls out readily. Loss of scalp, genital and beard hair may occur. Hair may be lost from the temporal aspects of the eyebrows but this sign may be present in other diseases. In men, the beard becomes sparse. The nails are thickened, brittle and striated. The non-pitting swelling is due to an abnormal accumulation of salts, mucopolysaccharides and protein in the interstitial spaces of the skin, with the consequent increase of water-binding capacity. Capillary permeability is augmented in hypothyroidism.

Tendon reflexes are slow, especially during the relaxation time, as a consequence of a decrease in the rate of muscle contraction. Patients with hypothyroid myopathy may presents with firm, large, well-developed muscles, especially in the arms and legs. More commonly, physical examination of muscles is unimpressive.

Cardiovascular signs include low pulse rate, diastolic hypertension with narrowing of pulse pressure, cardiomegaly and peripheral non-pitting oedema. The heart sounds may be diminished in intensity, due to pericardial effusion. Ascites is unusual in hypothyroidism and can occur in association with pleural and pericardial effusion.

Laboratory tests

The serum levels of creatine phosphokinase, aspartate and alanine aminotransferases, and lactate dehydrogenase may be increased.

Hypothyroidism reduces the basal metabolic rate. Synthesis and particularly degradation of proteins are decreased with the result that nitrogen balance is usually slightly positive. Due to reduced insulin degradation, sensitivity to exogenous insulin is increased but hypoglycaemia is rare. A variety of abnormalities in plasma lipid concentrations occur: triglycerides, phospholipids and low-density lipoprotein (LDL) cholesterol are elevated.

Anaemia is a common finding of hypothyroidism. It is usually mild and may be normochromic and normocytic, as a consequence of decreased production of erythropoietin and depression of bone marrow. Macrocytosis is a consequence of deficiency of vitamin B12 and folate, a typical feature of pernicious anaemia, which is usually associated with chronic autoimmune thyroiditis. An additional cause of anaemia is iron deficiency, resulting from blood loss due to menorrhagia and poor iron absorption secondary to achlorhydria. The most frequent defects in haemostasis are prolonged bleeding time, decreased platelet adhesiveness and low plasma concentrations of factor VIII and von Willebrand factor. The clinical relevance of these abnormalities is usually limited.

As a consequence of a mild decrease of renal blood flow and glomerular filtration rate, a slight increase of serum creatinine and uric acid can be present. Occasionally, minimal proteinuria is reported. The total body sodium content is increased, but its serum concentrations tend to be low.

Instrumental changes

Electrocardiogram changes include sinus bradycardia, prolongation of the PR interval, low amplitude of the P wave and the QRS complex, alterations of the ST segment and flattened or inverted T waves, which are all suggestive of myocardial ischaemia. Complete heart block is uncommon. Ventricular premature beats and ventricular tachycardia may occur. These changes disappear with thyroid hormone treatment. Echocardiographic findings include a prolongation of the pre-ejection time and pericardial effusion, which is more common and severe in long-standing, severe hypothyroidism.

Electroencephalographic changes include slow α-wave activity and general loss of amplitude. Cognitive tests of patients with moderate to severe hypothyroidism indicate difficulties in performing calculations, recent memory loss, reduced attention span and slow reaction time. Electromyography abnormalities are not specific.

Particular conditions of hypothyroidism

Hypothyroidism during pregnancy

Severe hypothyroidism is associated with stillbirth and prematurity. Gestational hypertension is two to three times more common in hypothyroid women and can cause premature delivery with low birth weight. Thyroid hormones are essential for brain development. Indeed, euthyroid neonates born to mothers who were hypothyroid during pregnancy achieve a lower intelligence quotient later in life [22] whereas fetal death and congenital abnormalities are not increased in properly treated hypothyroid pregnant women [23].

Hypothyroidism in the elderly

The clinical features of hypothyroidism described in younger patients are often absent and several symptoms and signs, including fatigue, weakness, cold intolerance, dry skin, hair loss, constipation, poor appetite, depression and/or mental deterioration, hearing loss, cardiomegaly and congestive heart failure, may be confused with changes of 'normal' ageing [24]. Neurological manifestations (syncope, seizure, impaired cerebellar function, carpal tunnel syndrome) and arthritic complaints are common. Due to the cardiovascular involvement, dyspnoea and chest pain are common. As a consequence of reduced appetite, some older hypothyroid patients lose weight. Neuropsychiatric symptoms are common and depression may be the presenting symptom of hypothyroidism.

Subclinical hypothyroidism

Subclinical hypothyroidism, particularly in the presence of TSH levels >10 mIU/L, has been associated with neuromuscular symptoms, increased cholesterol levels and other lipid abnormalities, cardiac alterations and vascular impairment. Subclinical hypothyroidism has been reported to be an independent risk factor for atherosclerosis and myocardial infarction in postmenopausal women [25] and in men [26]. However, other authors have reported that subclinical hypothyroidism does not alter mortality rate [27].

A large epidemiological study has shown that the upper limit of serum TSH in a population living in an iodine-sufficient area and with no evidence of thyroid autoimmunity does not exceed 2.5 mIU/L [28]. Thus the suggestion has been made by some but not all authors to consider 2.5 mIU/L as the upper limit of the normal range of TSH. As mildly elevated TSH may normalize over time, it is generally recommend to confirm this finding by a second determination.

Myxoedema coma

Myxoedema coma, a rare but feared event, is more common in older subjects and represents the extreme of hypothyroidism. It generally occurs in the winter months and can be precipitated by non-thyroidal illness, drugs, exposure to cold and stress. Cold intolerance, constipation to paralytic ileus, progressive deterioration of mental status to stupor and coma are the typical symptoms. Localized neurological signs, marked hypotension, bradycardia, periorbital oedema and dry skin are the usual signs. Laboratory findings include hypercapnia, hypoglycaemia, hypoxaemia, hyponatraemia and elevated creatine phosphokinase. Cardiac enlargement is present at thoracic radiography, with bradycardia, low voltage and non-specific ST waves changes at ECG. Echocardiography shows decreased left ventricular contractility and cardiac workload. The mortality rate is very high, unless vigorous treatment with thyroid hormones and supportive measures is given immediately.

Diagnosis

In primary hypothyroidism, low concentrations of thyroid hormones (thyroxine (T4) and tri-iodothyronine (T3)) associated with high levels of serum TSH identify

clinical hypothyroidism, whereas subclinical hypothyroidism is characterized by an isolated rise of TSH levels.

The thyroid gland and the serum thyroid hormone bound to specific plasma proteins represent the reserve of thyroid hormones. The thyroid gland produces all serum T4 and only 20% of serum T3. The remaining 80% of T3 is produced by deiodination of T4 in non-thyroidal tissues. T4 represents a prohormone for the production of the more active T3 and about 99.96% of circulating T4 is bound to specific serum proteins. The bound fraction of T3 is lower (99.6%). Since the concentrations of total thyroid hormones (TT4 and TT3) are in the nanomolar range and those of free thyroid hormones (FT4 and FT3) in the picomolar range, methods for the determination of total thyroid hormones were developed before those for the determination of free thyroid hormones. However, because only the free fraction of the thyroid hormones enters the cells and therefore is active and because many physiological and pathological conditions affect the concentration of TBG, measurement of the free fractions is actually the golden standard for measurement of thyroid hormones. It must be taken into account that the assays now available for determination of FT4 and FT3 are still characterized by some relevant flaws.

Thyroid-stimulating hormone is the most sensitive test of thyroid hormone action and its increase is correlated logarithmically with the decrease of T4. Non-radioactive immunometric assays (IMAs) for determination of TSH levels are able to identify the increase of TSH levels typical of hypothyroidism. Therefore measurement of TSH is the first-line test for the diagnosis of hypothyroidism. However, in conditions that modify the correlation between thyroid hormones and TSH (pituitary diseases, drugs and other conditions interfering with thyroid function and the syndrome of resistance to thyroid hormones), the sole determination of TSH can be misleading.

Serum FT4 is below the normal range in clinical hypothyroidism, and normal or close to the lower limit of normal range in subclinical hypothyroidism. In hypothyroidism, measurement of FT3 is less useful because FT3 can be normal even in presence of low levels of FT4. In addition, FT3 can be reduced in patients with non-thyroidal illness (NTI) (also known as 'low T3 syndrome').

Positive serum thyroid autoantibodies (TPOAb and thyroglobulin autoantibodies (TgAb)) and a hypoechogenic pattern on thyroid ultrasound are typical of autoimmune hypothyroidism [29].

TREATMENT

Treatment of surgical hypothyroidism

Replacement treatment is required in all patients after total thyroidectomy. In these patients LT4 at fully replacement doses must be started immediately after surgery.

Treatment of patients after partial thyroidectomy is less straightforward. In the presence of both clinical and subclinical hypothyroidism after partial thyroidectomy for Graves' disease or multinodular goitre, it is recommended to initiate replacement therapy at lower doses. Careful monitoring of thyroid function is required in these patients.

Treatment with thyroxine

Since it became available, synthetic levothyroxine has gradually replaced animal thyroid extracts for the treatment of hypothyroidism. The full replacement dose of LT4 is 6–15 µg/kg/day for infants, 5–6 µg/kg/day for children 1–5 years old, 4–5 µg/kg/day for children 6–12 years old, 1–3 µg/kg/day for adolescents, 1.6–1.8 µg/kg/day for young adults and 1.2–1.4 µg/kg/day for older adults (Table 32.1). The dose required is higher (approximately 2.0–2.2 µg/kg/day for young adults) when suppression must be attained, as in the postsurgical follow-up of patients with differentiated thyroid carcinoma. The dose decreases with age, paralleling the age-dependent reduction of lean body mass, which is its main determinant [30]. Women starting oral oestrogen replacement therapy may need to increase LT4 dose [31]. The replacement dose can augment because of treatment with drugs that increase LT4 metabolism or with drugs and dietary supplements that reduce LT4 absorption. Impaired acid secretion [32] and small bowel disease that induce malabsorption

have similar effects. Differences in LT4 preparation can also modify the required dose.

During infancy, rapid restoration of euthyroidism is essential. A full replacement dose of 37.5–50 µg/day should be given as starting dose. In children and adolescents the starting dose should be 25 µg/day and 50 µg/day, respectively. The dose should be increased by 25 µg increments at 4–8-week intervals until a normal circulating TSH level is obtained. Starting daily dose of LT4 in patients under 40 years should be 50–75 µg, with a reassessment of TSH and FT4 levels in 2–3 months. In patients over 40 years, the starting daily dose should be 25–50 µg, with increments of 25 µg every 3–4 weeks. In elderly patients, particularly with known or suspected coronary heart disease, the initial dose of LT4 should be very small (even 12.5–25 µg/day) and should be increased by 12.5–25 µg every 4–6 weeks, in order to reach the replacement dose in 3–4 months. In the presence of subclinical hypothyroidism, the required dose is lower and the treatment can be initiated at a lower level.

Thyroid hormone treatment aims to restore euthyroidism without inducing thyrotoxicosis. Normalization of circulating FT4 and TSH should be achieved, with a target range for TSH of 0.5–2.0 mIU/L. Low TSH levels should be avoided, particularly in older patients, in whom they are associated with increased risk of atrial fibrillation [33] and with hip and vertebral fractures in women [34]. After restoration of euthyroidism with LT4 treatment, patients should be followed up at intervals of 6–24 months, with careful monitoring of FT4 and TSH values.

Association of tri-iodothyronine with thyroxine

Current guidelines recommend LT4 monotherapy for the treatment of hypothyroidism since T4 is converted to its biologically active form, T3, in peripheral tissues. Oral LT4 administration ensures that T3 serum concentrations remain constant and avoids the non-physiological T3 surge and short effect that follow liothyronine (LT3) ingestion. These are the main considerations that provide the rationale for the preference of LT4 monotherapy over the combined treatment with LT4 and LT3.

However, the question is still open to debate and some considerations should be taken into account [35]. First, at least 20% of circulating T3 in normal individuals is secreted by the thyroid. Second, in some LT4-treated patients, normal serum TSH values can be obtained only

Table 32.1 Treatment of hypothyroidism.

	Dose (µg/kg/day)	Starting dose (µg/day)
Infants	6–15	25–50
Children (1–5 years)	5–6	25
Children (6–12 years)	4–5	25
Adolescents	1–3	50
Adults <40 years	1.6–1.8	50–75
Adults >40 years	1.6–1.8	25–50
Older adults	1.2–1.4	12.5–25

by maintaining elevated free T4/T3 serum ratio and serum FT4 values close to the upper limit of its normal range or frankly elevated. This condition probably results in thyrotoxicosis in some organs. Finally, incomplete recovery has been reported by some hypothyroid patients treated with LT4, despite normal hormonal profiles and lack of signs of thyroid hormone deficiency. On these grounds, combined treatment would seem logical. It was proposed in the 1970s, but quickly abandoned because of the adverse effects, which were mainly induced by the excessive doses of LT4 and LT3 used.

More recently, combined treatment has been reported to be more effective than LT4 alone for the control of psychiatric symptoms of hypothyroidism [36]. Other authors have failed to demonstrate such a benefit. Partial substitution of LT4 with LT3 in the treatment of hypothyroid patients might improve their perception of well-being and indeed, some recent studies reported that patients preferred combined treatment to monotherapy. This could be caused by an overcompensation of thyroid hormone deficiency in the tissues, resulting from a transient surge of serum T3 after oral administration of LT3. Thus a pharmacological effect of supraphysiological active hormone concentrations in tissues, rather than the optimization of the thyroid status, could be responsible for this result [35]. In addition, adverse cardiac and skeletal side-effects might result from mild thyrotoxicosis if treatment were prolonged.

In conclusion, current evidence indicates that combined treatment should not be recommended as a treatment of choice for hypothyroid patients until safety has been definitively proven.

Treatment of myxoedema coma

For treatment of myxoedema coma, an intravenous bolus of 500 μg of LT4, followed by a daily maintenance dose of 50–100 μg, is required. Before starting LT4 treatment, co-existent adrenal insufficiency must be ruled out and treated when present. In addition, hypoglycaemia and hyponatraemia need adequate treatment.

Treatment in pregnancy

Correct treatment during pregnancy is required to avoid the consequence of fetal hypothyroidism. In hypothyroid women of child-bearing age who are planning pregnancy, LT4 treatment should be adjusted in order to maintain a TSH value <2.5 mIU/L. The need for additional LT4

replacement therapy during pregnancy has been clearly established. The increment of dosage depends upon the aetiology. Seventy-six percent of women taking LT4 as replacement therapy for clinical hypothyroidism following surgery or ^{131}I therapy need to increase their dose, the mean increment of LT4 dosage being 52 μg/day. Conversely, only 30% of women who are taking LT4 as replacement therapy for subclinical hypothyroidism following surgery or ^{131}I therapy need to increase their dose [37]. The required daily dosage in overt hypothyroidism first diagnosed during pregnancy is usually 1.8–2.0 μg/kg/day. In all hypothyroid pregnant women treated with LT4, serum TSH levels should be monitored every 6–8 weeks and more frequently after a dosage change. However, in pregnancy, serum TSH falls, as a consequence of human chorionic gonadotrophin (HCG) secretion. The upper limit of normal values of TSH is reported to be 2.5 mIU/L in the first trimester and 3.0 mIU/L in the second and third trimesters of pregnancy [38].

During the first trimester of pregnancy, maternal FT4 surges and this increase is probably crucial for fetal neurodevelopment [39]. Therefore, substitutive treatment should be adjusted in order to maintain FT4 close to its upper normal limit, particularly during the first trimester of pregnancy. After delivery, the required dose usually returns to pregestational levels, particularly in surgical hypothyroidism.

Treatment of subclinical hypothyroidism

While the need for treatment of clinical hypothyroidism is unanimously accepted, that of subclinical hypothyroidism is under discussion. Based on the consideration that large randomized control trials showing benefit of treatment are lacking, a consensus panel has recommended against treatment of patients with subclinical hypothyroidism with serum TSH levels of 4.5–10 mIU/L [40]. These conclusions were challenged in a consensus statement from the American Association of Clinical Endocrinologists (AACE), the American Thyroid Association (ATA) and the Endocrine Society (TES), which considered that these recommendations were based on 'the lack of evidence for benefit rather than on evidence for a lack of benefit' [41].

There are indeed a number of observations that favour the opportunity to actively treat subclinical hypothyroidism. Serum TSH values are directly correlated with total and LDL cholesterol levels [42] and serum TSH determination is recommended when circulating cholesterol is elevated [43]. Effectiveness of treatment of subclinical hypothyroidism in normalizing total and/or LDL cholesterol levels and other lipid abnormalities has been reported in many, though not all studies. Similar results have been reported for other abnormalities associated with subclinical hypothyroidism, namely non-specific symptoms, cardiovascular dysfunctions and vascular impairments. Although still debated, based on clinical judgement, it would appear that treatment of subclinical hypothyroidism should be supported, or at least not discouraged [41,44].

References

1 Falk SA. Metabolic complications of thyroid surgery: hypocalcemia and hypoparathyroidism; hypocalcitoninemia; and hypothyroidism and hyperthyroidism. In: Falk SA (ed) Thyroid Disease; Endocrinology, Surgery, Nuclear Medicine, and Radiotherapy. Philadelphia: Lippincott-Raven, 1997: 717–38.

2 Toft AD, Irvine WJ, Sinclair I, McIntosh D, Seth J, Cameron EH. Thyroid function after surgical treatment of thyrotoxicosis. A report of 100 cases treated with propranolol before operation. N Engl J Med 1978; 298(12): 643–7.

3 Cusick EL, Krukowski ZH, Matheson NA. Outcome of surgery for Graves' disease re-examined. Br J Surg 1987; 74(9): 780–3.

4 Barsano CP. Other forms of primary hypothyroidism. In: Braverman LE, Utiger RD (eds) Werner & Ingbar's The Thyroid: A Fundamental and Clinical Text. Philadelphia: Lippincott-Raven, 1996: 768–78.

5 Miccoli P, Vitti P, Rago T, et al. Surgical treatment of Graves' disease: subtotal or total thyroidectomy? Surgery 1996; 120(6): 1020–4.

6 Kuma K, Matsuzuka F, Kobayashi A, et al. Natural course of Graves' disease after subtotal thyroidectomy and management of patients with postoperative thyroid dysfunction. Am J Med Sci 1991; 302(1): 8–12.

7 Matte R, Ste-Marie LG, Comtois R, et al. The pituitary-thyroid axis after hemithyroidectomy in euthyroid man. J Clin Endocrinol Metab 1981; 53(2): 377–80.

8 O'Brien T, Gharib H, Suman VJ, van Heerden JA. Treatment of toxic solitary thyroid nodules: surgery versus radioactive iodine. Surgery 1992; 112(6): 1166–70.

9 Bransom CJ, Talbot CH, Henry L, Elemenoglou J. Solitary toxic adenoma of the thyroid gland. Br J Surg 1979; 66(8): 592–5.

10 Sridama V, McCormick M, Kaplan EL, Fauchet R, DeGroot LJ. Long-term follow-up study of compensated low-dose 131I therapy for Graves' disease. N Engl J Med 1984; 311(7): 426–32.

11 Bertelsen J, Herskind AM, Sprogoe JU, Hegedus L. Is standard 555 MBq 131I-therapy of hyperthyroidism ablative? Thyroidology 1992; 4(3): 103–6.

12 Huysmans DA, Hermus AR, Corstens FH, Kloppenborg PW. Long-term results of two schedules of radioiodine treatment for toxic multinodular goitre. Eur J Nucl Med 1993; 20(11): 1056–62.

13 Nygaard B, Hegedus L, Gervil M, Hjalgrim H, Soe-Jensen P, Hansen JM. Radioiodine treatment of multinodular non-toxic goitre. BMJ 1993; 307(6908): 828–32.

14 Verelst J, Bonnyns M, Glinoer D. Radioiodine therapy in voluminous multinodular non-toxic goitre. Acta Endocrinol (Copenh) 1990; 122(4): 417–21.

15 Hancock SL, Cox RS, McDougall IR. Thyroid diseases after treatment of Hodgkin's disease. N Engl J Med 1991; 325(9): 599–605.

16 Shafer RB, Nuttall FQ, Pollak K, Kuisk H. Thyroid function after radiation and surgery for head and neck cancer. Arch Intern Med 1975; 135(6): 843–6.

17 Locatelli F, Giorgiani G, Pession A, Bozzola M. Late effects in children after bone marrow transplantation: a review. Haematologica 1993; 78(5): 319–28.

18 Martino E, Bartalena L, Bogazzi F, Braverman LE. The effects of amiodarone on the thyroid. Endocr Rev 2001; 22(2): 240–54.

19 Ward DL, Bing-You RG. Autoimmune thyroid dysfunction induced by interferon-alpha treatment for chronic hepatitis C: screening and monitoring recommendations. Endocr Pract 2001; 7(1): 52–8.

20 Marazuela M, Garcia-Buey L, Gonzalez-Fernandez B, et al. Thyroid autoimmune disorders in patients with chronic hepatitis C before and during interferon-alpha therapy. Clin Endocrinol (Oxf) 1996; 44(6): 635–42.

21 Desai J, Yassa L, Marqusee E, et al. Hypothyroidism after sunitinib treatment for patients with gastrointestinal stromal tumors. Ann Intern Med 2006; 145(9): 660–4.

22 Haddow JE, Palomaki GE, Allan WC, et al. Maternal thyroid deficiency during pregnancy and subsequent neuropsychological development of the child. N Engl J Med 1999; 341(8): 549–55.

23 Burrow GN, Fisher DA, Larsen PR. Maternal and fetal thyroid function. N Engl J Med 1994; 331(16): 1072–8.

24 Latrofa F, Pinchera A. Aging and the thyroid. Available at: www.hotthyroidology com.

25 Hak AE, Pols HA, Visser TJ, Drexhage HA, Hofman A, Witteman JC. Subclinical hypothyroidism is an independent risk factor for atherosclerosis and myocardial infarction in

elderly women: the Rotterdam Study. Ann Intern Med 2000; 132(4): 270–8.

26 Imaizumi M, Akahoshi M, Ichimaru S, *et al*. Risk for ischemic heart disease and all-cause mortality in subclinical hypothyroidism. J Clin Endocrinol Metab 2004; 89(7): 3365–70.

27 Parle JV, Maisonneuve P, Sheppard MC, Boyle P, Franklyn JA. Prediction of all-cause and cardiovascular mortality in elderly people from one low serum thyrotropin result: a 10-year cohort study. Lancet 2001; 358(9285): 861–5.

28 Hollowell JG, Staehling NW, Flanders WD, *et al*. Serum TSH, T(4), and thyroid antibodies in the United States population (1988 to 1994): National Health and Nutrition Examination Survey (NHANES III). J Clin Endocrinol Metab 2002; 87(2): 489–99.

29 Latrofa F, Pinchera A. Autoimmune hypothyroidism. In: Weetman AP (ed) Autoimmune Diseases in Endocrinology. Totowa, NJ: Humana Press, 2008: 136–74.

30 Santini F, Pinchera A, Marsili A, *et al*. Lean body mass is a major determinant of levothyroxine dosage in the treatment of thyroid diseases. J Clin Endocrinol Metab 2005; 90(1): 124–7.

31 Arafah BM. Increased need for thyroxine in women with hypothyroidism during estrogen therapy. N Engl J Med 2001; 344(23): 1743–9.

32 Centanni M, Gargano L, Canettieri G, *et al*. Thyroxine in goiter, Helicobacter pylori infection, and chronic gastritis. N Engl J Med 2006; 354(17): 1787–95.

33 Sawin CT, Geller A, Wolf PA, *et al*. Low serum thyrotropin concentrations as a risk factor for atrial fibrillation in older persons. N Engl J Med 1994; 331(19): 1249–52.

34 Bauer DC, Ettinger B, Nevitt MC, Stone KL. Risk for fracture in women with low serum levels of thyroid-stimulating hormone. Ann Intern Med 2001; 134(7): 561–8.

35 Pinchera A, Santini F. Is combined therapy with levothyroxine and liothyronine effective in patients with primary hypothyroidism? Nature Clin Pract Endocrinol Metab 2005; 1(1): 19.

36 Bunevicius R, Kazanavicius G, Zalinkevicius R, Prange AJ. Effects of thyroxine as compared with thyroxine plus triiodothyronine in patients with hypothyroidism. N Engl J Med 1999; 340(6): 424–9.

37 Mandel SJ. Hypothyroidism and chronic autoimmune thyroiditis in the pregnant state: maternal aspects. Best Pract Res Clin Endocrinol Metab 2004; 18(2): 213–24.

38 Glinoer D, Spencer CA. Serum TSH determinations in pregnancy: how, when and why? Nat Rev Endocrinol 2010; 6(9): 526–9.

39 Escobar G, Obregon MJ, Rey F. Maternal thyroid hormones early in pregnancy and fetal brain development. Best Pract Res Clin Endocrinol Metab 2004; 18(2): 225–48.

40 Surks MI, Ortiz E, Daniels GH, *et al*. Subclinical thyroid disease: scientific review and guidelines for diagnosis and management. JAMA 2004; 291(2): 228–38.

41 Gharib H, Tuttle RM, Baskin HJ, Fish LH, Singer PA, McDermott MT. Subclinical thyroid dysfunction: a joint statement on management from the American Association of Clinical Endocrinologists, the American Thyroid Association, and the Endocrine Society. J Clin Endocrinol Metab 2005; 90(1): 581–5.

42 Canaris GJ, Manowitz NR, Mayor G, Ridgway EC. The Colorado thyroid disease prevalence study. Arch Intern Med 2000; 160(4): 526–34.

43 Expert Panel on Detection, Evaluation, and Treatment of High Blood Cholesterol in Adults. Executive Summary of the Third Report of the National Cholesterol Education Program (NCEP) Expert Panel on Detection, Evaluation, and Treatment of High Blood Cholesterol in Adults (Adult Treatment Panel III). JAMA 2001; 285(19): 2486–97.

44 Pinchera A. Subclinical thyroid disease: to treat or not to treat? Thyroid 2005; 15(1): 1–2.

CHAPTER 33

Quality of Life after Thyroid Surgery

Alessandro Antonelli and Poupak Fallahi

Department of Internal Medicine, University of Pisa – School of Medicine, Pisa, Italy

Introduction

Patients affected with thyroid diseases, independently of hormonal status, also display significant impairment in health-related quality of life (HRQOL) when compared to the general population [1–6]. In fact, about one half of patients affected with thyroid diseases are limited in daily activities and report having social and emotional problems. The reasons for the quality of life (QOL) impairment in patients with thyroid disorders remain to be clarified. Since thyroid diseases may require drug treatment, surgery or radioiodine, exact knowledge of the impact of each treatment modality on the QOL of patients is important [7].

The QOL is defined as the perceptions of an individual regarding his or her position in life in the context of the culture and value systems in which he or she lives and in relation to his or her goals, expectations, standards and concerns [8]. HRQOL refers to a multidimensional concept that encompasses perception of negative and positive aspects of physical, emotional, social and cognitive functions, which could be affected by the disease or its treatment [8].

Patients with untreated thyroid disease suffer from a wide range of symptoms and have major impairment in most areas of HRQOL. For example, 22–35% of goitre patients, 18–66% of hyperthyroid patients,

7–99% of patients with thyroid-associated ophthalmopathy and 16–51% of hypothyroid patients experience limitations in usual activities during the untreated phase of their disease, and perceive their general health as impaired and have social and emotional impairment. Cognitive problems are also prevalent, as it is fatigue [7].

All the classic symptoms of hyperthyroidism appear to be consistently prevalent in hyperthyroid patients, whereas the classic symptoms of hypothyroidism are more variably present in hypothyroid patients. Persistent HRQOL impairment is very frequent among patients with both hyper- and hypothyroidism. Two-thirds are fatigued and about one-third are anxious and have cognitive as well as sexual problems. However, the association with actual thyroid status has not been addressed. According to the available literature, HRQOL impairment in patients with benign thyroid disorders is prevalent, both in the untreated phase and in the long term [7].

Few studies have investigated the QOL in patients udergoing thyroidectomy for different thyroid pathologies. In this paper we review the above-mentioned studies. Since the impact on QOL is obviously different in patients treated with thyroidectomy for thyroid cancer than in those affected by benign thyroid pathologies, we will treat these arguments separately.

Thyroid Surgery: Preventing and Managing Complications, First Edition. Edited by Paolo Miccoli, David J. Terris, Michele N. Minuto and Melanie W. Seybt.

Quality of life in patients treated with thyroidectomy for benign thyroid diseases

The report by Miccoli *et al.* first prospectively studied the impact of surgical treatment alone on QOL and psychiatric symptoms. The aim of this study was to investigate the course of both HRQOL and psychiatric symptoms in patients affected with thyroid diseases with surgical indication before and after thyroidectomy [9]. Forty-seven patients undergoing thyroid surgery (TS) were assessed before thyroidectomy (T0) and 37 also after surgery, ≥ 6 months after euthyroidism was achieved (T1): QOL and psychiatric symptoms were evaluated. Indications for TS were thyroid benign disorders in 39 patients, while only eight patients had differentiated thyroid cancer (DTC). QOL scores at T0 were compared with those of patients undergoing surgery for nonthyroidal disease and the Short Form 36 Health Survey (SF-36) scores were also compared with the normative Italian sample. HRQOL in TS patients before surgery was poorer than in the comparison group on the SF-36 mental component summary measure and social functioning. Mental health improved significantly after surgery but social functioning remained markedly impaired. A significant reduction in the severity of psychiatric symptoms was observed. These results indicate that even long after euthyroidism is achieved after surgery, patients show a significant improvement of mental health and a reduction of psychiatric symptoms. Nevertheless, patients continue to have a poorer QOL compared to the Italian normative sample [9].

Interestingly, it has been hypothesized that higher antithyroperoxidase antibody (AbTPO) levels would be associated with an increased symptom load and a decreased QOL in female euthyroid patients. This hypothesis has been evaluated in a prospective cohort study of 426 consecutive euthyroid female patients undergoing TS for benign thyroid disease [10]. Histology revealed Hashimoto's thyroiditis (HT) in 28/426 (6.6%) subjects, 47 patients with AbTPO > 121.0 IU/mL. The mean number of reported symptoms was significantly higher in patients with AbTPO levels > 121.0 IU/mL than in the other group. There were no differences in preoperative thyroid-stimulating hormone (TSH). Chronic fatigue, dry hair, chronic irritability, chronic nervousness, a history of breast cancer and early miscarriage, and lower QOL levels were significantly associated with AbTPO levels exceeding the cut-off point. The authors conclude that women with HT suffer from a high symptom load, and that hypothyroidism is only a contributing factor to the development of associated conditions [10].

The effects of treatments in Graves' disease (GD) patients were evaluated in a 14–21-year follow-up of 179 patients after randomized treatment with surgical, medical or radioiodine therapy. The authors found no difference among treatments; however, the HRQOL for Graves' patients was lower compared with a large age- and sex-matched Swedish reference population [11].

To evaluate whether QOL was related to the thyroid hormone status, 91 GD patients were studied. HRQOL does not seem to be influenced by the thyroid hormone levels of the patients, including subclinical thyrotoxicosis. The authors suggest that the personality of GD patients may be associated with both the initial appearence and development of GD, such as with lower HRQOL scores later on in life [12].

Quality of life in patients treated with thyroidectomy for thyroid cancer

Traditionally, the main outcome measure in oncology patients has been survival on tumour control, but recently it has been increasingly recognized that the diagnosis and management of cancer can have a major effect on every aspect of the QOL of patients [13]. The aims of cancer treatment became not only to increase survival but also to preserve QOL, and measuring these changes has been considered to be of paramount importance [13].

Patients with DTC, in general, have a very good prognosis, and overall long-term survival is higher than 90%, with variations in subsets of patients [13,14]. In DTC, surgery is the therapy of choice. Surgical options include lobectomy with isthmectomy or total thyroidectomy (TT) with or without neck lymph node dissection. The choice of procedure is affected by well-defined prognostic factors [15,16]. Ablative surgery of the thyroid and possible neck disease and postoperative radioactive iodine therapy (RIT) result in prolonged survival but may lead to voice alterations, dysphagia, sialadenitis, taste disturbance and xerostomia [17–19].

When thyroid cancers are 'cured' it is often assumed that the patients are able to resume their normal lives. However, this point is actually under debate. In a recent study, 150 consecutive patients with DTC (who had a history of TT followed by radioiodine ablation), free of metastatic disease and under levothyroxine treatment were evaluated for QOL [20]. Findings indicate that 'Vitality', 'Role – physical', 'Mental Health', 'Role – emotional' and 'Social functioning' were significantly impaired during the first year after diagnosis. Thereafter, QOL improves, correlating with the time since initial diagnosis. However, 'Vitality' and 'Role – emotional' remain permanently impaired in thyroid cancer patients [20].

Huang et al. studied 146 Chinese adult patients who had a thyroidectomy for cancer, by telephone interviews asking about sociodemographic variables, disease/treatment characteristics and social support [14]. QOL was measured by the Chinese version of the QOL Index. The regression model showed that patients at 19–36 months after operation had lower QOL compared with those within 18 months of operation. Current symptoms of fatigue and chills were negatively associated with QOL. Those who rated the impact of operational scar on activities as 'high' had lower QOL scores. Social support from families and friends had positive effects on QOL. The authors suggest that surgeons should consider types of operation in which the scar would be less likely to influence the patients' activities [14].

Tan et al. evaluated 152 DTC patients, who answered a self-administered questionnaire containing the SF-36 and assessing sociodemographic, disease and treatment-related status [13]. There was a statistically significant decrease in SF-36 scores between thyroid cancer survivors and the general population in all domains except for social functioning. Physical functioning was worse in those survivors who were aged 50 years or older. Mental health scores were better in those who had more than 12 years of formal education. Being employed had a positive influence on 'Role – physical' and 'Role – emotional' scores. The authors conclude that, even if most DTC survivors have near normal life expectancy, there is a significant decrease in their QOL, especially in the elderly and poorer educated. Returning to work should be encouraged to improve the QOL in DTC survivors [13].

Voice alterations after thyroidectomy can be found even with preserved function of laryngeal nerves. De

Pedro Netto et al. conducted a prospective non-randomized study of 100 patients who underwent TS and compared the results with a control group of 30 patients who underwent breast surgery [18]. Postoperative videolaryngoscopy showed larynx alterations in 28% of the thyroidectomized patients, without significant alterations in the control group. There were subjective voice changes in 29.7% of the patients without vocal fold immobility after TS and no statistically significant changes after breast surgery. Acoustic analysis showed significantly increased values in the voice turbulence index parameter in both groups, although it was higher in the thyroid group. In the voice handicap index assessment, voice complaints were more frequently registered in the thyroid group than in the control group. In summary, voice alterations were frequently observed after thyroidectomy even with preserved vocal fold mobility [18].

Swallowing alterations following TT, in the absence of recurrent nerve injury, were evaluated in 39 patients aged 21–65 years by Lombardi et al [19]. Preoperative and postoperative acoustic voice analysis and maximum phonation time scores did not differ significantly. The mean postoperative voice impairment scores were significantly higher than the preoperative score at 1 week and 1 month after TT but not 3 months after TT. The mean and swallowing impairment scores (SIS) were higher than the preoperative SIS at 1 week, 1 month and 3 months after TT. This study shows that transient voice and swallowing symptoms may occur following TT, and that mild symptoms may occur in the majority of operated patients [19].

Almeida et al. studied 154 patients submitted to thyroidectomy (1997–2006) who were evaluated using the University of Washington QOL questionnaire [21]. Patients 45 years or younger had better recreation scores than did patients older than 45 years. Thirty-eight patients were submitted to neck dissection. Patients submitted to modified radical neck dissection reported worse chewing and shoulder scores than did patients submitted to selective paratracheal lymph node dissection only and those without neck dissection. Patients who received more than 150 mCi of RIT reported significantly worse pain, swallowing, chewing, speech, taste, anxiety and composite scores. Co-morbidities showed significant effect on recreation, activity, speech, saliva and composite scores. In multivariate analysis, RIT is the only variable associated with a worse composite score. The authors conclude that, although QOL after treatment of thyroid cancer can be considered good for most patients, those submitted to RIT at doses higher than 150 mCi are at risk for poor QOL and, therefore, may need more intensive follow-up and treatment [21].

Damage to salivary gland function following external irradiation has been documented. In a first study, Malpani *et al.* showed that RIT produces a significant effect on salivary gland function that is dose related and becomes evident over a period of several months after treatment [22]. The role of raioiodine in determining salivary gland dysfunction has subsequently been confirmed in other studies [23–25]. In a recent study to evaluate side-effects of radioiodine therapy on salivary gland function, 182 patients were evaluated [26]. RIT had a strong association with decreased elimination counts by salivary gland scintigraphy. Patient age was the only variable associated with sialometry; age and the use of xerostomic drugs were strongly associated with decreased mean values of salivary flow. Dysphagia was strongly associated with RIT. These results show that patients subjected to RIT have more difficulty in draining saliva, mainly from the parotid glands, which is associated with clinical dysphagia in this subset of patients [26].

The psychological performance and QOL in patients with DTC, either during treatment with chronic suppressive doses of levothyroxine or during the withdrawal of levothyroxine needed to perform whole-body scanning with radioactive iodine, in comparison with those of appropriate healthy controls, were studied by Botella-Carretero *et al.* [27]. Eighteen women with DTC and 18 euthyroid age-matched healthy women were recruited. Patients were studied the day before levothyroxine withdrawal (when in chronic mild or subclinical hyperthyroidism), 4–7 days later (when most patients had normal serum free thyroxine (FT4) and free tri-iodothyronine (FT3) levels), and the day before scanning (when in profound hypothyroidism). In comparison with controls, patients showed impairment of several indexes during chronic suppressive levothyroxine therapy (total score, emotional, sleep, energy, mental health, general health and social scores). Also, QOL indexes, cognitive tests, and affective and physical symptoms visual mental scales worsened during profound hypothyroidism. QOL and cognitive performance were almost comparable with those of euthyroid controls when most patients had normal FT4 and FT3 levels. The authors conclude that QOL and psychometric functionality in patients with DTC are affected not only by withdrawal of levothyroxine but also by long-term treatment with supraphysiological doses of levothyroxine.

The HRQOL in patients with DTC with T_4 withdrawal in preparation for whole-body radioactive iodine scanning was also studied in a Chinese population by Chow *et al.* [28]. Seventy-eight patients with DTC completed the Functional Assessment of Cancer Treatment-General (FACT-G) questionnaire on weeks 0, 2 and 4 after T4 withdrawal with corresponding checking of serum TSH. Comparing FACT-G scores at weeks 0 and 4, 'physical', 'social' and 'emotional' aspects were lowered as well as 'total' HRQOL. Total HRQOL was affected early (in the first 2 weeks) in T4 withdrawal. The authors conclude that HRQOL declines with time of T4 withdrawal, and that the impact is more severe in the later period of T4 withdrawal [28].

To examine the relationship between optimism-pessimism and QOL in survivors of head and neck and thyroid cancers, Kung *et al.* evaluated 190 patients who completed the Minnesota Multiphasic Personality Inventory, used to assess explanatory style (optimism-pessimism) and to assess QOL [29]. For all 190 patients, optimism was associated with a higher QOL on both the mental and physical component scales. For patients with thyroid cancer, optimism was associated with higher QOL on both component scales and six subscales. Optimism was associated with a higher QOL in survivors of thyroid cancer and with the mental rather than physical QOL subscales.

The relationships among physical complaints, HRQOL, anxiety and depression were examined by Tagay *et al.* in 136 DTC patients under short-term hypothyroidism (on thyroid hormone withdrawal) for radioiodine administration [30]. Compared to the German general population, hypothyroid patients had significantly impaired HRQOL. Surprisingly, the prevalence of anxiety (62.5%) but not depression (17.9%) was much higher in hypothyroid DTC patients than in the general population. In multivariate analysis, depression and age were independently associated with the physical health score, but only psychological variables (depression, mood disturbance and anxiety) were associated with the mental health score. The authors conclude that HRQOL is severely impaired in DTC patients under short-term hypothyroidism. As potential predictors of generic HRQOL impairment, depression, anxiety and mood disturbance could be used to preselect the patients most needing psychiatric care.

In another study to assess the determinants of medium-term QOL after the initial therapy, 88 thyroid cancer patients received either recombinant human TSH or hypothyroid-assisted radioiodine ablation [31]. The results show that the use of radioiodine ablation does not seem to affect the medium-term QOL scores of patients. Medium-term QOL is mainly determined by preablation QOL. The authors conclude that assessment of baseline QOL might be interesting to evaluate in order to adapt the treatment protocols, preventive strategies and medical information to patients for potentially improving their outcomes [31].

Conclusion and perspective

Quality of life is impaired in patients affected by thyroid disorders. A number of different parameters may influence QOL in these patients, such as hypothyroidism, hyperthyroidism, the presence of thyroid autoimmunity, the presence of thyroid cancer, and the specific treatments for each disease. TS may influence voice change in patients without laryngeal nerve dysfunction. Radioiodine therapy in DTC patients is associated with dysfunction of salivary glands and swallowing.

In summary, the QOL of thyroid patients is substantially impaired over a wide range of aspects of HRQOL in the untreated phase and continues to be so in many patients in the long term. Studies systematically exploring the relative importance of these various aspects to thyroid patients are lacking, as is a comprehensive, validated thyroid-specific HRQOL questionnaire: further studies are needed [7].

A crucial aspect of QOL in patients experiencing thyroidectomy is an adequate substitution of thyroid function by thyroid hormone supplementation. However, when levothyroxine supplementation produces normal circulating values of FT4, FT3 and TSH, the physiology of thyroid metabolism is not reproduced. In fact, thyroid hormone production is regulated via pituitary thyrotropin modulation of T4 prohormone secretion by the thyroid gland, and regulation of active T3 production in peripheral tissues via metabolic events influencing activities of the iodothyronine monodeiodinase enzyme systems. Control at both levels is modified in serious non-thyroidal illness (trauma, infection, cancer, metabolic diseases, etc.), such by various types of drugs (β-blockers, amiodarone, etc.). There is a circadian rhythm of TSH secretion, with peak values at the onset of sleep and nadir concentrations during the afternoon hours. Peak and nadir concentrations differ by approximately +/− 50%. The effect on circulating T4 and T3 concentrations is slight because of the large size of the extrathyroidal T4 pool. Nutrition also has a minimal impact, except for variation in iodine intake [32]. This complex system that regulates thyroid metabolism is obviously altered during thyroid hormone substitution. Theoretically, thyroid transplantation could reproduce the normal physiology of thyroid metabolism, as previously hypothesized by Ferrini & Cremonesi [33]. Further studies will be necessary to explore this appealing hypothesis.

References

1 Gulseren S, Gulseren L, Hekimsoy Z, *et al*. Depression, anxiety, health-related quality of life, and disability in patients with overt and subclinical thyroid dysfunction. Arch Med Res 2006; 37: 133–9.

2 Giusti M, Sibilla F, Cappi C, *et al*. A case-controlled study on the quality of life in a cohort of patients with history of differentiated thyroid carcinoma. J Endocrinol Invest 2005; 28: 599–608.

3 Eustatia-Rutten CF, Corssmit EP, Pereira AM, *et al*. Quality of life in long-term exogenous subclinical hyperthyroidism and the effects of restoration of euthyroidism, a randomized controlled trial. Clin Endocrinol (Oxf) 2006; 64: 284–91.

4 Biondi B, Palmieri EA, Fazio S, *et al*. Endogenous subclinical hyperthyroidism affects quality of life and cardiac morphology and function in young and middle-aged patients. J Clin Endocrinol Metab 2000; 85: 4701–5.

5 Sgarbi JA, Villaça FG, Garbeline B, *et al*. The effects of early antithyroid therapy for endogenous subclinical hyperthyroidism in clinical and heart abnormalities. J Clin Endocrinol Metab 2003; 88: 1672–7.

6 Biondi B, Fazio S, Carella C, *et al*. Control of adrenergic overactivity by beta-blockade improves the quality of life in patients receiving long term suppressive therapy with levothyroxine. J Clin Endocrinol Metab 1994; 78: 1028–33.

7 Watt T, Groenvold M, Rasmussen AK, *et al*. Quality of life in patients with benign thyroid disorders. A review. Eur J Endocrinol 2006; 154: 501–10.

8 World Health Organization Quality of Life (WHOQOL) Group. Study protocol for the World Health Organization

project to develop a Quality of Life assessment instrument (WHOQOL). Qual Life Res 1993; 2: 153–9.

9 Miccoli P, Minuto MN, Paggini R, *et al.* The impact of thyroidectomy on psychiatric symptoms and quality of life. J Endocrinol Invest 2007; 30: 853–9.

10 Ott J, Promberger R, Kober F, *et al.* Hashimoto's thyroiditis affects symptom load and quality of life unrelated to hypothyroidism: a prospective case-control study in women undergoing thyroidectomy for benign goiter. Thyroid 2011; 21: 161–7.

11 Abraham-Nordling M, Törring O, Hamberger B, *et al.* Graves' disease: a long-term quality-of-life follow up of patients randomized to treatment with antithyroid drugs, radioiodine, or surgery. Thyroid 2005; 15: 1279–86.

12 Abraham-Nordling M, Wallin G, Lundell G, *et al.* Thyroid hormone state and quality of life at long-term follow-up after randomized treatment of Graves' disease. Eur J Endocrinol 2007; 156: 173–9.

13 Tan LGL, Nan L, Thumboo J, *et al.* Health-related quality of life in thyroid cancer survivors. Laryngoscope 2007; 117: 507–10.

14 Huang SM, Lee CH, Chien LY, *et al.* Postoperative quality of life among patients with thyroid cancer. J Adv Nurs 2004; 47: 492–9.

15 Mazzaferri EL. An overview of the management of papillary and follicular thyroid carcinoma. Thyroid 1999; 9: 421–7.

16 Bilimoria KY, Bentrem DJ, Linn JG, *et al.* Utilization of total thyroidectomy for papillary thyroid cancer in the United States. Surgery 2007; 142: 906–13.

17 Mandel SJ, Mandel L. Radioactive iodine and the salivary glands. Thyroid 2003; 13: 265–71.

18 De Pedro Netto I, Fae A, Vartanian JG, *et al.* Voice and vocal self-assessment after thyroidectomy. Head Neck 2006; 28: 1106–14.

19 Lombardi CP, Raffaelli M, d'Alatri L, *et al.* Voice and swallowing changes after thyroidectomy in patients without inferior laryngeal nerve injuries. Surgery 2006; 140: 1026–32.

20 Crevenna R, Zettinig G, Keilani M, *et al.* Quality of life in patients with non-metastatic differentiated thyroid cancer under thyroxine supplementation therapy. Support Care Cancer 2003; 11: 597–603.

21 Almeida JP, Vartanian JG, Kowalski LP. Clinical predictors of quality of life in patients with initial differentiated thyroid cancers. Arch Otolaryngol Head Neck Surg 2009; 135: 342–6.

22 Malpani BL, Samuel AM, Ray S. Quantification of salivary gland function in thyroid cancer patients treated with radioiodine. Int J Radiat Oncol Biol Phys 1996; 35: 535–40.

23 Newkirk KA, Ringel MD, Wartofsky L, *et al.* The role of radioactive iodine in salivary gland dysfunction. Ear Nose Throat J 2000; 79: 460–8.

24 Bushnell DL, Boles MA, Kaufman GE, *et al.* Complications, sequela and dosimetry of iodine-131 therapy for thyroid carcinoma. J Nucl Med 1992; 33: 2214–21.

25 Maier H, Bihl H. Effect of radioactive iodine therapy on parotid gland function. Acta Otolaryngol 1987; 103: 318–24.

26 Almeida JP, Sanabria AE, Lima EN, *et al.* Late side effects of radioactive iodine on salivary gland function in patients with thyroid cancer. Head Neck 2011; 33: 686–90.

27 Botella-Carretero JI, Galán JM, Caballero C, *et al.* Quality of life and psychometric functionality in patients with differentiated thyroid carcinoma. Endocr Relat Cancer 2003; 10: 601–10.

28 Chow SM, Au KH, Choy TS, *et al.* Health-related quality-of-life study in patients with carcinoma of the thyroid after thyroxine withdrawal for whole body scanning. Laryngoscope 2006; 116: 2060–6.

29 Kung S, Rummans TA, Colligan RC, *et al.* Association of optimism-pessimism with quality of life in patients with head and neck and thyroid cancers. Mayo Clin Proc 2006; 81: 1545–52.

30 Tagay S, Herpertz S, Langkafel M, *et al.* Health-related quality of life, depression and anxiety in thyroid cancer patients. Qual Life Res 2006; 15: 695–703.

31 Taieb D, Baumstarck-Barrau K, Sebag F, *et al.* Heath-related quality of life in thyroid cancer patients following radioiodine ablation. Health Qual Life Outcomes 2011; 9: 33.

32 Fisher DA. Physiological variations in thyroid hormones: physiological and pathophysiological considerations. Clin Chem 1996; 42: 135–9.

33 Ferrini O, Cremonesi G. [Total lingual ectopia of the thyroid gland: diagnostic and therapeutic aspects of a clinical case]. Arch Maragliano Patol Clin 1958; 14: 773–87.

Index

ABBA *see* axillo-bilateral
   breast approach
absorbable haemostatic agents 205–6
acceptable morbidity rates 4–7
acute hypoparathyroidism 231–3
acute parathyroid insufficiency *see*
   hypoparathyroidism
acute respiratory distress syndrome (ARDS) 194
adenomas
   paediatric patients 38
   pneumothorax 210
   upper mediastinal disease 100–1, 102
air leaks 214–15
airway management 195
AIT *see* amiodarone-induced thyrotoxicosis
alfacalcidiol 233
Allis clamps 47–8
alveolar-pleural fistulas 214–15
amiodarone-induced hypothyroidism 295–6
amiodarone-induced thyrotoxicosis
   (AIT) 179–87
   clinical features 183–4
   differentiation of two types 179, 183–5
   effects on abnormal thyroid glands 181
   effects due to molecular structure 181–2
   epidemiology 182
   iodine load 181
   monitoring during amiodarone therapy 182
   pathogenesis 182–3
   patients requiring amiodarone therapy 185
   patients requiring total thyroidectomy 185–7
   patients who do not require
      amiodarone 184–5
   pharmacology 180
   predictors of 182
   structure of amiodarone 180
   therapeutic approach 184
   thyroid function 180–1
   thyroid hormones tests 181, 183
anaemia 298
anaesthesia
   amiodarone-induced thyrotoxicosis 187
   bleeding 201
   emergence from 195

lateral neck dissection 81, 84, 85
pneumothorax 211, 213–14
recurrent laryngeal nerve 222–3
respiratory failure 195–6
thyroidectomy 46
upper mediastinal disease 98
angiography 164, 166
anhidrosis 239
anisocoria 238–9
anoxic brain injury 15
ansa cervicalis 261
anterior border dissection 81
anterior-to-posterior technique 81–2
anterior-to-superior technique 101
antibiotics 28, 242, 244
antithyroid drugs (ATD) 33
appetite 297
apraclonidine 239
ARDS *see* acute respiratory distress syndrome
Army-Navy retractors 55–6
arterial stents 164
arytenoid abduction 224
aspiration 212–13
assisted ventilation 211
ataxia 239
atherosclerosis 274
autolysis 242
autotransplantation
   hypoparathyroidism 24–5, 27
   parathyroid glands 139, 235
axillary endoscopic thyroidectomy 276
axillo-bilateral breast approach (ABBA) 54,
   277, 282
axonal regrowth 221
axonotmesis 221

BABA *see* bilateral axillo-breast approach
Bartlett test 9
benign multinodular goitre 22, 26
Bernard–Horner syndrome 237–40
Berry's ligament
   minimally invasive video-assisted
      thyroidectomy 58
   recurrent laryngeal nerve 120, 122, 124

reoperation 108
robotic thyroid surgery 64
thyroidectomy 50–1
bilateral axillo-breast approach (BABA) 54,
   277, 281–2
bilateral recurrent laryngeal nerve paralysis
   (BRNLP) 20, 24
bilateral vocal fold immobility (BVFI) 223–4
bleeding 199–207
   drain placement 204–5
   haemostasis 205–6
   implications 201–2
   laryngotracheal and oesophageal
      injuries 158
   lateral neck dissection 89
   major vessel injuries 161, 162–6, 167
   management 202–4
   medical malpractice 14–15
   minimally invasive video-assisted
      thyroidectomy 59, 281–2
   paediatric patients 34
   perioperative techniques 204
   presentation and diagnosis 202
   prevention 204–6
   recurrent laryngeal nerve 122
   reoperation 105
   risk factors 199–201
   thyroidectomy 51
   timing 199
blunt dissection
   lateral neck dissection 81
   minimally invasive video-assisted
      thyroidectomy 57
   pneumothorax 213–14
   reoperation 107–8
   robotic thyroid surgery 65
   thyroidectomy 47–8
   upper mediastinal disease 95–7
botulinum toxin 224
brachial plexopathy 285–6
brachial plexus 243, 282–3
brachiocephalic trunk 162
breast endoscopic thyroidectomy 276–7
breathiness 124–5

Thyroid Surgery: Preventing and Managing Complications, First Edition. Edited by Paolo Miccoli, David J. Terris,
Michele N. Minuto and Melanie W. Seybt.
© 2013 John Wiley & Sons, Ltd. Published 2013 by John Wiley & Sons, Ltd.

BRNLP *see* bilateral recurrent laryngeal
    nerve paralysis
broncho-pleural fistulas 214
bronchoscopy 154, 156
Brown–Forsyth test 9
BVFI *see* bilateral vocal fold immobility

calcitonin 35
calcitriol 35, 141–2, 231–5
    see also vitamin D
calcium metabolism 227–8, 230
calcium supplementation 17, 73, 232–4
cancer *see* malignancies; thyroid cancer
cardiovascular symptoms 296, 298
carotid artery
    lateral neck dissection 88, 171–2
    major vessel injuries 161, 165
    minimally invasive video-assisted
        thyroidectomy 274
    reoperation 105
carotid sheath violation 286–8
central compartment node dissection
    (CCND) 278
central neck dissection 67–77
    complications 73–4
    incidence and prevalence 68
    intraoperative considerations 70
    lymph node metastases 67, 68–72
    medical malpractice 17
    morbidity rates 5–7
    paediatric patients 37
    persistent/recurrent disease 72–3
    preoperative considerations 68–70, 72
    prophylactic CND 71–2
    reoperation 72–3
    risk-appropriate treatment 22, 23
    standard of care 67–8
    therapeutic CND 70–1
    thyroid cancer 67–74
    thyroidectomy 47
cephalosporins 244
cervical approach 275
cervical lymph nodes 170
cervical lymphadenopathy 69
cervical oesophagus 158–9
cervical plexus 173
cervical spine injury 243
cervical thyroid 93–4
chest tube placement 213–14, 215
chest wall hypaesthesia 288
chi-square test 9
choking 259, 265–6
chronic hypoparathyroidism 233–4
chronic occipital pressure ulcers 240
chronic pain 21
Chvostek sign 229–30, 251
chyle leak 84
chylous fistulas 249–50
closure procedures
    bleeding 204
    cosmetic complications 146–7, 148
    lateral neck dissection 89

minimally invasive video-assisted
    thyroidectomy 59
    patient positioning 242
    sternotomy 246
    thyroidectomy 50–1
cocaine 239
Cochran method 9
common carotid artery 88, 161, 165
common peroneal nerve 243
compressive haematoma 192–3
computed tomography (CT)
    central neck dissection 69–70, 72
    Horner's syndrome 240
    laryngotracheal and oesophageal
        injuries 154
    major vessel injuries 166
    pneumothorax 211
    reoperation 106
    respiratory failure 195
    robotic thyroid surgery 287
    sternotomy 245
    unilateral recurrent laryngeal nerve
        paralysis 25
    upper mediastinal disease 93, 97, 98, 100, 102
confidence intervals (CI) 11
conjunctival hyperaemia 238
consent *see* informed consent
continuous positive airway pressure
    (cPAP) 194
cosmetic complications 145–9
    closure procedures 146–7, 148
    drain placement 148–9
    hypertrophic or hyperpigmented
        scarring 146–8
    incision location 145–6
    minimally invasive video-assisted
        thyroidectomy 272–3, 275
coughing 133, 265–6
cPAP *see* continuous positive airway pressure
cricothyroid (CT) muscle 129–31, 133
cytokines 296

Dandy clamps 47
debridement 241–2, 245–6
delayed hypocalcaemia 250–2
DeMoivre–LaPlace law 9
desethylamiodarone (DEA) 180, 182
diabetes 20
diagnostic delays 15
diagnostic errors 14, 15
differentiated thyroid cancer (DTC)
    laryngotracheal and oesophageal
        injuries 154
    lateral neck dissection 80, 82, 84–5
    paediatric patients 35, 36–8
    quality of life 306–9
dihydrotachysterol (DHT) 233–4
dilation lag 238
diplopia 239
distant metastases 109
Doppler ultrasound (US) 166, 184
down and out position 48

Down's syndrome 243
drain placement
    bleeding 204–5
    cosmetic complications 148–9
    pneumothorax 213, 214
DTC *see* differentiated thyroid cancer
dysaesthesia pain 85
dysphagia
    respiratory failure 193
    superior laryngeal nerve 133
    upper mediastinal disease 94
dysphonia 193, 253–4, 262
Dysphonia Severity Index (DSI) 253–4, 262

EBSLN *see* external branch of the superior
    laryngeal nerve
ECG *see* electrocardiogram
ectopic parathyroid glands 102, 137
ectopic thyroid glands 167
EJV *see* external jugular vein
elderly patients 23, 298
electrocardiogram (ECG) monitoring 141, 298
electrocautery 62
electromyographic (EMG) monitoring
    patient positioning 242
    recurrent laryngeal nerve 125–6
    superior laryngeal nerve 132–3
    voice and swallowing dysfunction 262
electrothermal bipolar vessel-sealing
    system 205, 206
emergency treatment 193
EMG *see* electromyographic
endoscopy
    central neck dissection 72
    cosmetic complications 145, 147, 149
    laryngotracheal and oesophageal
        injuries 154, 156
    major vessel injuries 166
    recurrent laryngeal nerve 125, 224
    remote-access thyroid surgery 276–7
    reoperation 106
    respiratory failure 195
    robotic thyroid surgery 62
    upper mediastinal disease 94, 98
    see also minimally invasive video-assisted
        thyroidectomy
endotracheal tube (ETT) 192
energy devices 111–15
    literature review 113–15
    radiofrequency 111–12, 113–14
    tips and tricks 114
    see also Harmonic® technology
ePAP *see* expiratory positive airway pressure
esophageal *see* oesophageal
ETE *see* extrathyroidal extension
ex-ante analysis 7, 9
exogenous thyroid hormone 95
expiratory positive airway pressure (ePAP) 194
ex-post analysis 7, 9
external branch of the superior laryngeal
    nerve (EBSLN) 129–33
    late complications 253

minimally invasive video-assisted thyroidectomy 280
voice and swallowing dysfunction 258, 260, 262–3, 267
external jugular vein (EJV) 63, 81
external radiotherapy 295
extrathyroidal extension (ETE) 153
extubation
bleeding 204
pneumothorax 215–16
respiratory failure 191, 195–6

facial nerve monitoring 85, 87
familial hypocalciuric hypercalcaemia (FHH) 100
Farabeuf retractors 55–6
FHH see familial hypocalciuric hypercalcaemia
fibreoptic laryngoscopy 107, 125, 133
fibrin sealants 206
fine needle aspiration (FNA)
central neck dissection 71
medical malpractice 14, 15
paediatric patients 36
sternotomy 245
upper mediastinal disease 94
Fligner–Killeen test 9
floor of the neck 172
Floseal 206
flow-volume loops 94
FNA see fine needle aspiration
follicular thyroid cancer (FTC) 35, 67
fractured ribs 246
friction injuries 240–1
FTC see follicular thyroid cancer
Functional Assessment of Cancer Treatment-General (FACT-G) questionnaire 308

Galli-Curci, Amelita 129
GAN see greater auricular nerve
gas insufflation
complications induced by 282
minimally invasive video-assisted thyroidectomy 55, 276–7, 282
risk-appropriate treatment 28
robotic thyroid surgery 61–2
gasless transaxillary endoscopic thyroidectomy 277–9, 282
gastro-oesophageal reflux (GORD) 20, 265–6
GD see Graves' disease
GH see growth hormone
Glasgow–Edinburgh Throat Scale (GETS) 265, 266
globus 264–5
Glottal Function Index (GFI) 222
glucocorticoids 188
GORD see gastro-oesophageal reflux
Graves' disease (GD)
bleeding 205
late complications 250–2
paediatric patients 33–5

quality of life 306
radioactive iodine therapies 33, 34
reoperation 105, 106
risk-appropriate treatment 22
surgery 34–5
voice and swallowing dysfunction 258, 261
GRBAS grading of voice quality 262
great vessel injuries see major vessel injuries
greater auricular nerve (GAN) 63, 288
Grillo stitch 158
growth hormone (GH) 250

H&E see haematoxylin and eosin
haematoma formation
bleeding 200, 203–4
lateral neck dissection 84
medical malpractice 14–15
minimally invasive video-assisted thyroidectomy 271–2
reoperation 105
respiratory failure 192–3
risk-appropriate treatment 21, 28
haematoxylin and eosin (H&E) 169
haemophilia 200
haemorrhage see bleeding
haemostasis
bleeding 205–6
devices and agents 205–6
energy devices 113
lateral neck dissection 84, 88
minimally invasive video-assisted thyroidectomy 59
risk-appropriate treatment 28–9
thyroidectomy 50–1
Harmonic® technology 112–15
bleeding 205, 206
lateral neck dissection 89
risk-appropriate treatment 24, 28
robotic thyroid surgery 62, 64, 113
thyroidectomy 47
upper mediastinal disease 101, 108
Hartley test 9
health insurance 13
health-related quality of life (HRQOL) 305–10
hidden lymph nodes 88
high-resolution ultrasound (US) 68–9, 169–70
high-riding innominate artery 162–3
hoarseness 124, 259
hormone replacement therapy (HRT) 234, 303
Horner's syndrome 88, 237–40
HRT see hormone replacement therapy
hungry bone syndrome 228
Hurthle cell thyroid carcinoma 244
hydrocortisone 188
25-hydroxyvitamin D 228–9
hypaesthesia 288
hypercalcaemia 233–4
hypercarbia 282
hyperparathyroidism 99, 102
hyperpigmented scarring 146–8
hyperplasia 99
hyperthyroglobulinaemia 106

hyperthyroidism
amiodarone-induced thyrotoxicosis 179
late complications 251–3
paediatric patients 34, 38
quality of life 305
thyroid storm 179, 187–8, 252–3
upper mediastinal disease 94
hypertrophic scarring 146–8
hyperventilation 229
hypocalcaemia
delayed 250–2
medical malpractice 16–17
morbidity rates 6
paediatric patients 34
parathyroid glands 139–42, 228, 231–3
risk-appropriate treatment 21, 24, 28
thyroidectomy 250–2
hypomagnesaemia 231
hypoparathyroidism
acute 231–3
autotransplantation 24–5
biochemical and hormonal evaluation 229
central neck dissection 73
chronic 233–4
definition, causes and classification 228
evaluation and clinical manifestations 229
follow-up 234
identification 24–5
late complications 250
management 231
medical malpractice 14, 16–17
medical treatment 231–4
minimally invasive video-assisted thyroidectomy 280–1
morbidity rates 4, 6–7
paediatric patients 34–5, 36–7
parathyroid glands 137, 141–2
postoperative 229–31
prediction 25
predictive factors 229–31
preservation 24
prevention 231
risk-appropriate treatment 21, 22, 24–9
supplementation 25–6
surgical 228
symptoms and signs 229
hypothyroidism
amiodarone-induced thyrotoxicosis 181
quality of life 305, 308
see also iatrogenic hypothyroidism
hypoxaemia 192, 211

iatrogenic hypothyroidism 293–303
aetiology 293–4
clinical presentation 296–7
diagnosis 299
drugs 295–6
elderly patients 298
external and internal radiation 293, 294–5
instrumental changes 298
laboratory tests 298
myxoedema coma 299, 301

iatrogenic hypothyroidism (*cont'd*)
   overt hypothyroidism in adulthood 296–7
   physical findings 297–8
   pregnancy 298, 301
   subclinical hypothyroidism 299, 301–2
   surgical hypothyroidism 293–4, 300
   thyroxine treatment 300–1
   treatment 300–2
IBSLN *see* internal branch superior
   laryngeal nerve
immunocompromised patients 20
incision placement 46–7, 145–6
infections
   lateral neck dissection 89
   patient positioning 242
   risk-appropriate treatment 21, 28
   sternotomy 244–6
inferior laryngeal nerve injuries 4–6
inferior parathyroid 137–8
inferior thyroid artery (ITA) 124
informed consent 45
innominate artery 162–3, 165, 167
insurance premiums 13
internal branch superior laryngeal nerve
   (IBSLN) 129, 133–4
internal jugular vein (IJV)
   lateral neck dissection 88, 170–3
   major vessel injuries 165–6
   reoperation 105, 108
International Monitoring Study Group 16
intraoperative death 3
intraoperative neurophysiological monitoring
   (IONM) 16, 23, 132–3
intraoperative rapid parathyroid hormone
   (IOPTH) 141–2
inverse ptosis 238
iodine load 181, 187–8, 295
IONM *see* intraoperative neurophysiological
   monitoring
iopanoic acid 186
isthmus dissection 59, 64
isthmus transection 47
ITA *see* inferior thyroid artery

Kelley clamps 47–8
keloid scars 3, 23, 84, 89, 148, 273
Kern study 14, 17
Kocher incisions 81, 87–8
Kruskal–Wallis test 9

Langer's line 46–7
laryngeal cancers 14
laryngeal electromyography (LEMG) 222
laryngeal entry point 120, 123
laryngeal reinnervation 223
laryngectomy 158
laryngoscopy
   best practices 72, 94
   morbidity rates 5
   recurrent laryngeal nerve 125, 224
   reoperation 107
   risk-appropriate treatment 20–1, 23–4
   superior laryngeal nerve 133

laryngotracheal injuries 153–8
lateral cricoarytenoid (LCA) muscles 224
lateral neck disease 108–9
lateral neck dissection 79–91, 169–77
   anaesthesia 81, 84, 85
   anterior border dissection 81
   anterior-to-posterior technique 81–2
   cervical plexus and spinal accessory
      nerves 173, 174–6
   chyle leak 84
   complications 84–5, 87–9, 173–6
   deep surface of sternocleidomastoid
      muscle 81
   definitions 79–80
   differentiated thyroid cancer 80, 82, 84–5
   dysaesthesia, paraesthesia and pain 85
   exposure of major vessels 171–2
   extent of dissection 85–7
   floor of the neck and phrenic nerve 172, 173
   hidden lymph nodes 88
   historical development 79
   incision 171
   incision types 87–8
   indications 80–1
   level I nodes 86–7
   level II nodes 82–3, 85–6
   level III nodes 83
   level IV nodes 83, 88
   level V nodes 86, 88
   local complications 84
   medullary thyroid cancer 80–1
   nodes anterior to internal jugular vein 173
   papillary thyroid cancer 169–73, 176
   patient positioning 81
   posterior-to-anterior technique 83–4
   prophylactic 80–1
   skin incision 81
   spinal accessory nerve paresis or
      paralysis 84–5, 88–9
   technique 81–4
   thoracic duct 172–3, 176
   thyroid cancer 79–89
LCA *see* lateral cricoarytenoid
LDL *see* low-density lipoprotein
leak of chyle 249–50
LEMG *see* laryngeal electromyography
Levene test 9
levothyroxine 296
LigaSure™ 205, 206
litigation *see* medical malpractice
LNM *see* lymph node metastases
lobectomy
   minimally invasive video-assisted
      thyroidectomy 58–9, 275
   paediatric patients 36, 38
   risk-appropriate treatment 19, 21–2
lobectomy-hemithyroidectomy 294
local anaesthesia
   amiodarone-induced thyrotoxicosis 187
   pneumothorax 214
   thyroidectomy 46
   upper mediastinal disease 98
logistic regression 9

Lombardi Subjective Swallowing Evaluation
   Questionnaire 266
Lombardi Subjective Voice Evaluation
   Questionnaire 263
low-density lipoprotein (LDL)
   cholesterol 298, 302
lung disease 203
Lydiatt study 14
lymph node metastases (LNM)
   central neck dissection 67, 68–72
   laryngotracheal and oesophageal
      injuries 153
   lateral neck dissection 79–89, 169–73, 176
   major vessel injuries 165–6
   minimally invasive video-assisted
      thyroidectomy 54
   paediatric patients 36–7
   quality of life 306–7
   reoperation 105
   risk-appropriate treatment 22
   sternotomy 244
   upper mediastinal disease 97–8
lymphostasis 88

McFee incisions 87–8
magnetic resonance angiography (MRA) 166
magnetic resonance imaging (MRI)
   central neck dissection 69, 72
   energy devices 113
   Horner's syndrome 240
   laryngotracheal and oesophageal
      injuries 154
   reoperation 106
   upper mediastinal disease 100
major vessel injuries 161–7
   aberrant pathways 161–2
   anatomy of great vessels of the neck 161–2
   carotid artery rupture 165
   internal jugular bleeding 165–6
   intraoperative bleeding 162–4
   postoperative bleeding 164
   postoperative haemorrhage 164
   prevention of injury 166–7
   sentinel bleeding events 166
   tracheo-innominate fistulas 164–5, 166
malignancies
   central neck dissection 67–74
   laryngotracheal and oesophageal
      injuries 153–9
   lateral neck dissection 79–89, 169–73, 176
   major vessel injuries 165–6
   medical malpractice 14, 17
   paediatric patients 34, 35–8
   pneumothorax 209–10
   quality of life 306–9
   recurrent laryngeal nerve 221
   reoperation 105
   risk-appropriate treatment 19, 22, 23
   sternotomy 244
   upper mediastinal disease 97–8
malpractice *see* medical malpractice
malunion of the sternum 244
Mann–Whitney test 9

maximum phonation time (MPT) tests 253
MCT *see* medium chain triglycerides
medial arytenoidectomy 224
medialization laryngoplasty 223
mediastinitis 245
mediastinum 210
medical malpractice 13–18
    diagnostic delays 15
    hypoparathyroidism 16–17
    poor outcomes 14–15
    recurrent nerve injury 16
    study methods and results 14
medium chain triglycerides (MCT) 250
medullary thyroid cancer (MTC) 71, 80–1, 169
meta-analysis 10–11
metastatic thyroid carcinoma 209
    see also lymph node metastases
methimazole (MMI) 33, 34, 187, 253
methylene blue 24
MG *see* myasthenia gravis
midline sternotomy 96
minimally invasive video-assisted
        thyroidectomy (MIVAT) 53–60
    axillary endoscopic thyroidectomy 276
    axillo-bilateral breast approach 277, 282
    bilateral axillo-breast approach 277, 281–2
    bleeding 281–2
    brachial plexus injury 282–3
    breast endoscopic thyroidectomy 276–7
    carotid artery injuries 274
    cervical approach 275
    classification of techniques 53–4
    completion of lobectomy 58–9
    complications 271–4, 279–83
    extraction of thyroid lobe 58–9
    gas insufflation 276–7, 282
    gasless transaxillary endoscopic
        thyroidectomy 277–9, 282
    haematoma formation 271–2
    historical development 53
    hypoparathyroidism 280–1
    identification of RLN and parathyroid
        glands 57–8
    incision and access to thyroid region 55–6
    indications 54
    intraoperative management of
        complications 272
    patient positioning 278, 282–3
    patient and surgeon positioning 54
    postoperative management of
        complications 272
    recurrent nerve injury 279–80
    remote-access thyroid surgery 275–84
    risk-appropriate treatment 28
    robotic thyroid surgery 61
    section of the upper pedicle 55, 57
    skin damage and cosmetic
        issues 272–3, 275
    superior laryngeal nerve 132, 280
    suture of the access 59
    technique 54–9
    through the neck access 271–4
    through other accesses 275–84

tracheal injuries 273–4
    voice and swallowing dysfunction 265
Minnesota Multiphasic Personality
        Inventory 308
miosis 238
MIVAT *see* minimally invasive video-assisted
        thyroidectomy
MNG *see* multinodular goitres
morbidity rates 3–12
    acceptable rates of complications 4–7
    context 3
    hypoparathyroidism 4, 6–7
    inferior laryngeal nerve injuries 4–6
    meta-analysis 10–11
    recurrent nerve injuries 4–6
    reporting of complication incidence 4–6
    risk-appropriate treatment 19–21
    statistical and epidemiological analysis 7–8
    statistical power 7–10
mortality rates 3, 15
motor unit action potentials (MUAP) 222
MPT *see* maximum phonation time
MRA *see* magnetic resonance angiography
MRI *see* magnetic resonance imaging
MTC *see* medullary thyroid cancer
MUAP *see* motor unit action potentials
multinodular goitres (MNG) 94
muscular symptoms 297
myasthenia gravis (MG) 194–5
myxoedema coma 299, 301

neck pain 288
necrotic tissue 241–2
negative pressure pulmonary
        oedema 193–4
negative voice outcome (NVO) 254
nerve monitoring 16, 23, 132–3
nerve stimulation 49
neural electrophysiological monitoring 125–6
neurological symptoms 297
neuropraxia 16, 19–20, 221
neurotmesis 221
nodule evaluation 35–6, 38
nominal variables 9
non-inferiority tests 9–10
non-localized lesions 100
non-recurrent laryngeal nerve (NRLN) 121
NVO *see* negative voice outcome

O-silk sutures 46–7
oculosympathoparesis 237–40
odds ratios 9, 11
odynophagia 264
oesophageal injuries 153–5, 158–9
    minimally invasive video-assisted
        thyroidectomy 283
    robotic thyroid surgery 286–7
oesophagoscopy 154
omohyoid muscle 63
oncological diagnosis 14
optimal incision location 145–6
overt hypothyroidism in adulthood 296–7
oxidized regenerated cellulose 205–6

p-values 8
paediatric patients 33–42
    Graves' disease 33–5
    lateral neck dissection 84
    nodule evaluation 35–6, 38
    radioactive iodine therapies 33, 34, 37–8
    risk-appropriate treatment 23
    standard of care 37–8
    surgery 34–5, 36–7
    thyroid cancer 34, 35–8
pain
    Horner's syndrome 239
    iatrogenic hypothyroidism 297
    lateral neck dissection 85
    minimally invasive video-assisted
        thyroidectomy 275
    risk-appropriate treatment 21, 28
    robotic thyroid surgery 288
papillary thyroid cancer (PTC) 35
    central neck dissection 67–8, 70–2
    laryngotracheal and oesophageal injuries 153
    lateral neck dissection 80, 169–73, 176
paraesthesia 85, 283
parathormone 25
parathyroid glands 137–43
    acute hypoparathyroidism 231–3
    anatomy 99, 137–8
    anterior-to-superior technique 101
    autotransplantation 139, 235
    chronic hypoparathyroidism 233–4
    hormone replacement therapy 234
    hypoparathyroidism 137, 141–2
    indications for mediastinal
        dissection 99–100
    localized lesions 100–1
    major vessel injuries 162
    medical malpractice 13–18
    minimally invasive video-assisted
        thyroidectomy 57–8
    non-localized lesions 100
    physiology and calcium metabolism 227–8
    posterior mediastinal dissection 101
    postoperative complications 227–36
    postoperative hypocalcaemia 139–42
    postoperative hypoparathyroidism 229–31
    preservation during thyroidectomy 137, 138–9
    recurrent laryngeal nerve 122–3
    robotic thyroid surgery 64
    surgical hypoparathyroidism 228
    thyroidectomy 49
    upper mediastinal disease 99–102
parathyroid hormone (PTH) 17
    late complications 251–2
    parathyroid glands 137, 141–2
    physiology and calcium metabolism 227–8
    upper mediastinal disease 99
patient positioning
    complications from 240–3
    lateral neck dissection 81
    minimally invasive video-assisted
        thyroidectomy 54, 278, 282–3
    robotic thyroid surgery 286–7
    thyroidectomy 46, 237, 240–3

pectoralis flaps 156
PEEP *see* positive end-expiratory pressure
Pemberton's sign 94
percutaneous ethanol 108
peripheral nerve injury 242–3
perivisceral nerve plexus 260
permanent anaesthesia 21
permanent hypoparathyroidism 6–7, 142
  central neck dissection 73
  paediatric patients 37
  risk-appropriate treatment 21, 29
permanent unilateral recurrent laryngeal nerve
     paralysis (URLNP) 20–1, 29
persistent papillary thyroid cancer (PTC) 72
PET *see* positron emission tomography
phenylephrine 240
phospholipids 298
phrenic nerve 85, 172, 173
pitch of voice 259
platysmal skin flaps 109
pneumothorax 209–17
  air leaks 214–15
  blunt dissection 213–14
  clinical manifestations 210–11
  complications 215
  diagnosis 211
  discharge and follow-up 216
  drainage system/water seal/suction 214
  extubation 215–16
  gas insufflation 282
  management 211–12
  pathophysiology 209–10
  pleural drain and chest tube
    placement 213–14, 215
  Seldinger technique 213
  simple aspiration 212–13
  standard of care 212
  x-radiography 211, 215
positive end-expiratory pressure (PEEP) 194
positron emission tomography (PET) 69, 72, 106
postauricular incision 63, 65
posterior-to-anterior technique 83–4
posterior mediastinal dissection 101
posterior-to-superior technique 99
posterior transverse cordotomy 223
post-hoc analysis 8–9
postoperative death 3
post-thyroidectomy respiratory failure
    (PTRF) 191
pre-existing unilateral recurrent
    laryngeal nerve paralysis (URLNP) 23
prefabricated flaps 156–7
pregnancy 298, 301
pressure ulcers 240–2
primary spontaneous pneumothorax
    (PSP) 209, 211
primary substernal goitres 93–4
prophylactic central neck dissection 71–2
prophylactic lateral neck dissection 80–1
propylthiouracil (PTU) 33, 187, 253
PSP *see* primary spontaneous pneumothorax
PTC *see* papillary thyroid cancer

PTH *see* parathyroid hormone
ptosis 238
PTRF *see* post-thyroidectomy respiratory
    failure
pulmonary oedema 193–4
pupillary miosis 238
pyramidal lobe 50–1

quality of life (QOL) 305–10
  benign thyroid diseases 306
  thyroid cancer 306–9

radial nerve 243
radiation therapy 23, 295
radical neck dissection 210
radioactive iodine (RAI) therapies
  amiodarone-induced thyrotoxicosis 183–5
  central neck dissection 69
  iatrogenic hypothyroidism 293, 294–5
  late complications 251
  paediatric patients 33, 34, 37–8
  quality of life 306–9
  reoperation 107
  upper mediastinal disease 95
radiofrequency ablation (RFA) 108
radiofrequency devices 111–12, 113–14
radiography 211, 215
radionuclide studies 94
RAI *see* radioactive iodine
railroad tracking 148
RAT *see* robotic axillary thyroidectomy
recurrent laryngeal nerve palsy/paresis
    (RLNP) 193, 258
recurrent laryngeal nerve (RLN) 119–27
  anatomical landmarks 123–4
  anatomy of great vessels of the neck 161–3
  central neck dissection 72
  general identification principles 122
  gross surgical anatomy 119–21
  Horner's syndrome 239
  inferior approach 122
  intraoperative neural electrophysiological
    monitoring 125–6
  laryngotracheal and oesophageal injuries 153
  late complications 253
  lateral approach 123
  mechanisms of injury 124
  microanatomy 119
  minimally invasive video-assisted
    thyroidectomy 57–8
  non-recurrent laryngeal nerve 121
  pathophysiology 221
  postoperative complications 221–5
  rates of iatrogenic damage 121
  reoperation 105–6
  respiratory failure 193
  risk-appropriate treatment 19–20
  sternotomy 244
  superior approach 122–3
  thyroidectomy 49–50
  treatment of postoperative
    complications 222–4

upper mediastinal disease 94, 96
visualization and approach during
    surgery 121–2
vocal fold hypomobility 221–2
voice changes after injury 124–5
voice and swallowing dysfunction 258, 260,
    262–7
  see also bilateral recurrent laryngeal nerve
    paralysis; recurrent nerve injury; unilateral
    recurrent laryngeal nerve paralysis
recurrent nerve injury (RNI)
  anatomy of great vessels of the neck 161–2
  central neck dissection 72
  mechanisms of injury 124
  medical malpractice 16
  minimally invasive video-assisted
    thyroidectomy 279–80
  morbidity rates 4–6
  paediatric patients 35, 36
  respiratory failure 193
  upper mediastinal disease 98
  voice and swallowing dysfunction 124–5,
    260, 267
recurrent papillary thyroid cancer (PTC) 72
rehabilitation 134
reimplantation 25, 27
remote-access thyroid surgery
  axillary endoscopic thyroidectomy 276
  axillo-bilateral breast approach 277, 282
  bilateral axillo-breast approach 277, 281–2
  breast endoscopic thyroidectomy 276–7
  complications 279–83
  gas insufflation 276–7, 282
  gasless transaxillary endoscopic
    thyroidectomy 277–9, 282
  minimally invasive video-assisted
    thyroidectomy 275–85
  robotic thyroid surgery 289
renal insufficiency 20
reoperation 105–11
  anatomy 105–6
  benign disease 105, 106
  central neck dissection 72–3
  complications 109
  distant metastases 109
  indications 105
  investigations and evaluation 106–7
  lateral neck disease 108–9
  local/thyroid bed disease 107–8
  malignancies 105, 106
  paediatric patients 37
  risk-appropriate treatment 23
  surgical principles 107–9
  thyroid cancer 108–9
reporting of complication incidence 4–6
resection 154–8
respiratory failure 191–7
  aetiology 192–5
  airway management 195
  anaesthesia 195–6
  compressive haematoma 192–3
  extubation 191, 195–6

negative pressure pulmonary
    oedema 193–4
preoperative assessment 195
recurrent laryngeal nerve
    palsy/paresis 193
respiratory insufficiency 194–5
tracheomalacia 192
respiratory insufficiency 194–5
respiratory symptoms 296–7
retained thyroid tissue 286
retro-oesophageal lymphadenopathy 69
retro-oesophageal subclavian artery 161–3
retrosternal goitres 244
RFA *see* radiofrequency ablation
RFT *see* robotic facelift thyroidectomy
rib fractures 246
risk-appropriate treatment 19–32
    bilateral recurrent laryngeal nerve
        paralysis 20, 24
    central neck dissection 22
    haemostatic technologies 28–9
    hypocalcaemia 21, 24, 28
    hypoparathyroidism 21, 22, 24–9
    lobectomy versus total thyroidectomy 19,
        21–2
    local complications 21, 28
    minimizing risk of complications 23–9
    morbidity rates 19–21
    patient characteristics 23
    postoperative pain 21, 28
    scarring 21, 28
    surgical experience 23
    thyroid cancer 22, 23
    unilateral recurrent laryngeal nerve
        paralysis 19–21, 23–6, 29
    voice disorders 20–1
risk/benefit ratios 19
risk management 13–14
RLN *see* recurrent laryngeal nerve
RNI *see* recurrent nerve injury
robotic axillary thyroidectomy
    (RAT) 61–2, 285–8
robotic facelift thyroidectomy (RFT) 61, 62–5,
    285, 288–9
robotic thyroid surgery 61–6
    brachial plexopathy 285–6
    carotid sheath violation 286–8
    chest wall hypaesthesia 288
    complications 285–90
    energy devices 113
    greater auricular nerve hypaesthesia 288
    neck pain 288
    oesophageal injuries 286–7
    patient positioning 286–7
    patient selection 63
    RAT technique 61–2
    rationale for development 62
    remote-access thyroid surgery 289
    retained thyroid tissue 286
    RFT techniques 61, 62–5
    technique 63–5
    tracheal injury 286

saturated solution of potassium iodide
    (SSKI) 34, 252–3
scarring
    cosmetic complications 145–8
    hypertrophic or hyperpigmented 146–8
    incision location 145
    lateral neck dissection 89
    minimally invasive video-assisted
        thyroidectomy 275
    morbidity rates 3
    risk-appropriate treatment 21, 28
SCM *see* sternocleidomastoid muscle
secondary substernal goitres 93–4
segmental resection 156–8
Seldinger technique 213
sentinel bleeding events 166
sepsis 242
seroma 21, 283, 288–9
serotonin 24
SF-36 questionnaire 306–7
short chain triglycerides 250
shortness of breath 210, 211
significance tests 9
simple aspiration 212–13
single photon emission computed tomography
    (SPECT) 100, 102
skin complications
    iatrogenic hypothyroidism 296, 297
    minimally invasive video-assisted
        thyroidectomy 272–3
    see also cosmetic complications; scarring
SLN *see* superior laryngeal nerve
SNS *see* sympathetic nervous system
solitary nodules 22
somatostatin 250
SPECT *see* single photon emission computed
    tomography
spinal accessory nerve 84–5, 88–9, 170, 173,
    174–6
SSKI *see* super saturated potassium iodine
STA *see* superior thyroid artery
statistical power 7–10
sternoclavicular joint 88
sternocleidomastoid muscle (SCM)
    laryngotracheal and oesophageal
        injuries 101
    lateral neck dissection 81, 170–2
    minimally invasive video-assisted
        thyroidectomy 277–8, 280
    parathyroid glands 140
    reoperation 108
    robotic thyroid surgery 63
sternocleidomastoid myoperiosteal
    flaps 156
sternothyroid muscles 261
sternotomy
    major vessel injuries 163
    postoperative complications 243–6
    upper mediastinal disease 96, 99
stroboscopy 133, 261
subclavian artery 161–3
subclinical hypothyroidism 299, 301–2

submandibular gland 87
submandibular incisions 87–8
submandibular nodes 88
submental nodes 88
subplatysmal skin flaps 47–8, 87, 96
substernal goitres 93–9
    anaesthesia 98
    anatomy 93–4
    malignancies 97–8
    postoperative complications 98–9
    presentation and evaluation 94
    surgical management 95–8
    technique 96–7
    treatment 94–5
suctioning 214
super saturated potassium iodine (SSKI) 34,
    252–3
superior laryngeal nerve (SLN) 129–35
    anatomical variation 130–2
    anatomy and physiology 129–30
    injuries 133–4
    late complications 253
    minimally invasive video-assisted
        thyroidectomy 280
    nerve monitoring 132–3
    rehabilitation 134
    surgical approach 133
    voice and swallowing dysfunction 258, 260,
        261, 262–3, 267
superior parathyroid 137–9
superior pole 48–9, 122–3
superior thyroid artery (STA) 129, 133
supernumerary parathyroid glands 137
surgical experience 23
surgical hypothyroidism 293–4, 300
Sutherland classification 19
swallowing
    aetiology 260, 265
    evaluation and management 265–6
    nature of the impairment 264–5
    principles, prevalence and anatomy 263–4
    quality of life 307
    recurrent nerve injury 125
    superior laryngeal nerve 133
    thyroidectomy 253–4, 257, 260, 263–6
swallowing impairment scores (SIS) 265–6, 307
sympathetic nervous system (SNS) 237–40

TA *see* thyroarytenoid
tachycardia 282
temporary hypoparathyroidism 6, 73
tension pneumothorax 210–11
tests for therapeutic equivalence 9–10
tetra-iodothyronine 296
therapeutic central neck dissection 70–1
therapeutic equivalence, tests for 9–10
thionamide drugs 253
thoracic cavity 93–4
thoracic duct 172–3, 176
thoracotomy 96
thyroarytenoid (TA) muscles 224
thyroglobulinaemia 106

thyroid cancer
central neck dissection 67–74
laryngotracheal and oesophageal
injuries 153–9
lateral neck dissection 79–89
major vessel injuries 165–6
nodule evaluation 35–6, 38
paediatric patients 34, 35–8
quality of life 306–9
radioactive iodine therapies 34, 37–8
reoperation 108–9
risk-appropriate treatment 22, 23
standard of care 37–8
sternotomy 244
surgery 36–7
thyroid lobe 58–9
thyroid receptor antibodies (TRAb) 33
thyroid-stimulating hormone (TSH)
amiodarone-induced thyrotoxicosis 181,
183, 185
iatrogenic hypothyroidism 293, 295,
299–301
late complications 250
quality of life 303, 306
thyroid-stimulating immunoglobulins
(TSI) 33
thyroid storm 179, 187–8
aetiology 187
late complications 252–3
management 187–8
presentation and diagnosis 187
thyroid suppression 95
thyroidectomy
amiodarone-induced thyrotoxicosis 185–7
Berry's ligament, haemostasis and
closure 50–1
best practices 45–51
bleeding 51, 200–2
chylous fistulas 249–50
cosmetic complications 146–9
delayed hypocalcaemia 250–2
iatrogenic hypothyroidism 294
identification of RLN and parathyroid
glands 49
imaging studies 45–6
incision placement 46–7
informed consent 45
intraoperative considerations 46–51
isthmus transection 47
late complications 249–55
medical malpractice 15–17
mobilization of lower pole vessels 49
morbidity rates 3–7
paediatric patients 36
parathyroid glands 137, 138–9
patient positioning 46, 237, 240–3
pneumothorax 210
postoperative considerations 51
preoperative considerations 45–6
quality of life 305–10
raising skin flaps and mobilizing strap
muscles 47–8

risk-appropriate treatment 19, 21–2, 28
superior laryngeal nerve (SLN) 132
superior pole dissection 48–9
thyroid storm 252–3
tubercle of Zuckerkandl dissection 49–50
voice and swallowing dysfunction 253–4,
257–68
see also minimally invasive video-assisted
thyroidectomy; robotic thyroid surgery
thyroiditis 179
thyroplasty 25
thyrotoxic osteodystrophy 251
thyrotropin 35
thyroxine 35
thyroxine treatment 300–1
TIF see tracheo-innominate fistulas
tissue necrosis 241–2
tissue transfer reconstruction 167
TNM classification system 37–8
tortuous vessels 161
total parenteral nutrition (TPN) 250
total thyroidectomy
amiodarone-induced thyrotoxicosis 185–7
iatrogenic hypothyroidism 294
paediatric patients 36
parathyroid glands 139
pneumothorax 210
risk-appropriate treatment 19, 21–2
toxic adenomas 38
TPN see total parenteral nutrition
TRAb see thyroid receptor antibodies
tracheal injury
minimally invasive video-assisted
thyroidectomy 273–4
pneumothorax 210
robotic thyroid surgery 286
tracheo-innominate fistulas
(TIF) 164–5, 166
tracheomalacia 98–9, 192, 193–4
tracheostomy 191, 192, 204
transaxillary endoscopic
thyroidectomy 277–9, 282
transcervical mediastinal dissection 99–100
transient hypoparathyroidism 6, 22, 34–5
transient unilateral recurrent laryngeal nerve
paralysis (URLNP) 20–1
triangle of Miccoli–Berti 58
triglycerides 250, 298
tri-iodothyronine 296, 300–1
Trousseau sign 229–30, 251
TSH see thyroid-stimulating hormone
TSI see thyroid-stimulating
immunoglobulins
tubercle of Zuckerkandl
recurrent laryngeal nerve 123, 124
reoperation 105–6
thyroidectomy 49–50
type II errors 7–10
tyrosine kinase inhibitors 296

UADS see upper aerodigestive symptoms
ulnar nerve 243

ultrasound (US)
amiodarone-induced thyrotoxicosis 184
central neck dissection 68–9, 72
energy devices 112–14
lateral neck dissection 80, 169–70
major vessel injuries 166
medical malpractice 15
paediatric patients 35–6
pneumothorax 213
reoperation 106
thyroidectomy 45–6
unilateral recurrent laryngeal nerve paralysis
(URLNP) 19–21, 23–6, 29
unilateral vocal fold paralysis (UVFP) 222–3
upper aerodigestive symptoms
(UADS) 263–4
upper mediastinal disease 93–103
anaesthesia 98
anatomy 93–4, 99
anterior-to-superior technique 101
complications 101–2
indications for mediastinal
dissection 99–100
localized lesions 100–1
malignancies 97–8
non-localized lesions 100
parathyroid glands 99–102
posterior mediastinal dissection 101
postoperative complications 98–9
presentation and evaluation 94
substernal goitres 93–9
surgical management 95–8
technique 96–7
thyroid glands 93–9
treatment 94–5
upper pedical dissection 57
URLNP see unilateral recurrent
laryngeal nerve paralysis
urogenital symptoms 297
UVFP see unilateral vocal fold paralysis

vagus nerve 81–2, 171–2, 173
Valsalva manoeuvre 204, 215, 249
ventilation impairments 4
vertical hemilaryngectomy 158
vertigo 239
videofluoroscopic swallowing study
(VFSS) 265
videolaryngoscopy 195, 307
videolaryngostroboscopy (VLS) 261, 265
visceral injury 286
vitamin D
late complications 251–2
paediatric patients 35
parathyroid glands 137, 141, 232–4
risk-appropriate treatment 25–6
VLS see videolaryngostroboscopy
vocal cords 130, 193, 259
vocal fold hypomobility 221–2
vocal fold synkinesis 221
Vocal Performance Questionnaire
(VPQ) 262

voice disorders
  aetiology 260–1
  evaluation and management 261–3
  morbidity rates 4
  nature of the impairment 259
  principles, prevalence and
    anatomy 257–8
  quality of life 307
  recurrent nerve injury 124–5
  risk-appropriate treatment 20–1
  thyroidectomy 253–4, 257–63
Voice Handicap Index-10 (VHI-10) 132, 222,
    262–3, 307
von Willebrand's disease 200

water seal devices 214
WESTLAW database 14
Wharton's duct 87
widened scarring 147
Wolff–Chaikoff effect 181, 252–3, 295

x-radiography 211, 215